MW00609784

Synopsis of

# Clinical cancer

# Synopsis of Clinical cancer

Condict Moore, M.D.

*Professor of Surgery (Oncology), Associate in Pathology,*
*University of Louisville School of Medicine;*
*Director of Tumor Clinic, Louisville General Hospital, Louisville, Kentucky;*
*Chairman, Cancer Coordinating Committee of the Kentucky Medical Association;*
*Chairman, Cancer Liaison Fellows for Kentucky of the American College of Surgeons;*
*former trainee of the National Cancer Institute and of the American Cancer Society*

**Second edition**

With 37 illustrations

The C. V. Mosby Company

Saint Louis 1970

*First edition published privately by Dr. Condict Moore*

*Printed in the United States of America*

*Standard Book Number 8016-3472-5*

*Library of Congress Catalog Card Number 70-104975*

*Distributed in Great Britain by Henry Kimpton, London*

*To*

Virginia, Martha, and Michael

# Preface

This summary of clinical cancer information originates from twenty years of learning, teaching, and practice in the field of oncology. It results from the study of cancer in many aspects: cancer in the patient at first diagnosis, cancer at the operating table, cancer under radiotherapy treatment, cancer in the gross and microscopic pathology laboratory, cancer in the follow-up clinic or office, cancer in laboratory animals and in statistical follow-up analyses, cancer in the family and social setting, and the cancer patient undergoing rehabilitation. Notes for lectures, talks, and seminars for medical students and practitioners, generally well received, have been expanded and updated. The wide scope of training given at the Memorial Hospital in New York City enabled me to begin work in cancer some years ago from an unusually broad base of knowledge about many types of cancer, and with an enthusiasm for the diagnosis and treatment of cancer considered naive by many. In retrospect the sum total of advances made in cancer during the past two decades justifies much of this enthusiasm.

In spite of undoubted advances a defeatist mythology persists about cancer in the minds of most doctors. I hope to help dispel this myth by the broad scope of the book, inclusion of very recent data, clear expression, condensation, separation of basic from trivial information, and emphasis on similarities among the various cancers, and by placing cancer in better perspective within the field of medicine.

Medicine seems to advance by steps. One consists of discoveries by superspecialist investigators; another step is the communication of newly discovered knowledge so that all may understand and use it. Physicians who feel responsible for communicating cancer information work, as a rule, in isolated specialties and in large institutions where they see only complicated or advanced cancers. The busy practicing physician who recognizes and controls localized cancers has little time to report his experience; he passes on quickly to more pressing problems. Communications that encompass the whole field from experience are, therefore, rarely achieved.

This volume is an attempt to perform a communications task that seems to need doing. Most of this material has already proved its appeal and usefulness for medical students, house staff, and practitioners in our local area. I hope it serves as an introduction to cancer, a first reference, or a handy review for students and physicians in all specialties. I also hope it will prepare the reader to use recent and future discoveries in the emerging area of cancer prevention, an area destined to become an increasingly productive part of medical practice.

No one individual can be an expert in all fields of clinical cancer. I gratefully acknowledge the willing cooperation and careful, detailed criticism given by colleagues on the faculty of the University of Louisville School of Medicine during the preparation of this volume. Mention of these individuals does not necessarily mean that they approve all the ideas expressed herein. There are many controversial areas in clinical medicine, particularly in the field of cancer, where few individuals exactly agree. Nevertheless, without the unselfish cooperation of the following physicians this work would not have been possible: Drs. Marion F. Beard, William M. Christopherson, Marcine Davies, Ellis A. Fuller, Laman A. Gray, Douglas M. Haynes, James W. Harkess, William W. Johnson, Donald R. Kmetz, Roderick Macdonald, Fitzhugh Mullins, Rudolf J. Noer, Herbert T. Ransdell, Ralph M. Scott, Donn L. Smith, and Beverly T. Towery.

The excellent volume on cancer by Drs. Lauren V. Ackerman and Jual A. del Regato, edition 3, has been used extensively as a reference in nearly every chapter.

Mrs. Catherine Bauscher, medical artist, has brought unusual skill and experience to the preparation of the illustrations. A considerable debt is due the reference librarians, Mrs. Ruth Atwood and Miss Nancy Lorenzi, of the Kornhauser Health Sciences Library, University of Louisville. Dr. H. R. Pascoe of St. Louis contributed to an extensive revision of the chapters on lymphoma and leukemia. Dr. Lawrence W. O'Neal, also from St. Louis, gave valuable criticism of the chapter on the adrenal gland. The preparation of the manuscript has been most ably handled by Miss Edna Henderson, Miss Jean Fortwengler, and Mrs. Patricia McWilliams.

The early preparation of this synopsis was supported in part by Grant No. T-12-CA-8011, a clinical cancer training grant to the University of Louisville School of Medicine from the Department of Health, Education and Welfare, U. S. Public Health Service, Washington, D. C.

**Condict Moore, M.D.**

# Contents

Synopsis of

# Clinical cancer

Chapter 1

# Introduction

Most physicians realize the fundamental changes taking place today in our approach to cancer; we are beginning to study causes rather than being content to describe effects. Next to pathologists, treatment specialists have led in the development of oncology; but surgery and radiation today have nearly reached their limit of effectiveness. We need surgeons and therapists more than ever, but other groups are now able to participate at the forefront. Chemotherapy has entered the picture and, although generally unsuccessful, it is a modality that all can use and one that compels us to undertake the biologic study of basic growth phenomena. We might reasonably predict that, as in other fields, the control of cancer will come from those who study basic mechanisms.

For these reasons, and because molecular biology and chemistry have given us new conceptual tools and new laboratory methods, the field of neoplasia is finding a firm foundation and a unification. Unifying trends appear in several areas: (1) we now accept neoplasia as a single field of study; (2) we can now recognize the outline of similar types of phenomena that precede many anatomically different tumors; for example, the same chemical carcinogen may produce different tumors in different organs and species at different times, but probably by the same basic process; (3) we can easily visualize the mechanisms of metastasis common to many diverse tumors; (4) we can apply a single method of early tumor detection, cytology, to different tissues of the body; (5) we find similar "precancerous" changes in different tissues when we seek them intently; (6) we often find that one drug inhibits growth in different types of tumors, whereas a single type of tumor responds to several different drugs. Until these and other ideas coincided, cancer reports treated each type of tumor as an isolated syndrome rather than as an example of a common growth disorder.

James Ewing drew all tumors together into a single field for study in 1919 by his monumental book, *Neoplastic Diseases*. However hard he sought a unifying thread, Ewing actually featured the differences among cancers, so painstakingly did he review all publications and so carefully did he eschew irresponsible speculation. Recent fairly reliable data, both clinical and laboratory, now make some responsible speculation possible. Neoplasia begins to take form in our minds as a *universal tissue response*. The peculiar combinations of cancer's antecedent circumstances (environmental, genetic, and metabolic) are as multiple and variable as are the morphologic growth patterns that result; but the fact remains that nearly all tissues develop tumors.

Traditional "mechanistic" concepts of tumor growth, with emphasis on gross and microscopic morphology, size, and anatomic relationships, although fundamental to a complete picture of neoplasia, now run second in importance to our growing understanding of cell and tissue growth processes, cell differentiation, and growth control mechanisms. The anatomic relations of a tumor, so vital to the therapist, soon fail the modern diagnostician as a basis for progress. Seeing the success of cervical cytology, the practitioner realizes that tomorrow's cancer control depends on recognition of minor tissue changes long before gross anatomic alteration takes place.

The strong need exists to emphasize neoplasia as a unique field of study, just as one studies infectious diseases, metabolic diseases, and trauma. No longer does the traditional assignment of tumors to traditional departments satisfy fundamental concepts of neoplasia. In the past some tumors were considered medical, others were considered surgical, and still others radiologic. Other tumors were parcelled out to various anatomically oriented specialties. Today all specialties must deal with cancer. Cancer is a truly multidisciplinary, interdepartmental disease complex. Only its consideration as a single, although complicated, pathologic process can give the beginning clinician a proper platform upon which to build future knowledge integrated with future experience.

## RATIONALE FOR A SYNOPSIS

Comprehensive textbooks on cancer must necessarily be bulky because of the many volumes of publications they attempt to cover. Increasingly difficult revisions due to the rapid pace of new discoveries, make each new edition larger and less up-to-date. Few students will purchase such expensive texts as collateral or unrequired reading without a scheduled, required course on tumors in the medical school curriculum. Few of these courses, texts, or students exist. The student will pick up spotty information on tumors in medical and surgical tomes while hoping to get his turn at a cancer text in the library. If he writes a paper, he will rely on highly detailed journal reviews, abstracts, indexes, and library retrieval systems. The comprehensive text is the best starting point for a study of a particular tumor, but where does each beginner get enough reliable, basic information about neoplasia in general, related to each tumor in particular, to prepare for a meaningful clinical experience? He needs an accurate clinical sketch at the start and always at hand for check and review. He needs a basic orientation about tumors in general, a fundamental pattern into which he can fit each tumor patient to supplant memorization of a hundred or so isolated tumor syndromes.

A synopsis of clinical cancer information may be one answer to this problem. It can supplement any clinical departmental teaching program, can serve as a "starter" in courses with heavy tumor content, and can act as a "refresher" for practitioners. The reader of such a synopsis will have contact with data carefully selected by physicians who have had wide clinical experience with many types of neoplasia. Most clinicians have a limited experience with a variety of cancers and perhaps an in-depth experience with only one. It is natural to view the world through one's own glass.

A recent remark by a family physician who had practiced for 40 years in a rural town illustrates the extreme of this situation. When a woman with breast cancer whom he had referred for treatment was returned with a good prognosis for 5-year survival (80%), he stated that if she were alive and well in 5 years he would be very much surprised because she would be the first such person he had seen in his entire medical practice. He had seen a great deal of advanced breast cancer and believed that he knew about cancer in general—it was invariably fatal.

On the other hand, most basic laboratory scientists have little clinical orientation. Although they contribute much to our basic concepts, they are unable to bring these to the bedside. Thus bridging the gap between the burgeoning biologic sciences and highly specialized and departmentalized clinical medicine to produce an integration of clinical and laboratory knowledge is necessarily slow. Beginning clinicians need to know how to make a start in such an integrative process and to realize their responsibility for carrying the process ever further during their professional lives.

A synopsis may mislead by oversimplifying, thus demeaning the importance of a field of study; it may select data poorly; or it may prevent the student from developing deep interest by seeming to sanction the adequacy of superficial review. However, the advantages of a carefully prepared condensation seem to us to outweigh these possible drawbacks. In addition to what we have said above, all of us are only too aware of the confusion and profusion of journal reports that flood us and threaten to inundate us every month. Any reasonable attempt to select and condense this material pays dividends to the student or physician beginning to review. In considering medical school curricula the new "core" curriculum nearly abolishes the lecture type of presentation of material to a large group of students. No effective opportunity remains for imparting the heart of cancer information to an entire group, but it must be done. Furthermore, with the advent of audiovisual aids and programed teaching to the learning process, codification of data in each discipline will eventually be required. A synopsis could constitute the first step toward programed teaching.

We do not suffer the delusion that we can present for clinicians the best possible synthesis of laboratory and clinical information about cancer. We merely present an effort at such a synthesis at this time. We urge the clinician to examine it and, after careful study and reflection, to improve upon it.

## SPECIAL EMPHASES

In this résumé we aim at the student, resident, or young practicing general clinician, not the training specialists expert in one technique of therapy. We will not give lengthy descriptions of treatment. Several treatment modalities and the principles of treatment for each particular regional cancer are mentioned in each section, but detailed discussions of therapy will merely distract from our purpose —understanding cancer. We will try to emphasize the similarities of the neoplastic process wherever possible. Mechanisms of origin will be mentioned wherever they seem well founded. An attempt will also be made to reflect the more recent realistic attitudes toward clinical cancer that have arisen because we have gained greater experience with this disease.

Now that the increasing possibilities of cancer control with our present knowledge of therapy become apparent, a general attitude of cautious optimism begins to replace an older, uncritical pessimistic approach. The concept of control rather than cure stands today as the real aim of cancer treatment. Prompt and vigorous rehabilitation of cancer patients is becoming more widespread. Wider appreciation of the importance of environmental agents in cancer causation promises real benefit in terms of cancer prevention and control; thus the growing wish of the medical profession to accept its responsibilities for the practice of preventive medicine is becoming possible in an increasing number of cancers.

When a point of information is controversial, simple mention of this will have to suffice without lengthy justification. The largest amount of space has been allotted to those cancers of which knowledge of etiology, diagnosis, and treatment has advanced enough to reward clinicians' efforts in terms of numbers of patients salvaged. Cancers that kill most patients, such as those in the esophagus, are not accorded extra space merely because of high mortality. In the résumé we seek to give a balanced importance to the three disciplines primarily involved in cancer—pathology, surgery, and radiology—without showing bias for one or the other. Such an even balance is seldom attainable, but our intention is to treat them equally.

## CLASSIFICATION

Much as we are devoted to unifying the various clinical cancers, we have not tried to impose unity by attempting a new classification of cancers; far wiser men have tried and failed. Traditional classification by gross anatomic site gives us little information about tumor behavior. On the other hand, grouping of tumors by the function of the tissue of origin, although basic and enlightening, becomes confusing when followed to its logical conclusion. For example, small bowel mucosa acts like a lining tissue and produces a garden variety of gastrointestinal adenocarcinomas; it also acts like a secreting, absorbing, glandular tissue and produces carcinoid tumors of most unusual behavior.

Two fundamental points about tumor classifications bear emphasis: (1) structure and function (they always go together) of the tissue of origin exert great influence on the behavior of the cancer that develops from that tissue; and (2) tissues of basically similar structure and function occur in widely separate organs all over the body, whereas quite different tissues occur side by side in the same organ. Cancers of the mouth and anus behave in basically similar ways according to the similarity of the squamous epithelium in the two locations. However, the kidney produces two cancers that behave in dissimilar ways—the parenchymal cells of the collecting tubules and the lining cells of the kidney pelvis have considerably different structure and function. If we expect gross anatomy to correlate with tumor behavior, we court confusion. But if we study the tissues and cells of origin from the viewpoint of microscopic structure and detailed physiology and embryology, a picture begins to form of basically consistent tumor types arising from similar tissues.

Throughout we will endeavor to emphasize "early" cancer. However, under sections on natural history of the various cancers, descriptions of "late" disease will be included for contrast and background. We have included a section on "precancerous" lesions in many chapters. The term is properly in disrepute among pathologists and other experts on neoplasia because proof is lacking of the inevitable advancement of any of these lesions to invasive cancer. But we badly need some term to convey the idea that in most cancers there are tissue changes indicating preparation for invasive cancer, changes that mean a predisposed tissue. The more we look for these changes, the more we find them. We do not imply that a "precancerous" condition inevitably becomes cancer, but only that the *strong probability* exists.

Benign tumors will be given attention equally with the malignant tumors in some chapters; in other chapters they will only be mentioned among the differential diagnoses. Because benign tumors play a large role in diagnostic thinking at some sites and a small role in others, they will be treated somewhat irregularly. Emphasis throughout the synopsis will be on malignant neoplasms.

The volume is designed to be useful clinically, not as a reference book. A few references appear at the end of each chapter so that the reader may begin to compose a bibliography by consulting these references.

## STATISTICS

We include a short chapter on end result reporting. Numerical data, necessarily part of the clinical lore of each regional cancer, appear in the text as approximate percentages only to confer a general idea of their value. Exact percentages of patients salvaged, for example, are of limited accuracy and of limited clinical value despite the extreme emphasis accorded them in cancer publications. Data on the incidence of each regional cancer are expressed as relative proportions of the total number of cancers. Absolute rates on incidence, prevalence, and mortality do not appear because imperfect reporting systems make the majority of such figures too suspect to be worth a student's concentrated effort at the beginning of the study of cancer. There is no section on the increasingly contributive field of cancer epidemiology; the sections on incidence, distribution, and etiology will note important epidemiologic data. When interesting geographic variations in the incidence of some cancers are mentioned, this does not necessarily imply hereditary, genetic, or racial basis for such distribution.

## THE GOOD PHYSICIAN

The good physician is a rare human being. The most difficult activity of the human mind is a good physician's job—to analyze the multiple biologic variables of illness and to correlate basic scientific data with the individual needs of an ailing human being. It is a rare mind indeed that optimally responds to the emotional and physical illness of a patient with a fruitful mixing of his own scientific knowledge, sympathy, and logical deductive powers. Each physician aims for this optimum. Cancer offers him a special challenge—absolute cure is often possible, the disease is frequent, and it is inevitably devastating if nothing is done.

The good physician begins to develop when he first enters the physician-patient relationship. He must realize the value of this relationship from the start. Here he first has a chance to practice the analysis of the multiple biologic variables in solving the problem of illness, an analysis requiring a more intimate blending of rigidly critical judgment and intuition than perhaps any other human activity. For this valuable analytical situation an outline, at least, of clinical background information about disease is essential. Without a minimum fund of clinical information to begin with, the clinician cannot take the first step toward understanding the process and component types of activity involved in the complex doctor-patient interaction. The learning doctor, who is an "applied" scientist, must have some guide to reliable clinical correlations as a background to apply before he can get the feel of the new vital role he is beginning to explore. In this regard, carefully prepared synopses of clinical information may be of help.

The qualities of a good physician are probably inherent and cannot be instilled at the graduate student level. Most aspiring clinicians possess these qualities and need only to have them stimulated. Some of the basic qualities, such as intellectual curiosity, intellectual honesty, deep concern for the individual human and his physical and mental health, and a real desire to be of service, can be fertilized by observing what facets and facts of human disease an older teacher selects as important and which ones he rejects. Here, again, some indications of this process may be evident from a synopsis.

**REFERENCES**

Atchley, D. W.: The role of the patient in medical education, J.A.M.A. **185:**396-398, 1963.

Easson, E. C.: Cancer and the problem of pessimism, CA **17:**7-14, 1967.

Ewing, J.: Neoplastic diseases, ed. 4, Philadelphia, 1942, W. B. Saunders Co.

Harrell, G. T.: Trends in education—practice and organization of health service, J.A.M.A. **196:**334-338, 1966.

Leaf, A.: Changing needs in medical education, Med. Opinion Rev., pp. 18-22, Feb., 1967.

Chapter 2

# Glossary of terms

Physicians dealing with neoplasia have evolved special meanings and usages for common words to describe more easily the material in their field. We will attempt a simple definition of some of these terms.

**anaplastic** Similar to the term undifferentiated, describes a tumor whose cells uniformly lack special cell characteristics.

**benign tumor** Neoplasm of partially controlled growth character that will not metastasize and will rarely cause death.

**biopsy** Strictly defined, the whole diagnostic process of securing a tissue specimen *plus* the interpretation by the pathologist; commonly used more loosely, the technical maneuver of taking the tissue specimen from the patient.

- **excision biopsy** Narrow removal of a whole lesion for diagnosis, not for treatment.
- **negative biopsy** Biopsy showing no cancer.
- **positive biopsy** Biopsy showing cancer.
- **wedge biopsy** Excision of a portion of a lesion for diagnosis.

**cancer** Any malignant neoplasm, regardless of histogenesis.

**capsule** Condensation or thin layer of compressed tissue at a growing tumor edge or the wall of cystic neoplasms, sometimes found with benign and malignant tumors. It was formerly considered a barrier to cancer spread. A better term for a cancer capsule is pseudocapsule, which implies a lack of any real function as a barrier to spread.

**carcinoma** Malignant neoplasm of epithelial origin.

**chemotherapy** Usually means treatment with a nonhormonal, cytotoxic drug.

**cobalt 60** Radioactive source emitting the same general types of rays as x-ray machines and thus used for treatment of neoplasms.

**cocarcinogen** Agent that enhances the cancer-producing action of another agent.

**cure** Complete arrest of growth of cancer cells, primary and metastatic. It is, of course, the ultimate aim of treatment. This word must be used with circumspection because recurrences sometimes develop after many years. If a patient's survival is such that his calculated life expectancy equals that of the general population of the same age and sex, then this amounts to clinical cure. "Five-year cure" merely means 5-year survival without evidence of cancer.

**differentiated** Cells with characteristic features that correlate with specialized function.

**direct extension** Spread of cancer by continuous, invasive growth in contrast to spread by metastasis.

**five-year survival** Appropriate yardstick of successful management in many cancers, implying the probability of cure, while admitting the possibility of later recurrence. (In some other cancers, 10-year survivals may be more appropriate—breast melanoma, and lymphoma.)

**gland** Organ of internal or external secretion, as distinct from a lymph node.

**grade** Histopathologic class (usually I through IV) sometimes assigned to tumors by pathologists to help determine prognosis.

**growth rate** An imprecise expression dependent on clinical impressions. Precise measurements and comparisons of growth rates in human tumors have seldom been made. True growth rate depends upon concepts of cell population kinetics (Chapter 3).

**initiator** Agent that can start the first essential phase of the carcinogenic sequence.

**irradiation** Maneuver of using special rays, such as x-ray, to treat tissues and cancers.

**latent period (latency)** Time between the application of a carcinogenic agent and the clinical appearance of cancer.

**leukemia** Malignant overgrowth of blood cells.

**local recurrence** Reappearance of tumor at the primary site in the area of tissue treated or operated on.

**local surgery** Removal of all tissue around, and including, the primary tumor.

**lymphoma** Malignant neoplasm of lymphogenous origin.

**malignant tumor** Neoplasm with uncontrolled growth behavior, usually with the capability of metastasizing and the potential of killing the host.

**margin** Width of cancer-free tissue at the edges of a specimen.

**megavoltage** Very high energy x-rays (1000 kilovolts or more).

**metastasis** Established, spontaneous graft of malignant cells that takes place by embolization of cells in lymph or blood or by free-floating transport in a cavity.

**distant metastasis** Any metastasis beyond the tumor region at a more remote site in the body.

**neoplasm** New growth, lacking normal growth controls.

**node** Lymph node.

**negative node** Lymph node *without* metastasis on histologic examination.

**positive node** Lymph node *with* metastasis on histologic examination.

**regional nodes** Collection of lymph nodes nearest to the primary tumor.

**orthovoltage** X-rays of medium energy (200 to 400 kilovolts).

**palliation** Treatment aimed at symptomatic relief or prolongation of useful life only, without expectation of cure.

**precancerous** Tissue and cell changes that *probably,* but not necessarily, will progress to cancer if given enough time.

**primary** Original cancer at its original site.

**promoter** Agent that cannot initiate but can push forward the carcinogenic sequence once it has begun. (Sometimes we cannot distinguish between promoter and cocarcinogen.)

**rad** Commonly used unit of x-ray dosage, expressed as the amount of radiant energy (100 ergs) absorbed per gram of tissue.

**radiation** General phenomenon of x-ray production from natural and man-made x-ray sources. Used improperly sometimes to mean treatment by x-rays.

**radical surgery** Usually a complete removal, in more or less one block, of all local tissue and regional nodes that might contain cancer; usually done with intent to cure.

**recurrence** Clinical reappearance of cancer after its disapperance under treatment. It represents microscopic *residual* cancer that finally grows to a grossly detectable size.

**regional node dissection** One of the standardized operations for removal of nodes in the largest collection nearest the primary tumor (neck, axilla, groin, pelvis, retroperitoneum, or mediastinum).

**sarcoma** Malignant neoplasm of mesodermal origin.

**second primary** New, distinctly separate cancer developing from a new, separate carcinogenic process.

**stage** Degree of clinical spread of a cancer in the body (Chapter 31).

**survival rate**

**crude survival rate** Simply the proportion of all patients seen who were alive at a given time interval after the last patient was admitted to the study.

**relative survival rate** More accurate; the effect of cancer on longevity by adjusting for age and for the "natural" attrition of deaths from other causes.

**tumor** Any swelling or lump.

**tumor progression** Tendency of most cancers to gain, as time passes, increasingly malignant characteristics.

**undifferentiated** Describes cells lacking nearly all characteristic specialized features.

**x-rays** One of a number of types of rays produced by therapy machines used to treat neoplasms.

## REFERENCE

Martin, H. A.: Proposed glossary of cancer, Arch. Surg. **87**:534-537, 1963.

Chapter 3

# Carcinogenesis

To begin a consideration of the origin of tumors, we may assume that cancer comprises a large group of apparently diverse pathologic conditions that can be considered different manifestations of a single basic process. Cancer appears to arise from a uniquely complex set of biologic circumstances that must coincide and interrelate in certain ways, each of which is essential to the final outcome of cancer and therefore each qualifies as a contributory cause of cancer. One might further characterize neoplasia as a tissue response to a peculiar combination of biologic circumstances that is common to all living tissues; the contributing circumstances are multitudinous, variable from tissue to tissue and species to species, and substitutions may be made in any particular combination during the carcinogenic process. But any cell that divides may be subject to it.

The cancer-causing circumstances nearly always involve four classes of events: (1) action of an external agent (chemical, viral, or physical), (2) adequate dosage of this agent, (3) an internal predisposition (dietary deficiency, hormonal imbalance, immunologic defect, heritable genetic abnormality, etc.), and (4) the passage of relatively long periods of time. These four basic necessary elements seem commonly applicable to most mammalian tumors. One may object that we have couched these four elements in such general terms that any pathologic condition, not merely neoplasia, could be said to have such a theoretic background. We will try, in our following remarks, to sharpen these concepts sufficiently so that they may apply more specifically to cancer.

Investigators working with chemical carcinogens, carcinogenic viruses (identifiable only in animals), and radiation all agree that any theory of overall causes and mechanisms, to be complete, must encompass every factor operating to produce the various cancers. Therefore a single "cause" in the strict sense is an outmoded concept. The very multiplicity of interacting factors makes the aim of determining a "carcinogenic threshold dose" of a chemical or radiation and the establishment of a consistent dose-response relationship with a particular agent goals of doubtful attainment. For example, a certain dose of 3,4-benzpyrene given to one species of laboratory animal by one route will give a certain percentage of tumors in a definite period of time. But alterations of any one of many biologic factors in this system may cause a marked difference in the tumor result. In short, the problem of cancer is extremely complex, requiring the analysis of multiple variables.

## THEORETICAL FORMULA FOR MECHANISM OF CARCINOGENESIS

The first useful idea in the formulation of cancer theory arose from studies on skin carcinogenesis with aromatic hydrocarbons. This is the two-stage concept of *initiation* and *promotion* (Berenblum). Recent investigators have attacked this as unduly simplified and not universally applicable, but it helps us get around the unmanageable complexities of the problem. Briefly, Berenblum states that some external agents can initiate the cancerous sequence, but at low dosage these agents will not carry it to completion by themselves. Then other substances or factors, incapable of initiating cancer alone, can promote the process to clinical cancer. Most initiators do not need promoters, but all promoters need initiators. (Another term, *cocarcinogen,* indicates a weak initiator that enhances the action of a strong one.) In terms of skin cancer, benzpyrene exemplifies an initiator and croton oil a promoter. The whole process is vastly more complicated, but it helps to try to classify factors into the two major groups: (1) factors that alone start and complete the cancerous process and (2) factors that can push the process along but need the first group to begin it. This two-stage concept fits well with the following simple formula that uses our four basic factors, which we mention here again for emphasis. The formula serves to begin our thinking about cancer mechanisms:

$$\text{External factor} + \text{Adequate dosage} + \text{Internal predisposition} + \text{Time} \rightleftharpoons \text{Precancer} \rightarrow \text{Cancer}$$

Here the *external factor* is often the initiator. *Internal predisposition* is the term we choose to represent all the many biologic and metabolic derangements of organisms that might promote cancer. The almost limitless combinations of internal derangements (hormonal, immunologic, nutritional, genetic) defy description here. Suffice it to say that they appear to play a key promoting role in the cancer formula. (Internal agents, such as hormones or metabolites from liver or kidney, may initiate cancer, but solid evidence for their initiating action, except in bladder cancer, is meager.)

*Adequate dosage* cannot be defined accurately, but a range of threshold doses undoubtedly exists for each tissue, individual, species, and externally applied carcinogen. *Time* (latency), like dose, varies widely and the two are often interdependent. Often an inordinately long latent period elapses before clinical cancer appears. The time needed from inception to the full development of cancer is longer than we have ever before realized—up to 60 years for some cancers. If time and complexity of developmental process can be equated, and if we remember that the gestation time of the human fetus is only 9 months, then it is small wonder that we have not solved the riddle of cancer. Neoplasia usually takes years to develop from its first "stage setting" events and may be, in terms of cell biology and cytogenetics, as complex as fetal development. Our justification for including *precancer* in a basic theory may be questioned. We believe it is necessary on the grounds that precursor lesions occur more and more often in all tissues in which they can be properly sought.

To explain this theoretic framework for our cancer thinking further, we quote from a recent statement in a scientific advisory committee's report to the President: "The problem of carcinogenesis is probably one of individual carcinogens, very likely weakly carcinogenic, acting in combination, or with one mediating its effects through another, over a long period." We would add to this that there must be prepared, innately susceptible cells—the *target tissue*—and we would broaden the concept of an external carcinogen to include anything not manufactured or found naturally in the body. Under this definition external carcinogens would include viruses. The variety of tumors resulting in hamsters from a single virus, the polyoma virus (Stewart), expand the possibility of cancer-causing environmental substances into the whole field of virology. (Although no virus has been demonstrated to cause a human cancer, recent laboratory studies have yielded strong evidence that a virus may be the initiating agent in human leukemia and especially in Burkitt's lymphoma. A government organized and sponsored task force, composed of outstanding basic scientists and clinical researchers, is now exploring these leads intensively.)

The reader must remember not to rely slavishly on the previous simple formula. It will not bear the detailed scrutiny of the laboratory scientist; its categories will break down and merge into each other. But if we are to think at all, this will do for a starter.

## IMPORTANCE OF EXTERNAL CARCINOGENS

Emphasis on external chemical carcinogens naturally arises because of the hundreds of such substances that have been found to cause cancer in animals and because they are the known essential factors in some human cancers that we can control. They give us a "handle" on the disease, even though detailed basic mechanisms are obscure. Several major addresses at the Ninth International Cancer Congress in Tokyo (1966) stressed our ability to control them as the greatest hope for cancer progress; more than 200 papers were given at this meeting on chemical carcinogens.

Cancer-initiating compounds have been chemically identified for the last 50 years; the strongest and most studied are three polycyclic hydrocarbons—methylcholanthrene (MCH), benzpyrene (BP), and dimethylbenzanthracene (DMBA). Human contact with many carcinogenic chemicals occurs frequently today in many occupations: (1) those involving soots, tars, and creosotes, (2) those dealing with catalytically cracked oil residues, fuel oil, cutting oils, and shale oils, (3) those using dye intermediates, such as $\beta$-naphthylamine and 4-aminobiphenyl, and (4) certain ore and metal industries, especially those handling nickel, beryllium, cobalt, asbestos, and chromates.

In addition to industrial exposure, contact with substances of unknown biologic action polluting our atmosphere and with new pesticides, as well as with food additives, drugs, and industrial wastes, and with new food preservation and preparation substances is being forced upon the entire population every day. Many of these substances are produced by the burning of organic material at high temperatures. It might be speculated that whenever organic matter undergoes incomplete combustion at volatilizing temperatures, the likelihood exists of creating carcinogens (tobacco smoke, gasoline engine exhausts, and coal furnace fumes). We do not have well-established bioassays for the cancer-producing properties of new compounds, and we certainly lack adequate regulations for the unknown compounds being constantly introduced into our environment. For example, there is strongly suggestive clinical evidence linking cancer of the paranasal sinuses with employment and exposure in a furniture (woodworking) industry. Yet safeguards are said to be lacking.

It is further enlightening to remember the various ways in which external carcinogenic agents may impinge on body tissues. (1) They may make *direct contact* with "target" tissues, such as the sun's ultraviolet rays on skin and radioactive dust that settles directly on the bronchial mucosa of radioactive mine workers. (2) Ingested substances are metabolized and *excreted* or temporarily stored in tissues in which contact is prolonged; in this manner the bladder mucosa undergoes an effective application of commercial dye metabolites that have been ingested, changed, and then excreted in the urine. (3) *Permanent* body *storage depots* may develop cancer, such as when radioactive strontium 90 is ingested and stored permanently in bone marrow. The location of various cancers in various tissues may thereby be linked to external agents by noting which tissues act as reservoirs, places of stasis, or storage sites for ingested and excreted substances or for the metabolized products of potentially carcinogenic ingested substances.

While discussing external carcinogens, it may be well to try to summarize the theories about the action of these compounds. In one theory, discussed below, somatic mutation has been considered to result from interaction of an external chemical compound and the deoxyribonucleic acid (DNA) molecules. Another theory of action, proposed by Abell and Heidelberger, describes deletion of enzymatic growth control factors by chemical binding between the carcinogenic hydrocarbon and these enzymes or other repressor substances. The deleted factor may be a ribonucleic acid (RNA) molecule. A third theory postulates that altered antigenic properties of the cell may be caused by a combination of chemical compound and cell protein. Last, latent viruses may be activated as a result of deletion of repressor or controlling factors by the foreign chemical substance. These theories do not necessarily mutually exclude each other, and none of them has been proved.

## IMPORTANCE OF SOMATIC MUTATION

The "final common pathway" of most modern cancer theories involves a genetic change in the developing cancer cell, a somatic mutation. One must distinguish this from germ-cell mutation that is heritable from generation to generation, even though the genetic alteration may be very similar in either case. Nearly all investigators find inescapable the inclusion of genetic and chromosomal alteration at some point in the carcinogenic sequence of events. However, we have not included it in our simplified four-element formula, outlined above, because it may be a result of the carcinogenic change rather than a cause. Whether somatic mutation is cause or effect or whether it is the core of the problem, it usually appears as a notable feature of the cancerous change. However, germ cell mutation does play an important role in the development of certain rare human cancers, notably retinoblastoma of infants and familial multiple polyposis of the colon. In these conditions heritable defects in germ cells express themselves as cancers quite predictably. So strongly does the genetic abnormality favor cancer in these families that other external and internal factors do not alter the emersion of the tumor trait to any noticeable degree.

## IMMUNOLOGY

Several attractive theories involve immunologic alteration as their salient feature in determining whether or not clinical cancer will develop. The initial event in these mechanisms, however, is the impingement on the gene by an external agent and thus the creation of a foreign antigen. Modern immunology and cytogenetics contribute much to our thinking. Tyler's immunogenetic theory, which draws the analogy very convincingly between transplantation disease and cancer, deserves study, if only to review the complexity of multiple factor interaction that is possible and the ingenuity needed for integration of all major factors into a coherent single theory.

Immune responses consist of two main kinds—cellular and humoral. Cellular responses seem to come largely from lymphocytes and typically cause delayed hypersensitivity such as the tuberculin response and homograft rejection; humoral responses stem from immunoglobulins and typically account for antibacterial defenses. The homograft rejection mechanism assumes importance in explaining one basic factor that influences cancer metastasis. On the basis of many laboratory and some clinical studies we can begin to form a picture of the process. Lymphocytes constantly move in and out of nodes, lymphatics, and the bloodstream. When a sensitized lymphocyte meets a particular foreign antigen, the lymphocyte begins to divide and proliferate. Thus, according to the clonal selection theory of acquired immunity, a sensitized clone of lymphocytes appears, especially in the node, which enlarges. If a tumor specific antigen begins this process, regional nodes first enlarge and regional tumor graft rejection appears; then, later, systemic tumor graft rejection develops as more distant nodes develop clones. However, it may happen that continued primary tumor growth throws off excessive tumor antigen that overwhelms the sensitized clones; in this event nodes diminish, immunity wanes, and graft tolerance appears. Applying this concept to embolizing cancer cells, we can easily see how cellular immunity could prevent the cancer graft of cells from "taking" at first, then fail to prevent "take" later on, and allow metastasis to occur.

Metastasis of normal and benign tumor cells probably does not occur, except for the phenomenon of endometriosis, because of another mechanism, cell contact inhibition, a property possessed by normal cells but not by cancer cells (see below). Many other mechanisms probably also affect metastasis. The possibility exists that clinical cancer only develops when the tumor can overwhelm the immune defenses of the host. The long latent period in most cancers may result from antibodies produced during the preclinical stages. At present we cannot measure tumor immunity in man; it seems to be a generally weak and unreliable

**Table 1.** Chronic irritation and carcinogenesis*

| Substance | Irritation of skin | Cancer incidence |
|---|---|---|
| Coal dust | Most marked | Nil |
| Blast furnace pitch | Marked | Nil |
| Gas-tar pitch | Slight | High |
| Tar | Very slight | Marked |
| Soot | Absent | Most marked |

*From Ross, H. C.: Occupational cancer, J. Cancer Res. **3**:321, 1918.

clinical defense so far, but immunologists are diligently seeking ways to strengthen it.

## ROLE OF IRRITATION IN CARCINOGENESIS

Stimulated by suggestive clinical observations, chronic irritation has been invoked by many students of carcinogenesis as a common basic factor in the process. There is little laboratory evidence to support the idea that chronic irritation alone can initiate cancer. That it may act like a promoter, allowing more intimate contact between external initiating agents and target cells, cannot be denied. However, chronic irritation seems to play a minor role as Table 1 shows. It illustrates the inverse relation between the irritative quality and the carcinogenic power of various common substances.

## OTHER CONTRIBUTIONS

Embryology is doing much to focus our attention on basic processes regulating tissue growth, tissue organization, cell differentiation and dedifferentiation, and changes in injury, repair, and aging. Investigators are working out the biochemistry of tissue growth regulators, repressors, and evocators; one group finds cell differentiation is caused by a single nucleotide. This nucleotide undoubtedly is controlled by a specific gene, and hence we are speaking basically again of alteration involving somatic mutation.

A number of investigators working along the same lines of tissue growth regulators have reported extracts of various tissues, and of tumors themselves, that possess tumor-inhibiting properties. These extracts have not yet been chemically identified. Szent-Györgyi and associates believe that a cell proliferation inhibitor exists, probably an aldoketone methylglyoxal, whose action can be stopped by a "glyoxalase" enzyme system. If a cell loses the ability to bind and control glyoxalase, uncontrolled cell growth could result.

Some recent workers describe the specific chemical messengers that control the normal process of cell division as *chalones,* which are specific for certain tissues but identical in a number of different species. They probably represent the mechanisms whereby chemical messages are sent out, received, and acted on and are essentially the same for most forms of vertebrate life. If chalones carry messages necessary to normal growth control, alteration of the structure of such messengers by outside substances could lead to cancer.

Other investigators in the new field of *cell population dynamics* study patterns and mechanisms of tumor growth. Central to this study is the growth fraction concept of Mendelsohn; this concept postulates that a neoplasm, and, indeed normal tissue as well, is composed of a fraction of cells in the actively proliferating, mitotic-cycling stage, and another fraction of cells in a resting stage. Thus growth rate depends mainly on the *proportion* of proliferating cells to the whole cell population, including resting, inactive cells. In normal tissue only a tiny percentage of cells, if any, proliferate at any one time; this percentage varies from tissue to tissue and increases markedly with injury and repair. In neoplasms a much larger but variable percentage of cells proliferate, and so the tumor eventually outgrows the normal tissue bed around it and becomes clinically detectable as a lump.

Several other factors complicate the measurement of neoplastic growth: (1) the stroma of some cancers constitutes their main bulk and is composed, not of malignant cells released from normal growth controls, but of normal cells reacting to the cancerous ones; (2) the fraction of proliferating cancer cells can change frequently; (3) cell loss occurs—a varying percentage of cancer cells dies, sloughs off, and disappears; and (4) some cells apparently reach an absolutely nonproliferative stage in which they live on but never divide. We can readily appreciate, therefore, the complexity of any explanation of human cancer growth rate. Yet if a cancer were composed entirely of actively dividing cells that constantly doubled their number every 4 days, without cell loss, the patient would probably die in less than 4 months with over 1 trillion cancer cells present, beginning with one cell. Some acute leukemias may approach this rapid a course.

The concept of cell *contact inhibition* describes a process of intercellular control and communication among normal cells not possessed by cancer cells. Perhaps related is the fact that cell membranes are less mutually adhesive in cancer cells than in normal cells. When the normal cell contacts another normal cell, it inhibits its behavior so that coordinated, organized tissue results. Cancer cells do not have this contact inhibition between one another, and consequently this method of growth restraint fails, resulting in uncoordinated, abnormal tissue accumulation (neoplasia).

Genetic studies further elucidate mechanisms pertaining to carcinogenesis. A gene mutation may be spontaneous; it may also be induced by radiations (causing chromosomal breaks), by carcinogenic chemicals (combining with DNA), or by viruses (replacing or redirecting activity of genetic material). More recently theories of gene regulation, affecting expression or nonexpression of genetic traits, have been hailed as promising. These concepts involve regulator genes, operons, and structural genes. Others have elaborated this theory to postulate reversibility in the early stages of cancer with consequent hope for development of a cure along this line. Thus malignant change may involve a rearrangement in the normal sequence of genetic messages.

Analogies between cancer and infection have been used to advantage. The one that seems most appropriate today compares our present degree of advancement of basic knowledge about cancer, and our degree of control of the disease, with the situation in infectious diseases 20 years ago. At that time penicillin effectively controlled most staphylococcic and streptococcic infections before the basic mechanisms of action were known. (The mechanisms still are not clear.) So, too, we may have the tools for the control and prevention of cancer actually in hand today, although we do not have basic understanding and detailed knowledge of its causes. The most obvious tool is the potential control of external carcinogenic agents.

## COMMON CHARACTERISTICS OF MANY CLINICAL CANCERS

As our knowledge increases in diverse disciplines, each one contributing to some facet of the cancer problem, we become more aware of the features that many cancers possess in common and that make them an ever more unified group. In the field of histopathology it has long been known that hyperchromatism, aneuploidy, increased nuclear-cytoplasmic ratio, increased nuclear mass, and increased numbers of mitoses characterize cancerous—as opposed to normal—cells. The grading of cancerous tissues according to degree of anaplasia is in general related to the speed of growth and the aggressive invasiveness of the cancer. In the field of cell physiology all types of cancer cells possess in common a loss of contact inhibition, a lack of normal cohesiveness, increased ameboid motility, lowered calcium content, increased membrane permeability, and an increase in cytolytic effects. Clinical cancer is really defined by the common ability of diverse types to shed viable cells into the lymph stream, into the bloodstream, or into serous cavities. These emboli tend to concentrate at points of trauma regardless of the type of cancer. Tumors also possess in common the capacity to invade and destroy surrounding normal tissue.

As may have been evident from our remarks in the discussion on the importance of external carcinogens, many tumors are localized in the tissues of the body by factors influencing the dosage of the external carcinogen applied to the susceptible cell. Here concepts of stasis, concentration, and storage depots play a key role. In further thinking of the localization of cancer, susceptible tissues of a mammalian body seem to be those of the *very young organism;* for example, neonatal tisues are vastly more susceptible to carcinogens than adult tissues; also tissues undergoing quick turnover, change, frequent mitoses, those undergoing repair and replacement, and tissues in which two different types of cells lie adjacent seem more susceptible.

A further similarity among cancers appears when we compare various precancerous stages. Such stages have been described and well documented in the cervix, endometrium, breast, mouth, lung, skin, bladder, and vulva, and undoubtedly other regional cancers will have their precancerous stages characterized in the future. These various precursor stages all tend to look much alike. There also seems to be a similar pattern of action and response of the many different cancers to radiation and radiomimetic chemotherapeutic drugs. The mechanisms seem to be similar regardless of the different tissues of origin of these cancers. Furthermore, cancers all tend to be focal, local diseases at inception. A great deal of evidence indicates that all the initial steps in the carcinogenic sequence take place in a local area; whether it is one cell, multiple foci of single cells, a single group, or multiple small local groups of cells, the process seldom blossoms in widely scattered foci simultaneously. Even in the lymphomas and leukemias, it would seem logical to assume that the early stages are focal. Last, and perhaps most important, Greenstein has shown that the enzyme patterns of malignant tumors from different tissues with different normal patterns tend to converge toward a common cancer pattern. True, the difference is more quantitative than qualitative, but the common trend of a malignant cell away from specialized, different patterns toward a common enzymatic pattern seems established. Modern cell biology may ultimately succeed in identifying a fundamental error of intracellular (or intercellular) metabolism—an enzymatic defect, for example—that characterizes the cancerous cell in all cancers and precedes clinical cancer in most cases. This would free us from our present traditional morphologic definition of cancer, which so often misleads, confuses, or fails fully to explain cancer and which has probably been developed to its limit of usefulness as a diagnostic and therapeutic guide.

## SUMMARY

A crude formulation of the process of carcinogenesis might take the following form: some foreign agent that can closely affect or combine with the genetic or essential growth-regulating mechanisms of cells impinges on a tissue and initiates a focal, abnormal sequence of development in one small area of the tissue. Such an agent may be a chemical carcinogen, ionizing radiation, ultraviolet sunlight, or a virus, but it is definitely foreign to the normal physiology of the tissue.

At the cellular level the alteration may be virus activation, which then replaces normal genetic expression; it may be genetic or enzymatic deletion, resulting from the combination of DNA with the external agent; it may take the form of mitochondrial damage; it may be chemical message interference within the nucleus, between nucleus and cytoplasm, within the cytoplasm, or between cells; or it may be the creation of a new antigen. It may be variable combinations of these or something entirely different. However, it is a peculiar and specific alteration for this particular group of cells. Some cells may die as a result; other cells will survive as abnormal. The initiating agent must be applied over a proper period of time and in proper dosages, perhaps supported by other cocarcinogens or promoters. It avoids total cell population death and causes some abnormal function of the tissue above normal responses. This may theoretically be conceived of as a stimulus to the tissue to "overperform" its function. The response is seldom 100% in all cells and is highly conditioned by the "ground" state of the tissue. The promoter factors conditioning the tissue arise from an abnormal internal metabolic milieu and will run the gamut from imbalance in hormones to abnormal oxygen transport mechanisms, from altered inorganic mineral metabolism to excess mitotic excitants. However, in most cases the initiator, the foreign substance, will be an obligatory factor in the process, and this first change will be irreversible.

Then time needs to elapse, usually many years, for promoters to work, for natural selection of potentially cancerous clones to take place, for clones to proliferate and to dedifferentiate—time to overcome local and regional immunologic, chemical, and physical defense mechanisms. The first morphologic change we can detect is often called dysplasia. This is reversible. With continued unfavorable conditions, such as persistence of the carcinogenic external and internal circumstances, carcinoma in situ develops. This stage may or may not be reversible. After 6 to 10 years more of carcinoma in situ (the average for such change in the cervix), clinical cancer finally appears. By this time the tumor is invading surrounding normal tissues, single cells or clumps of cells may be breaking off from the parent tumor, and these cells are in a position to embolize via lymph or blood vascular channels. Whether any of these embolizing cells are vigorous enough to survive or will find suitable soil for growth and thereby establish regional or distant metastases is dependent on many local, regional, and systemic conditions. Usually by the time invasive cancer appears, the possibility of such metastasis exists, but a short period of some months to a few years generally elapses before actual metastases become established. It is as though invasive cancer needs time to "get up steam" for overcoming barriers to metastasis. This relatively short time interval gives the clinician his main chance to control invasive cancer. The interval gives real value to the term *early diagnosis;* it means diagnosis before spread.

We are in danger of being stifled by the multiplicity of physical and chemical systems that the human mind has created to explain the origin of cancer. We must try to simplify, but the problem is innately so complex that simplification amounts to distortion. A combination of laboratory investigation and clinical epidemiologic study will be required in the future if the many and various promoting factors in the carcinogenic process are to be found. Also we must identify the high-risk persons in any clinical approach to the cancer program. This can be as rewarding as finding an initiator or a regulator gene and as important to the final outcome as the discovery of an immunologic defect. Some of the complex biologic processes that enter into carcinogenesis can only be fully characterized by clinical observation and painstaking clinical tabulation.

**REFERENCES**

Abell, C. W., and Heidelberger, C.: Interaction of carcinogenic hydrocarbons with tissues, Cancer Res. **22**:931-946, 1962.

Abstract of Papers, Proceedings of Ninth International Cancer Congress, Tokyo, Oct., 1966, Berlin, 1967, Springer-Verlag.

Bendich, A.: Progress Report XVII, Sloan Kettering Institute for Cancer Research, April, 1967, p. 69.

Berenblum, I.: The cocarcinogenic action of croton resins, Cancer Res. **1**:44-48, 1941.

Cancer: Current concepts and research trends, a source paper: "Report to the President," Washington, D. C., 1966, U. S. Public Health Service.

Cole, L. J., and Nowell, P. J.: Radiation carcinogenesis: the sequence of events, Science **150**: 1782-1786, 1965.

Crile, G., Jr.: A biological consideration of the treatment of breast cancer, Springfield, Ill., 1967, Charles C Thomas, Publisher.

Gellhorn, A.: Thoughts on cancer research, Ann. Intern. Med. **59**:251-257, 1963.

Greenstein, J. P.: Biochemistry of cancer, ed. 2, New York, 1954, Academic Press, Inc.

Hueper, W. C., and Conway, W. D.: Chemical carcinogenesis and cancers, Springfield, Ill., 1964, Charles C Thomas, Publisher.

Iverson, O. H.: Discussion on cell destruction and population dynamics in experimental skin carcinogenesis in mice., Progr. Exp. Tumor Res. **4**:169-206, 1964.

Kark, W.: Synopsis of cancer, Baltimore, 1966, The Williams & Wilkins Co.
Mendelsohn, M. L.: The kinetics of tumor cell proliferation. In Cellular radiation biology, Baltimore, 1965, The Williams & Wilkins Co., pp. 498-513.
Miller, A. J., and Kimsey, L. S.: Biological inhibitor of transplantable mouse tumors, Cancer **20:**471-477, 1967.
Miller, J. A., and Miller, E. C.: Natural and synthetic chemical carcinogens in the etiology of cancer, Cancer Res. **25:**1292-1304, 1965.
Pitot, H. C.: Some biochemical essentials of malignancy, Cancer Res. **23:**1474-1482, 1963.
Potter, V. R.: Biochemical perspectives in cancer research, Cancer Res. **24:**1084-1098, 1964.
Raven, R. W., and Roe, F. J. C.: The prevention of cancer, New York, 1967, Appleton-Century-Crofts.
Ross, H. C.: Occupational cancer, J. Cancer Res. **3:**321, 1918.
Rous, P., and Kidd, J. G.: Conditional neoplasms and subthreshold neoplastic states: study of tar tumors of rabbits, J. Exp. Med. **73:**365-390, 1941.
Schmeer, M. R.: Mercenene: growth-inhibiting agent of Mercenaria extracts—further chemical and biological characterization, Ann. N. Y. Acad. Sci. **136:**211-218, 1966.
Smithers, D. W.: A clinical prospect of the cancer problem, London, 1960, E. & S. Livingstone, Ltd.
Stewart, H.: Experimental cutaneous carcinoma. In Homberger, F., editor: The physiopathology of cancer, ed. 2, New York, 1959, Paul B. Hoeber, Inc., pp. 3-17.
Stewart, S. E.: Symposium Proceedings, American Association for Cancer Research, June, 1960, p. 669.
Szent-Györgyi, A.: Cell division and cancer, Science **149:**341-344, 1965.
Szent-Györgyi, A., Egyud, L. G., and McLaughlin, J. A.: Keto-aldehydes and cell division, Science **155:**539-541, 1967.
Tyler, A.: A developmental immunologenetic analysis of cancer. In Henry Ford Hospital International Symposium, Biological interactions in normal and neoplastic growth, New York, 1962, Little, Brown & Co., pp. 533-571.

Chapter 4

# Cancer of the skin

## Excluding melanoma

### INCIDENCE AND DISTRIBUTION

Cancers of the skin comprise about 18 to 20% of all cancers, but the large number of such cancers treated without any histologic verification precludes an accurate incidence figure. The male to female ratio is 2:1. Approximately 20% of all male cancers occur in the skin, exceeded only by cancers of the digestive system, whereas 11% of all female cancers are of skin origin, exceeded by three others—breast, digestive system, and female genital organs. They are three times as common in the southern half of the United States as in the northern half. Distribution frequency is a product of climate and susceptible skin type.

### ETIOLOGY

#### External initiating agents

The major external agent is *ultraviolet sunlight* (radiations in the range of 2500 to 3500 Å). These rays are absorbed by the epidermis. Stimulation toward cancer depends on the cumulative effect of repeated exposures, not on isolated episodes of intense exposure.

Less frequent causes of skin cancer are *ionizing radiations* (x-rays, etc.), various oils, coal tar, pitch, creosote, paraffins, beryllium, nickel, and arsenical compounds encountered in industrial or occupational pursuits. The three strongest of the chemical carcinogens are polycyclic hydrocarbons derived from coal tar—methylcholanthrene, dimethylbenzanthracene, and benzpyrene. Over 500 chemical compounds show laboratory effects that suggest they would be carcinogenic to human skin.

#### Predisposing factors

Blond, fair, blue-eyed, thin-skinned, dry-skinned persons of Nordic and Anglo-Saxon background, who are older and often freckled, comprise the common phenotype of persons with skin cancer. Skin cancer is also an occupational hazard, threatening particularly persons working constantly in sunlight, such as farmers, sailors, and sportsmen. The list includes, of course, workers in industries contacting any of the long list of carcinogenic chemical compounds, a few of which are mentioned in Chapter 3.

## PATHOLOGY

There are two major types of skin carcinoma—basal cell and squamous or epidermoid. Both occur mainly on exposed skin surfaces. (Melanoma is discussed in Chapter 5.)

*Basal cell carcinoma* comprises about 80% of all skin cancers and is found commonly on the upper half of the face and head. Basal cell carcinoma almost never metastasizes. It appears as a pale, pearly, raised nodule that slowly enlarges and later develops a central ulceration. It can contain pigment and suggest melanoma.

*Squamous* or *epidermoid carcinoma* differs in being less common, is found on the lower face and dorsum of the hands, and will metastasize to regional lymph nodes. Grossly, it is also a raised firm nodule and is hard to distinguish from basal cell carcinoma. Epidermoid carcinoma grows faster than basal cell, may not develop a central ulcer crater, but rather develops a wider, irregular ulcerated surface in later stages.

*Basosquamous carcinoma* is sometimes diagnosed by the pathologist. This interesting variant behaves clinically like a basal cell carcinoma.

*X-ray skin carcinoma,* occasionally seen, often has spindle cells, is less differentiated than the two major types, and occasionally metastasizes quickly and widely.

*Kaposi's hemorrhagic sarcoma* is a rare, nonmetastasizing, aggressive skin tumor developing at multiple sites and whose origin is relatively mysterious.

*Xeroderma pigmentosum* is a hereditary condition of skin hypersensitivity to all sorts of radiation, especially sunlight, wherein multiple basal and squamous cancers develop in early childhood.

*Mycosis fungoides* constitutes a multicentric, fatal, malignant skin condition with systemic manifestations akin to the lymphomas.

### Precancerous lesions

The more common skin conditions that are known to become invasive cancers, frequently or occasionally, are listed:

*Senile keratosis* (actinic keratosis)—flat, scaly plaques on exposed skin

*Cutaneous horn*—grotesque piling up of keratin with cancer occasionally at the base

*Leukoplakia*—a flat, white plaque due to hyperkeratosis on various mucous surfaces

*Arsenical dermatosis*—a tiny, raised nodule from chronic trivalent arsenic ingestion, usually on palms and soles of the feet

Any *chronic dermatosis* or *isolated papules*—in a worker in a carcinogenic chemical industry

*Burn scars*—any that do not heal (Marjolin ulcer)

*Lupus vulgaris*

*Chronic skin ulcers*—from varicosities of legs, decubiti, or draining infected sinuses

*Bowen's precancerous dermatosis*—a true, in situ, intraepithelial carcinoma resembling psoriasis, on covered portions of the body, nearly always becoming invasive in time

*Keratoacanthoma*—a fast-growing lesion, often on the face, resembling skin cancer; its pseudoepitheliomatous hyperplasia under the microscope occasionally misdiagnosed as squamous cancer (This lesion is essentially benign and will usually regress spontaneously in a period of months, but cancer may develop in it on rare occasions.)

## NATURAL HISTORY

*Basal cell carcinoma* grows slowly over a period of years, invades and destroys local tissues, including bone, and causes serious morbidity and mortality by destruction of eyes, nose, and ears, and even invades the calvarium. Secondary infection with pain then occurs, and the use of drugs begins. Loss of appetite, weight loss, inanition, and finally death can occur. Death usually results essentially from starvation.

*Squamous carcinoma* also usually grows slowly and destroys locally much like a basal cell. In addition, in the later stages of the neglected, untreated cancer, it will often metastasize by lymphatic emboli to the regional lymph nodes and still later metastasize by blood-borne emboli to various organs and regions in distant parts of the body. It causes death by inanition and starvation if pneumonia does not supervene. A few squamous carcinomas are fast growing from the start.

## DIAGNOSIS

**History.** The only reasonably early symptom of a skin cancer is the feeling by the patient of a firm, raised nodule in the skin. This is also the only early sign. The pearly raised border with central ulceration characterizes a basal cell carcinoma. X-ray films and laboratory studies play no part in diagnosis.

**Biopsy.** Regardless of the treatment method, biopsy must always be carried out, since no clinician's judgment is infallible (15% error among experts). Melanomas or rare benign lesions simulate carcinomas. Also, biopsy prevents precancerous lesions from being overtreated. If the nodule is small, less than 1 cm., complete excision is done or in larger lesions a wedge biopsy can be done to satisfy the requirements of accurate diagnosis.

### Differential diagnosis

The multiplicity of skin lesions and new growths make up a long and varied list, many of which do not closely mimic the common skin cancers. Students who are in doubt about the nature of a skin lesion can and should resort to simple biopsy for their own education and the patient's welfare. We will not try to characterize in this section the previously mentioned precancerous lesions; suffice it to say that the most common differential the student faces is between precancer and very early invasive cancer.

Other differential lesions commonly encountered are as follows:

*Pyogenic granuloma*—soft, recent

*Sclerosing hemangioma*—very hard and pigmented, on thighs and legs

*Seborrheic keratosis*—greasy, soft, pigmented, and warty, on covered surfaces

*Psoriasis*—flat, scaly, on extensor surfaces of limbs
*Cavernous hemangioma*—bluish, soft, compressible, and detected first in youth

## PREVENTIVE MEASURES

A number of simple measures will occur to the reader to protect the skin from sunlight and from potentially carcinogenic chemicals. Newer suntan lotions and creams have an ability to filter out ultraviolet rays. Outdoor workers need to wear broad-brimmed hats and gloves to shield their faces and hands from the sunlight. Precancerous dermatoses can be easily removed by insistence on periodic medical check-ups for older people. Protective gloves and sunlight and air filters are being used more and more in industry.

## TREATMENT PRINCIPLES

1. Local wide eradication comes first in these slow-growing, localized cancers. A margin of 1 cm. suffices for surgical excision in most small lesions (Fig. 1). Both surgery and irradiation offer curative methods when skillfully applied because tumors are superficial and accessible and have easily defined margins. Surgery must be used for radiation skin cancers, very large lesions and lesions involving bone or cartilage. One usually prefers irradiation for lesions around and on the nose and eyelids.
2. Cosmetic result can always be taken into account with skin cancer, since the cure rate is so high.
3. Permanent cure should always be attained, except in a few long-neglected, advanced situations. Local recurrences do not preclude cure.
4. Cautery for precancerous lesions and curettement followed by electrocautery for small tumors are widely used with success by dermatologists. The technique is specialized, however, and like many others requires study, training, and clinical skill in recognition of gross pathology. Lack of pathologic control of margins constitutes a drawback.
5. Skin cancer arises in a large, highly predisposed tissue. Constant surveillance of the skin through the life of the patient must be a rule if the second, third, and subsequent skin cancers are to be recognized and treated early.
6. Pathologic studies for margins should be a rule.

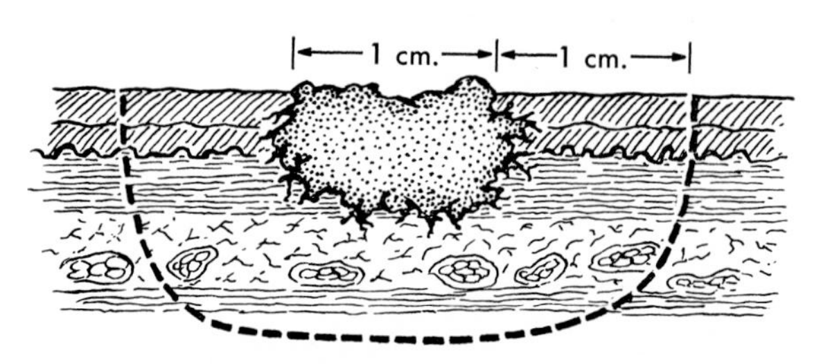


**Fig. 1.** Basal cell carcinoma of the skin; dotted line shows reasonably safe amount of tissue to be resected or volume of tissue to be irradiated for the size of this lesion.

7. Regional nodes are treated only if proved to be metastatic; then they are treated by surgery.

## COMMON ERRORS

Ackerman and del Regato ascribe failure to cure skin cancer to these five factors, listed in order of importance:

1. No skill by treating physician
2. Use of a single method for all lesions
3. Lack of pathologic control of margins
4. Lack of posttreatment study of suspicious areas
5. Failure to receive careful follow-up

## PROMISING DEVELOPMENTS FOR THE FUTURE

1. Klein has found that a delayed hypersensitivity response, an anamnestic reaction, when induced in a skin cancer patient with a nonspecific antigen (a dilute anticancerous drug), can cause disappearance of basal and squamous cancers in the skin and of benign lesions in mucous membranes.

2. Some dermatologists are using topical applications of chemotherapeutic agents to treat precancerous dermatoses and tiny skin cancers.

3. Cryosurgery for these same lesions demands future attention because the margin of tissue necrosis is sharper and more controllable than with electrocautery. Liquid nitrogen causes the tips of special instruments to freeze for this technique.

4. Fluorescence studies of tumors under special lights hold promise for accurately delineating margins.

## PROGNOSIS

The outlook for the absolute cure of skin cancer is *excellent*—92%. No one needs to die of squamous or basal cell skin cancer. Subsequent multiple, new primary cancers of the skin provide the real threat to these patients so that follow-up for life is mandatory. Physicians do not know much about controlling xeroderma pigmentosum, Kaposi's sarcoma, or mycosis fungoides, but these are extremely rare neoplasms. Basal or squamous cancers get out of control and cause death when inadequate initial treatment allows the neoplasm to recur and invade the mucous membranes of the nose or the bones of nose and face. Cancers arising from improperly irradiated skin and cancers in burn scars behave in treacherous aggressive and unpredictable ways. Fortunately, they are not common.

### REFERENCES

Ackerman, L. V., and del Regato, J. A.: Cancer, ed. 3, St. Louis, 1962, The C. V. Mosby Co., pp. 167-210.

Byrne, J. J.: Kaposi's sarcoma, New Eng. J. Med. **266:**337-338, 1962.

Davis, J.: Precancer of skin, New York J. Med. **66:**2923-2935, 1966.

Glass, R. L., Spratt, J. S., and Perez-Mesa, C.: The fate of inadequately excised epidermoid carcinoma of the skin, Surg. Gynec. Obstet. **122:**245-248, 1966.

Hueper, W. C., and Conway, W. D.: Chemical carcinogenesis and cancers, Springfield, Ill., 1964, Charles C Thomas, Publisher.

Kingery, F. A. J.: The self-healing "cancer," J.A.M.A. **193:**143-144, 1965.

Klein, E.: Delayed hypersensitivity reaction for carcinoma of the skin, paper delivered at monthly meeting of the New York State Medical Society, January, 1966.

Lund, H. Z.: Tumors of the skin. In Lund, H. D., editor: Atlas of tumor pathology, Sect. I, Fasc. 2, Washington, D. C., 1957, Armed Forces Institute of Pathology.

Statistics on cancer, Ca. Bulletin—publication of the American Cancer Society **17:**34-43, 1967.

Vickers, H. R.: The management of malignant tumors of the skin, Practitioner **196**(supp.)**:** 81-86, 1966.

Chapter 5

# Melanoma

## INCIDENCE AND DISTRIBUTION

Melanoma is not common, constituting only 1% to 2% of all cancers. It commands an important position in clinical cancer because of its aggressive metastasizing ability in many cases and because it occurs at younger ages than do most other cancers. It is unusual in Negroes. Males and females fall victim in equal proportion.

## ETIOLOGY

### External initiating agents

Ultraviolet rays are strongly suspected of playing a role in the origin of melanoma, but no convincing evidence exists for this as it does with ultraviolet light in skin cancer. Trauma to benign moles receives a great deal of blame for melanoma incitement on very flimsy clinical evidence. In the present state of our knowledge, no external agent plays a definite part in causation.

### Predisposing factors

White persons have twice as many melanomas as do Negroes. Redheads, especially, and blonds seem more susceptible than brunettes; many of the same skin characteristics that predispose to skin cancer seem to predispose to melanoma as well. Sex hormones were once believed to be important influences in the origin and perpetuation of melanoma because they definitely affect normal pigment metabolism (increased pigmentation of nipples and nevi occurs during pregnancy, and melanoma seldom metastasizes before the age of puberty). Hormones now receive little attention. Melanoma apparently does not depend on them for stimulation. Endocrine ablative operations yield no benefit, and even therapeutic abortion, once considered mandatory, has been abandoned in the presence of melanoma. The place of the hypophyseal factor (melanin-stimulating hormone, MSH) in melanin pigment metabolism seems definite, but the relation of MSH to melanoma remains obscure.

## PATHOLOGY

Melanomas occur on all areas of skin and occasionally in oral and rectal mucosa (same locations as nevi). The reported cases of small bowel melanoma are probably metastatic lesions from undetected skin primaries. The commonest sites are the skin of back, legs, feet, face, and scalp.

Classification by degree of dermal invasion correlates directly with curability. Many so-called early melanomas with minimal dermal invasion are now being found and the "cure" rate of any series depends largely on percentages of these early cases.

*Superficial melanoma* (lentigo maligna) seems to be a less aggressive, highly curable type.

*Juvenile melanoma* (spindle cell nevus) is a definite histopathologic type that is usually found at prepubertal and pubertal ages. Its identification merits attention because it is a *nonmetastasizing* neoplasm, requiring only wide local removal, but it resembles adult melanoma in most gross and microscopic characteristics.

*Amelanotic melanoma* is a type in which no pigment appears in the cancerous cells (10% to 15% of melanomas).

Varying degrees of microscopic differentiation occur in melanomas, which roughly correlate with the degree of aggressive biologic behavior in the patient. The degree of pigmentation bears no such relation, however. At present we believe the biologic behavior pattern lies inherent in the tumor from its inception and is not imposed on a uniform initial tumor pattern by outside circumstances such as trauma.

### Precancerous lesions

Melanomas generally arise from benign, true *nevi.* The skin of most persons contains 15 to 30 nevi, most of them pigmented, some invisible. With experience they can be clinically distinguished from keratoses, warts, and freckles. Nevi arise apparently from the epidermal melanocyte; these cells play the main role in tyrosine pigment metabolism and are responsive to the pituitary hormone MSH. So few nevi become cancerous relative to their frequency (perhaps 1 in 10 million) that it is somewhat misleading to call them precancerous.

Four types of nevi exist, which are divided into two classes:

1. *Never premalignant*
   a. *Intradermal nevus*
   b. *Jadassohn (blue) nevus*
2. *Possibly potentially malignant*
   a. *Junctional nevus*—nevus cells clustered at the junction of epidermis and dermis (The "junctional" change is a histologic criterion of primary melanoma. Nevi on soles, palms, perineal areas, and external genitalia are usually junctional in type.)
   b. *Compound nevus*—a combination of intradermal and junctional nevus, a common type in children

## NATURAL HISTORY

Fifteen percent of melanomas exhibit extremes of biologic behavior, such as rapid progression to widely disseminated disease in a few months or extremely indolent behavior in apparent symbiosis with an asymptomatic host for 15 years or more. Rare instances of spontaneous regression, related to immunologic factors, occur. The vast majority fall between the extremes in the following general pattern.

A long-standing, flat, light brown mole is one day noted to be darker; later it is nearly black and slightly raised above the skin level. Its edges appear irregular and it enlarges in all dimensions. If rubbed in washing, it may bleed. It grows at a moderate rate, perhaps tripling in size in 6 months. Tiny *satellite* black spots may appear around the lesion in the skin. After 9 to 12 months or longer a firm, enlarged regional node is palpable in two thirds of the patients. In the other one third the first sign of metastasis is from blood-borne emboli to lungs, distant skin, or distant nodes. After 1 to 3 years one or all three of the distant sites may be involved. When skin is involved distantly, a characteristic melanoma syndrome of myriad subcutaneous, 3 to 6 mm., pigmented nodules may spring up as though the patient had been peppered with buckshot. Appetite and weight begin to drop off. The primary lesion ulcerates and becomes secondarily infected; unilateral limb edema may occur from massive groin or axillary lymphatic and nodal growth. After these late stages, death gradually approaches, as with most advanced malignant tumors, through a sequence of discomfort leading to analgesic drugs, then to no food intake, then to a bedridden degree of weakness and consequent inanition, after which terminal pneumonia occurs.

## DIAGNOSIS

**History.** The only symptom noticed by the patient is the appearance of a *dark, raised, pigmented* lesion on the skin, or similar change in a mole. Itching or bleeding may or may not occur. The only signs are exactly the same. Every such change does not indicate a positive diagnosis of melanoma; false positive guesses are, and should be, frequent if we are to discover melanoma in its early, first stage.

**Biopsy.** Biopsy is best accomplished by an *excision* of the suspicious mole with a narrow but definite margin of normal skin. If the lesion is over 3 cm. or is on the face, one takes a tiny wedge at the edge, being careful not to infiltrate much skin with anesthetic nor to cause much bleeding. When in doubt about a mole, excise it. X-ray films are of no help.

**Laboratory studies.** Melanuria may appear in the later stages of disease. Unpigmented melanoma differs from other spindle cell cancers by showing positive dopa and tyrosine reaction tests. These uncomplicated histochemical tests demonstrate the pigment melanin in melanoma cells.

### Differential diagnosis

In addition to the true nevi listed above, many skin lesions can suggest early melanomatous change. These will confuse all of us some of the time; the most experienced clinician cannot distinguish every one of these lesions from melanomas without excision.

*Keratosis, seborrheic and senile*
*Pigmented verrucae (warts)*
*Sclerosing hemangioma*
*Intracutaneous and subungual hematomas (from trauma)*

*Cafe au lait spots of neurofibromatosis*
*Infected hemangiomas*
*Pyogenic granulomas*
*Pigmented basal cell carcinomas*
*Congenital verrucoid nevi*

## PREVENTIVE MEASURES

Obviously, preventive medicine must be practiced with common sense and a compromise with the ideal. One cannot excise every nevus nor even every junctional nevus. The best compromise consists in educating people to observe their moles once a month and to report to their physicians any moles *changing color, enlarging, becoming raised* or *thicker,* as well as those receiving chronic trauma from clothing, weight bearing, etc. These merit excision as a prophylactic and diagnostic measure. Dark, raised nevi in prepubertal children deserve excision also, since they may be juvenile melanomas that are believed able to change into adult metastasizing melanomas after puberty if left in place.

The dictum that one must *never cauterize* a mole to destroy it still stands as a reliable rule of thumb. The danger of missing a histologic diagnosis by cautery is probably the main reason for this rather than the unsupported assumption that electrocautery may alter the biologic potential of a nevus cell from benign to malignant.

## TREATMENT PRINCIPLES

1. One performs a narrow excision for diagnosis (0.5 cm. margin). The physician infiltrates the skin with local anesthetic a little distance away from the edge of the mole, but not into the mole itself. Much infiltration of a melanoma may open lymphatic spaces and risk spread. One excises larger lesions under general anesthesia for the same reason.

2. Do not insist on frozen section diagnosis. Allow the pathologist time to think and consult.

3. *Surgery alone constitutes adequate treatment.* X-ray therapy and drugs play no part in initial, curative treatment.

4. If the diagnosis is melanoma, as a *second procedure* one performs a wide excision of the healing wound followed by plastic repair (a split graft or local flap). This separate, second procedure needs to be done within 10 to 14 days of the first.

5. *Wide excision* implies a margin at least 5 cm. wide of the wound on the skin and 9 cm. wide in fate and fascia. Deep fascia overlying muscle should be removed to ensure an adequate deep margin. Some compromise with this scheme is forced on us by melanomas occurring on the face and forehead.

6. *Regional node dissection,* unless the melanoma is extremely superficial and small, is advocated by most authorities. (We recognize the controversy over this step. Opponents of this "radical" procedure point to "mutilation" and theoretic impairment of body defense mechanisms. We believe that simultaneous, especially in continuity, node dissections in negative node situations result in slightly better survival rates than with wide local removal only. Dissections do not appear to

harm chances for survival, and, if properly executed, result in relatively minor disability.)

## COMMON ERRORS

1. Reliance on only one pathologist when the lesion is a borderline case.

2. Insistence on carrying out full surgical treatment at one time, in one stage, on the basis of a clinical impression that the lesion "looks real bad." Almost invariably this results in too much surgery if benign, too little surgery if malignant.

## PROMISING DEVELOPMENTS FOR THE FUTURE

1. The combination of *regional isolation perfusion,* using appropriate anticancer drugs, with conventional, radical surgery for limb melanomas may add 5% to 10% to the 5-year survival figures. (At present, systemic chemotherapy offers little in melanomas at any stage of the disease.)

2. Cases exist of authentic spontaneous regression of melanoma; also, in a few instances medical maneuvers designed to stimulate immunologic mechanisms against the patient's melanoma have succeeded. These together constitute basis for hope that something akin to a cancer vaccine for certain specific types of tumors may yet be discovered.

## PROGNOSIS

The outlook is fairly good for a 5-year survival in melanoma. In all cases of Stage I and Stage II disease (without or with regional node metastases but still theoretically curable), most large clinics and groups report about *40%* of patients alive and well at 5 years. A 3% erosion per year, because of the occurrence of late metastases, reduces the figure to 25% by 10 years. As with most other aggressive human cancers, localized disease without any regional metastatic deposits carries a good prognosis; 70% of patients are alive and well at 5 years and 60% at 10 years. However, regional node involvement (Stage II) constitutes a group with dismal outlook—20% at 5 years and 12% at 10 years. So few patients survive when regional nodes are positive that some physicians tend to believe curative efforts are not worthwhile in this circumstance; a review of such figures as the above, however, reminds us that a small but definite number of people with positive nodes do survive when operated on for cure.

### REFERENCES

Allen, A. C., and Spitz, S.: Malignant melanoma, Cancer **6:**1, 1953.

Allyn, B., Kopf, A. W., Kahn, M., and Witten, V. H.: Incidence of pigmented nevi, J.A.M.A. **186:**890-893, 1963.

Creech, O., Jr., and Krementz, E. T.: Regional perfusion in melanoma of limbs, J.A.M.A. **188:**855-858, 1964.

Daland, E. M.: Malignant melanoma, New Eng. J. Med. **260:**453-460, 1959.

Fitzpatrick, T. B., Seiji, M., and McGugan, A. D.: Melanin pigmentation, New Eng. J. Med. **265:**328-332, 374-378, 430-434, 1961.

Fortner, J. G., Barber, H. J., and Pack, G. T.: Results of groin dissection for malignant melanoma in 220 patients, Surgery **55:**485-494, 1964.

McNeer, G., and dasGupta, T.: Melanoma survival, Surgery **56:**511-518, 1964.

Nicol, F. Z., Mathews, W. H., and Palmer, J. T.: Treatment of malignant melanomas of the skin, Arch. Surg. **93:**209-214, 1966.

Pack, G. T., Gerber, D. M., and Scharnagel, I. M.: End results in the treatment of malignant melanoma, Ann. Surg. **136:**905-911, 1952.

Pack, G. T., Scharnagel, I. M., and Morfit, M.: The principle of excision in continuity for primary and metastatic melanoma of the skin, Surgery **17:**839-866, 1945.

Southwick, H. W., Slaughter, D. P., Hinkamp, J. S., and Johnson, F. E.: The role of regional node dissection in the treatment of malignant melanoma, Arch. Surg. **85:**63-69, 1962.

Statistics on cancer, Ca. Bulletin—publication of the American Cancer Society **17:**34-43, 1967.

Stehlin, J. S., Jr., and Clark, R. L.: Melanoma of the extremities, Amer. J. Surg. **110:**366-383, 1965.

Stehlin, J. S., Jr., Hills, W. J., and Rufino, C.: Disseminated melanoma, Arch. Surg. **94:** 495-501, 1967.

Chapter 6

# Lip cancer

## Vermilion border of lip

Cancers on the lip occupy a peculiar position halfway between skin cancer and mouth cancer and possess some features of both. They constitute 1% to 2% of all cancers, and thus are common enough to demand our attention. Many of their features are covered in Chapters 4 and 7 and repetition would be superfluous. We will mention only their special characteristics.

Lip cancer involves *tobacco* as well as ultraviolet sunlight as external initiating agents. It occurs almost always in white males who smoke or engage in outdoor occupations. Nearly always located on the lower lip, the cancer presents as a whitish, raised plaque or a fissure with firm, raised edges and erythematous surrounding tissue. It is *always squamous* or *epidermoid* in type. Leukoplakia frequently precedes or accompanies cancer of the lip. These cancers are frequently multicentric and multiple.

Other lesions occur on the lip—*precancerous leukoplakia, mucous cysts* (bluish, soft, transient), *perlèche* (fissuring at commissures), *herpes simplex, pyogenic granuloma,* and *traumatic ulcers.*

Diagnosis and treatment follow the same outline for squamous cancer of the skin; biopsy precedes either surgery or irradiation, depending on size of the cancer and the talent available. It is important to remember, however, that occasional lip cancers behave in a most aggressive way by metastasizing to submental and submaxillary lymph nodes rather promptly after the primary tumor appears. Appropriate surgery for neck nodes succeeds if performed on first real suspicion of abnormally hard, enlarged nodes.

A good prognosis of about 80% 5-year survivals obtains in lip cancer. Since all the lip cancers are squamous or epidermoid, the outlook remains below the good results with skin cancer, where basal cell carcinoma, the nonmetastasizing cancer, predominates.

**REFERENCE**

Ackerman, L. V., and del Regato, J. A.: Cancer, ed. 3, St. Louis, 1962, The C. V. Mosby Co., pp. 258-283.

Chapter 7

# Cancer of the mouth

## Includes tongue, floor of mouth, gum, buccal mucosa, palate

### INCIDENCE AND DISTRIBUTION

Cancers in the above locations of the oral cavity comprise 4% to 5% of all cancers in western countries, and the male to female ratio of occurrence is 4:1. They show no predilection for one race over another, but certain southeast Asian countries (India and Ceylon) count mouth cancer as the most frequent of all cancers (40%). This high incidence is directly related to the betel quid habit—a quid containing several substances including tobacco.

### ETIOLOGY

#### External initiating agents

Most studies show a significant correlation between *tobacco* and cancers in the mouth at all sites (as well as cancers in the pharynx, larynx, lung, and probably esophagus). By tobacco we mean all forms reaching the mouth—cigarettes, cigars, pipes, chewing tobacco, snuff, and betel quid. Despite the lack of positive indictment of tobacco as a cause of mouth cancer by the exhaustive and excellent document, *Smoking and Health,* by the Surgeon General's Advisory Committee in 1964, more recent mouth cancer studies constitute a sufficiently definite designation of tobacco as the causative agent to serve as a guide to practicing physicians. Tobacco can be considered the external initiator in 90% of the instances; in a few patients other substances must be sought, since careful histories reveal no tobacco contact. These few exceptions, usually women, are to be expected in any biologic system of response as universal as neoplasia. An average of *30 years* of tobacco exposure precedes mouth cancer in the United States, the same average interval as with lung cancer.

The common location of mouth cancer varies in different countries (United States—tongue and floor; India and Ceylon—buccal mucosa). This variety itself points toward an external causative agent rather than internal factors. The most common site of oral cancer in each country seems to correspond with the oral site

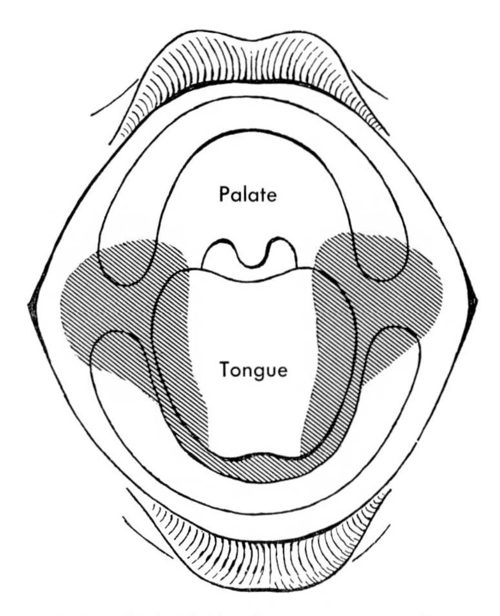


**Fig. 2.** Areas in the mouth in which 80% of cancers occur in western countries—floor of mouth, lateral and under surface of tongue, retromolar trigone, lower anterior tonsillar pillar, and posterior buccal mucosa—the "cancer-prone horseshoe." (From Moore, C.: Southern Med. Bull. **54:**15-22, 1966.)

most highly exposed to tobacco and tobacco smoke condensate. And each such oral site, in turn, reflects the way tobacco is used by different peoples. When smoking habits predominate, tobacco smoke condensate suspended in saliva apparently achieves highest contact with oral mucosa in the deep sulcus beneath the tongue and on the sides of the tongue.

### Predisposing factors

A moderate to high alcoholic intake seems, with present evidence, most likely a promoter of mouth cancer as well as throat and esophageal cancers. Alcoholism carries dietary inadequacies with it, and these undoubtedly play a part, especially deficiencies of vitamins A and B. It follows, of course, that 50% of mouth cancer victims exhibit laboratory evidence of liver impairment of some type. The typical patient is of low socioeconomic status, a male, a chronic alcoholic, 55 years of age on the average, a heavy smoker, poor eater, unmotivated, and unable to alter his habits. An interesting syndrome seems to predispose Scandinavian women to mouth, throat, and esophageal cancer—the Plummer-Vinson syndrome (atrophic glossitis, dysphagia, and anemia). Atrophic glossitis from any cause may be a precursor; this condition often accompanies pernicious anemia, tertiary syphilis, etc.

## PATHOLOGY

Ninety-two percent of malignant mouth tumors are *squamous* or *epidermoid* types, which have developed from the stratified squamous epithelium that lines the oral (and pharyngeal) cavity. Four percent of tumors are *adenocarcinomas* or *malignant mixed tumors* from mucous glands or minor salivary submucosal glands. These usually occur in and around the hard and soft palate. Lymphomas may present as mouth tumors, generally in or near the tonsils.

Rare mouth neoplasms include granular cell myoblastoma (benign), ameloblastoma (a nonmetastasizing tumor), osteogenic sarcoma of the mandible or maxilla, and occasionally a metastatic lesion to the mandible from elsewhere.

Three clinical varieties of squamous mouth cancer develop—the *exophytic,* the *verrucous,* and the *ulcerated* infiltrative. The first two varieties have a much better prognosis than the third, which unfortunately is the most common. The more differentiated, less biologically aggressive growths generally occur in the anterior mouth, whereas the less differentiated, more aggressive cancers grow in the posterior portions and structures. For example, many base of tongue cancers are so poorly differentiated that they almost constitute a different tumor syndrome from those cancers in the anterior, oral part of the tongue.

Oral cancer invades adjacent structures readily, such as the gum, palate, or cheek. When it infiltrates the muscles of the "root" of the tongue or the pterygoid musculature medial to the posterior lower jaw, the limits of extension elude clinical detection and treatment seldom succeeds. Attachment to, and invasion of, the bone of the mandible occurs often; when this invasion reaches the medullary canal of this bone, spread along the entire hemimandible is unobstructed and often rapid.

Metastases usually occur in most cancers over 3 cm. in diameter via the rich network of mouth-to-neck lymphatics. Metastases reside in the various and many neck nodes, usually along the jugular chain of nodes; the first-involved nodes depend on the location of the primary cancer (Fig. 6). Blood-borne metastases may develop late in the course of the disease.

### Precancerous lesions

*Erythroplasia,* a velvety, red change in the mucosa, is often associated with carcinoma in situ. This intraepithelial malignant change is found increasingly as physicians and dentists look for it as such, and it definitely precedes and presages invasive cancer.

*Leukoplakia,* if in thick, plaquelike concentrations, may generally be regarded as a precursor of cancer. Perhaps 15% to 20% of such plaquelike areas will develop into squamous carcinoma if not removed.

These lesions do not progress steadily; they grow by fits and starts, often with long periods of quiescence.

## NATURAL HISTORY

Cancer of the mouth usually grows at a moderate rate. Considerable variety characterizes its growth pattern. Many cancers have a doubling time of 3 or 4 months.

Typically, a small white or red patch on the lateral border of the posterior tongue, opposite the retromolar space, ulcerates and becomes secondarily infected on the surface, and thus is slightly sore. After several months the ulcer will have doubled in size. Pain on talking or swallowing develops and advances to persistent dull aching. The tongue seems stiff. Soon the patient finds the jaw stiff and unable to open widely. After several more months a hard lump appears in the middle of the neck and then a second deeper one appears below the ear. The cancer is now moderately advanced.

Forty percent of tongue cancers and 30% of cancers in the floor of the mouth, gum, and cheek have neck node metastases when first diagnosed. Crossing lymphatics yield 5% of *first* involved neck nodes in the opposite side of the neck. Blood-borne or venous emboli result in distant metastases in lungs, brain, and spine very late in the natural course of the disease.

The many painful, late complications of a large invading tumor in the mouth with nodes in the neck can easily be imagined. Teeth fall out from gum and mandible invasion or the mandible undergoes a pathologic fracture; dysphagia, trismus, oral-to-cheek fistula, and hemorrhage occur, depending on tumor location. Then the preterminal sequence begins—pain leads to use of drugs and then to inadequate caloric intake, followed by weight loss, weakness, a bedridden state, and finally a terminal pneumonia.

## DIAGNOSIS

**History.** The most common sites for cancer are the lateral borders of the tongue and the floor of the mouth. Very early symptoms are nonexistent when cancers are tiny. Slight soreness comes only after ulceration and infection. Otalgia (pain referred to the ear) often presages early cancer in the posterolateral tongue or posterior floor of the mouth. Only persons who examine their own mouths in a mirror or with their fingers find the small, whitish hard spot before symptoms occur.

**Physical examination.** Early signs correspond to a small firm or hard spot or plaque, usually in the lateral tongue or floor of the mouth and a reddish area, occurring in a mouth with leukoplakia. A lump in the neck may be the first sign

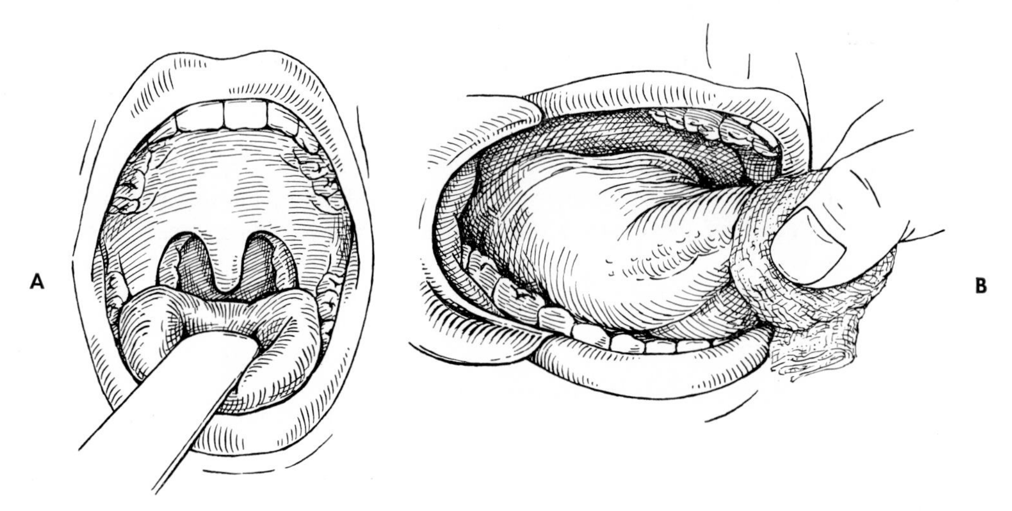


**Fig. 3. A,** Wrong and, **B,** proper method of examining mouth to reveal cancers or precancerous lesions. **A** shows how a tongue blade can flatten the tongue and hide most cancers.

or the cancer may be so asymptomatic or tiny that it can be found only after careful examination.

*Mouth examination* must include palpation and also the maneuver of retraction of cheek outward and forceful stretching of the tongue in the opposite direction to expose the posterolateral tongue and floor of the mouth where cancers occur frequently (Fig. 3). An effective six-step mouth and throat examination for soft tissue abnormalities runs as follows: (1) right alveololingual sulcus, (2) left alveololingual sulcus, (3) anterior floor of the mouth, (4) palate, gums, and cheeks, (5) mirror examination of the pharynx and larynx, and (6) palpation of the base of the tongue.

**Oral cytology.** A somewhat unreliable role is played by oral cytology. Scrapings done with a curette or other sharp instrument from suspicious areas of mucosa can alert one to follow this up with a formal biopsy. Oral cytology is not diagnostic, but only an adjunct to biopsy.

**Biopsy.** Wedge biopsy can easily be performed in the office with local, or even only topical, anesthesia. One needs a sharp-biting forceps and a silver nitrate applicator to control bleeding. Biopsy of any doubtful mouth lesions without delay forms a good rule of thumb. (Excision is appropriate only for lesions of known character.)

**X-ray studies.** An adjunctive role in the patient's work-up is played by x-ray studies of the mandible or maxilla to determine the extent of invasion of the tumor.

**Laboratory studies.** Liver impairment and positive serology (10% of mouth cancers) are revealed by laboratory studies, thus giving help peripherally.

## Differential diagnosis

More variety in pathologic lesions appears in the mouth than in any equal area of the body. Precancerous lesions simulating cancer have been considered above. Other lesions to be differentiated are as follows:

*Pyogenic granuloma*—soft and recent
*Papilloma*—wartlike and superficial
*Mucocele*—bluish, smooth, sharp edges, with clear fluid inside
*Geographic tongue* (glossitis migrans)—not a true disease, just redness inside irregular, red-white serpiginous lines
*Median rhomboid glossitis*—a diamond-shaped, developmental, isolated area of fibrous tongue tissue exactly in the midline of the tongue, just in front of the V of the circumvallate papillae (cancer seldom occurs in this location)
*Torus palatinus* and *torus mandibularis*—common bony lumps, like arthritic spurs, with normal overlying mucosa
*Gum granulomas*—soft, at the gum edge, sharply demarcated, noninfiltrating
*Hemangioma*—red or bluish, soft, compressible
*Lichen planus*—occurs on buccal mucosa commonly; resembles the same lesion on skin
*Tuberculous ulcer*—soft, rare, usually associated with open pulmonary tuberculosis
*Ranula*—soft cyst of the floor of the mouth under normal mucosa
*Fibroma*—smooth, discrete, round, in the cheek

*Lipoma*—unusual, yellow, soft, smooth

*Inflamed exfoliate papillae*—red, edematous, and tender tongue papillae at the lateral border of the tongue where the anterior pillar joins (cancer is also frequent here, and biopsy is often needed to differentiate)

*Tumors and cysts of jaws*—x-ray films needed for accurate diagnosis

## PREVENTIVE MEASURES

Selected high-risk persons must quit tobacco. These measures may effectively prevent second primary mouth cancers in patients cured of a first primary, whereas many patients who continue to use tobacco acquire second mouth or throat cancers in 5 to 6 years. Heavy smokers will never get rid of leukoplakia or other precancerous "mucoses" unless they quit smoking. Once the leukoplakia patient quits, then surgical eradication of thick areas of leukoplakia and erythroplasia is worthwhile.

Regular follow-up mouth examinations for high-risk persons on a regular schedule—every 4 to 6 months—and advice about mouth self-examination deserve a place in the routine of every physician's office practice.

## TREATMENT PRINCIPLES

1. Every patient with mouth cancer needs to be individualized. The mouth contains much complicated anatomy and function. Both surgery and irradiation can achieve approximately equally good results with small primary cancers.

2. Irradiation takes longer, has no pathologic control, but causes less interference with functions of swallowing, talking, and cosmetic appearance than does surgery.

3. A treatment conference between a skilled surgeon and a skilled radiotherapist is necessary on every case because combinations and sequences of therapy are so often needed.

4. Surgery is the most reliable method for controlling neck node metastases, which occur in half of the cases.

5. The time-honored dictum that "irradiation should come first, followed by surgery if this fails" is risky to apply universally because of the difficulty in early detection of postx-ray recurrences.

6. Bone invasion by cancer usually requires surgical treatment.

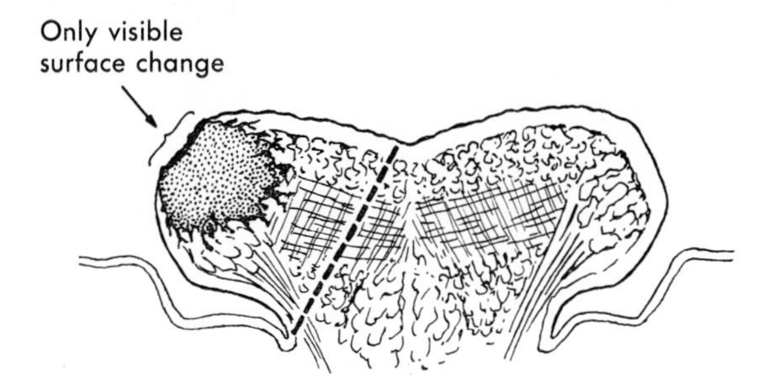


**Fig. 4.** Tongue cancer. Dotted line indicates a reasonably safe estimate of tissue to be removed or irradiated for eradication of a cancer of this size and in this typical location.

## COMMON ERRORS

1. *One mode of therapy* applied to all.

2. *Office excision* of cancer-suspicious lesions as a diagnostic procedure. Unless the lesion is tiny, this is too much surgery for a good biopsy and too little surgery for the treatment of a cancer. It risks acceleration of spread because it disturbs the delicate balance at the tumor edge where advancing tumor may be held in check by tissue defense mechanisms. Excision to avoid the danger of "cutting into" cancer almost always does cut through cancer inadvertently because of distortion of the edges of the growth by the infiltration of local anesthetic and by inadequate visualization from bleeding. Wedge biopsy serves best for diagnosis.

3. *Inadequate follow-up* to detect early recurrences, metastatic neck nodes, and new primaries, all of which may still be curable.

4. *Timid suggestions,* rather than strong insistence, about quitting tobacco.

5. Failure of the patient to follow the treatment plan.

## PROMISING DEVELOPMENTS FOR THE FUTURE

1. Planned *preoperative irradiation* in a carefully outlined combination of irradiation and surgery promises improved results in treating mouth cancer.

2. Methods of mouth and *jaw reconstruction* may yet be developed so they are safely performed immediately.

3. *Alteration* of *smoking tobacco* to eliminate carcinogenic chemical compounds may offer some future help.

4. Effective *smoking filters* for the removal of tobacco tars would seem worthwhile.

5. Universal acceptance and use of a uniform staging method for mouth cancer (and other cancers), called the *TNM method,* developed by the American Joint Committee for Cancer Staging and End Results Reporting, will go a long way toward providing intelligent interspecialty cooperation in managing mouth cancer. This method relates prognosis easily and directly with the anatomic extent of tumor and neck node metastases.

6. Increasing awareness by physician and patient concerning the great risk of second primary cancers in the upper alimentary and respiratory tract may salvage more patients in the future.

## PROGNOSIS

Generally the outlook in mouth cancer is fair. Sixty percent to 70% of patients with small cancers—1 to 2 cm. in greatest diameter—survive 5 years. At sizes of 2 to 4 cm., survivals drop to 40%. An overall rate of about 40% represents achievements of most large clinics. As with other cancers, undifferentiated and anaplastic types carry a poor prognosis when compared to well-to-moderately differentiated ones. Neck node metastases cut survival rates by one half as a general rule.

### REFERENCES

Ackerman, L. V., and del Regato, J. A.: Cancer, ed. 3, St. Louis, 1962, The C. V. Mosby Co., pp. 283-357.

Fayos, J. V., and Lampe, I.: Radiotherapy of squamous cell carcinoma of the oral portion of the tongue, Arch. Surg. **94:**316-321, 1967.

Frazell, E. L., and Lucas, J. C., Jr.: Cancer of the tongue, Cancer **15:**1085-1099, 1962.

Kinsey, D. L., and James, A. G.: Evaluation of failures in the treatment of lingual carcinoma, Arch. Surg. **84:**90-93, 1962.

Kreshover, S. J., and Salley, J. J.: Predisposing factors in oral cancer, J. Amer. Dent. Ass. **54:**509-514, 1957.

MacComb, W. S., and Fletcher, G. H.: Cancer of the head and neck, Baltimore, 1967, The Williams & Wilkins Co., pp. 89-151.

Martin, H. E.: Cancer of the head and neck, J.A.M.A. **137:**1306-1315, 1366-1376, 1948.

Moore, C.: Smoking and cancer of the mouth, pharynx and larynx, J.A.M.A. **191:**283-286, 1965.

Moore, C.: Cancer of the mouth, Southern Med. Bull. **54:**15-22, 1966.

Rush, B. F., Jr.: Combined procedures in the treatment of oral carcinoma, Curr. Probl. Surg., pp. 1-40, May, 1966.

Smoking and health, report of the Advisory Committee to the Surgeon General, Public Health Service Publication no. 1103, Washington, D. C., 1964, U. S. Department of Health, Education & Welfare.

Statistics on cancer, Ca. Bulletin—publication of the American Cancer Society **17:**34-43, 1967.

Strong, E. W., Henschke, U. K., Nickson, J. J., Frazell, E. L., Tollefson, H. R., and Hilaris, B. S.: Pre-operative x-ray therapy as an adjunct to radical neck dissection, Cancer **19:** 1509-1516, 1966.

Yashar, J. J., Guralnick, E., and McAuley, R. L.: Multiple malignant tumors of the oral cavity, respiratory system and upper digestive system, Amer. J. Surg. **112:**70-75, 1966.

Chapter 8

# Cancer of the throat

## Oropharynx, hypopharynx, larynx

Since the epithelium of the throat, as well as the impinging external and internal influences, is the same as in the mouth, basic clinical data on cancer of the mouth and throat have many similarities. We hope not to repeat them. If omissions occur in this chapter, the reader may assume that the data on the various throat locations resemble those in the mouth.

### INCIDENCE AND DISTRIBUTION

*Three percent* of all cancers arise in these anatomic locations, roughly grouped under the lay term *throat.* Males acquire four times as many cancers as females, a ratio similar to that in the mouth. Throat cancers occur in countries and geographic areas where smoking is common; in contrast to cancers of the mouth, they bear little relation to "chewing" or "quid habits."

### ETIOLOGY

#### External initiating agents

The Surgeon General's report on smoking and health found statistical evidence for a causal relation between *smoking* and cancer of the *larynx.* This seems definitely settled. The data are sparser regarding smoking and pharyngeal cancers. Clinical experience and what data appear all support the close connection between smoking and pharyngeal cancer. We have never personally seen a patient with hypopharyngeal cancer (epidermoid or squamous of the pharyngeal wall or hypopharynx or supraglottic larynx) who did not smoke. Evidently chewers are exempt from this regional cancer; either the burned tobacco products suspended in smoke are required for throat cancer, or the tobacco juices from chewing do not impinge long or strong enough on pharyngeal and laryngeal tissues.

#### Predisposing factors

As with mouth cancer, *alcoholism,* concurrent *poor diet,* as well as *cirrhosis* of the liver seem to play an important promoting role in th throat, probably even a stronger role than they play in the mouth.

## PATHOLOGY

As one would expect from the character of the epithelium, *90%* of these cancers are *squamous, epidermoid,* or its variants—lymphoepithelioma, transitional cell carcinoma, or undifferentiated carcinoma. Lymphoepithelioma and transitional cell types are common in the nasopharynx and oropharynx. All of these tumors arise in and on the stratified squamous epithelium of the pharynx and from squamous metaplasia of the columnar respiratory epithelium of the glottis or endolarynx.

Eight percent are lymphomas arising in the tonsils or the juxtatonsillar lymphoid collections of Waldeyer's ring.

*Adenocarcinomas* of minor salivary gland origin or submucosal tumors arising in the deep lobe of the parotid glands are occasionally present in the oropharynx.

Poorly differentiated epidermoid cancers frequently occur in the various throat locations. Since they are more anaplastic and aggressive than most oral cancers, they metastasize early to the jugular chain of neck nodes. Malignant tumors in the base of the tongue are included in the oropharynx. They differ from most anterior tongue cancers by their anaplasticity, quick invasiveness, and rapid growth pattern.

*Vocal cord* (glottic) cancers provide an exception to the above; they are usually squamous, well differentiated, slowly invasive, low grade, and late metastasizing tumors.

Collections of lymphocytes often characterize oropharyngeal cancers. They represent either a true body defense mechanism or inclusion of normal components of Waldeyer's lymphocytic ring in the neoplasm. Tumors with many such collections seem more curable.

### Precancerous lesions

As in the mouth, *leukoplakia* may precede invasive cancer. It occurs mainly on the vocal cords or endolarynx. Hyperkeratoses, called pachyderma laryngis, and papillomas of the cords can all be considered premalignant. The unusual case of papillomatosis of the larynx, occasionally seen in youngsters, may develop cancer. A leukoplakia or erythroplastic reaction representing carcinoma in situ is seldom seen in the oropharynx or hypopharynx in contrast to the mouth where such lesions are relatively common. The hypopharynx is not easily visible; this may account for cancers there appearing to arise de novo, without a precursor lesion.

## NATURAL HISTORY

We must treat each of the following sections in this chapter in two parts: (1) cancer of the vocal cord and (2) cancers of all other locations. Vocal cord cancer differs markedly from the poorly differentiated majority of cancers in other throat sites

**Vocal cord cancer.** A small thickness on one cord causes early hoarseness, grows slowly, and in 1 to 2 years fixes one cord and one side of the larynx by invasion of the cartilage, the musculature, or the anterior commissure. Hoarseness worsens, the breathing "chink" or opening narrows after another year or so, and the growth involves and fixes the opposite cord. "Stridor," a wheezing on inspiration, commences, and finally dyspnea on exertion from laryngeal obstruction becomes so severe that only an emergency tracheostomy can prevent death from suffocation. Metastases are unusual and very late.

**Supraglottic and pharyngeal cancers.** Vague discomfort appears and persists and gradually worsens for 2 to 4 months, always on the same side of the throat. Soon swallowing becomes troublesome from pain and increasing tumor bulk; the patient begins to lose weight. After 6 months constant pain begins, often referred to the ear, and the patient may begin to aspirate fluids and secretions; then a lump may appear in the lateral neck at the hyoid bone level. This lump is nontender and enlarges noticeably in 1 month. Other masses in the neck may develop above and below the first. In a few more months swallowing becomes so painful and difficult from involvement of the tongue or of the pharyngeal constrictor muscles that the patient gives up eating altogether, becomes weak, and addicted to narcotics. Hoarseness from endolaryngeal invasion commences, the patient "takes to his bed," and he finally succumbs to starvation and terminal pneumonia from uncontrolled aspiration of secretions.

These tumors grow rapidly, involve adjacent structures quickly, and attain a 3 to 4 cm. size before producing much in the way of symptoms, especially those in the piriform sinuses. Metastases to neck nodes and to the retropharyngeal nodes occur early, and distant metastases are frequent to spine, lungs, and brain.

## DIAGNOSIS

**Vocal cord cancer.** The patient notes *hoarseness* early because any tiny irregularity on the cord reflects itself in an altered air column with phonation. The sign of cancer is the rough ulcer on one cord or at one commissure that appears on mirror laryngoscopy. *Biopsy* follows in the hospital under direct laryngoscopy, using care to take just enough tissue to secure much of the abnormal area, but not so much as to damage the cord permanently if the tissue proves benign. X-ray films and chemistry studies do not help in these cases.

**Supraglottic and pharyngeal cancers.** Patients experience *no early symptoms.* When the cancer grows to 2 cm. or more and ulcerates, secondary infection produces recurring or persistent sore throat and pain on swallowing, especially with hot or spicy liquids. Lump in the neck (metastasis) may present as the first symptom. Soon dysphagia, weight loss from reduced caloric intake, cough from spillover into the larynx, and otalgia may appear.

Signs of early cancer are subtle and minor; if one examines the throat for some unrelated complaint or at routine examination, one may find a small reddish or whitish, rough patch on the aryepiglottic fold or in the piriform sinuses, or on one of the surfaces of the epiglottis. Palpation of the tonsils or base of the tongue may reveal a hard lump that cannot be seen. When tumors enlarge further, diagnosis becomes easier; fetid breath, ulcer in the pharynx or tonsil, edema or a whitish, and necrotic slough on one side of the larynx (seen by mirror) all quickly impress the examiner. One can seldom see the whole cancer in the mirror image at indirect laryngoscopy; usually only one edge shows so that the impression of a reddened edematous smooth mass—as asymmetry—alone alerts the physician to pursue diagnosis further.

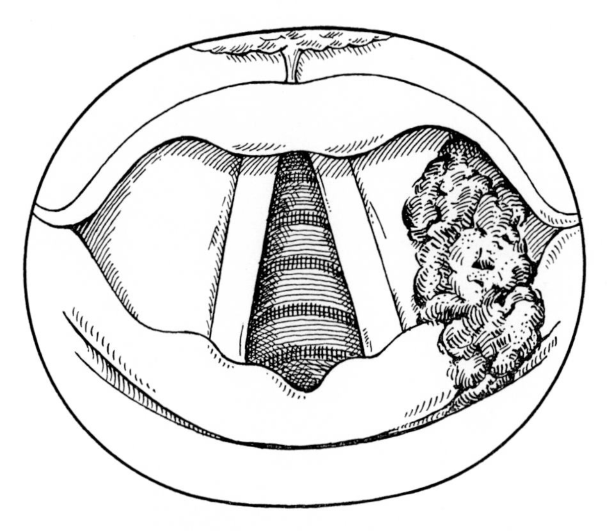

**Fig. 5.** Common type of noncordal cancer of the larynx, involving both inner and outer aspects (glottis and aryepiglottic fold).

**Biopsy.** Office biopsy lends itself to visible oropharyngeal lesions; those lesions on the cords in the hypopharynx and supraglottic larynx generally require hospitalization and direct laryngoscopy. Several biopsies at different sites and repeated biopsies are sometimes needed.

**Metastasis.** Lump in the neck (metastasis) tends to distract the physician from the main job, the search for the primary tumor in the pharynx, larynx, or base of tongue. *Needle aspiration biopsy* of a neck mass is appropriate if throat examination is negative. Because of consequent scarring and interference with later treatment, one avoids operative removal of the neck mass for diagnosis except as a last resort, unless it suggests lymphoma.

**X-ray studies.** Special x-ray films help considerably in defining the exact anatomic locations of growths in the supraglottic larynx and pharynx (soft tissue studies, frontal tomograms, laryngograms). If one suspects cancer, x-ray films done before biopsy yield truer information. *Chemistry studies* help estimate liver damage in alcoholic patients. Some liver impairment obtains in half of these patients.

### Differential diagnosis

**Vocal cord cancer.** The following vocal cord lesions all can mimic cancer: polyps, singer's nodes, granulomas, hypertrophies, tuberculosis, and fibroma.

**Supraglottic and pharyngeal cancers.** Few lesions in the adult supraglottic larynx and pharynx occur except cancer. The following conditions may occur: (1) hypertrophied lymphoid collections, (2) inflammations and abscesses, (3) lipomas, (4) fibromas, (5) tuberculosis, and (6) gummas.

## PREVENTIVE MEASURES

In addition to the obvious need for the high-risk smokers to quit, the necessity exists for an increasing campaign against teen-agers beginning to smoke. We must also improve our basic understanding of the emotional patterns involved in habit dependency. Another approach is the practical one aimed at creation of harmless habits that may substitute for tobacco.

High-risk persons may be detected by widespread routine health examinations that include mirror laryngoscopy of the throat. Any hyperkeratosis noted constitutes sufficient warning that this particular individual tissue may at some future time undergo cancerous change.

## TREATMENT PRINCIPLES

### Vocal cord cancer

1. Surgeon-radiotherapist conference.

2. Generally supervoltage radiation for smaller cancers, surgery for larger ones. It requires extensive experience for a surgeon to decide when partial laryngectomy can safely be done, instead of total laryngectomy.

### Supraglottic and pharyngeal cancer

1. Surgeon-radiotherapist conference.

2. Supervoltage radiation serves best for base of tongue and tonsillar cancers. Surgery yields the best results for supraglottic larynx, pharyngeal wall, piriform sinus neoplasms, and neck metastases, if the primary cancer is curable. The occasional small supraglottic lesion lends itself to partial laryngectomy by an expert.

3. Lymphomas respond best to irradiation; surgery seldom plays a part.

## COMMON ERRORS

1. A single treatment consultant or a single method of treatment for all of these tumors results in far less than optimum salvage.

2. Reliance on a single negative biopsy, when clinical suspicion should be high, results in serious delay of treatment.

## PROMISING DEVELOPMENTS FOR THE FUTURE

1. Preoperative irradiation for selected lesions, perhaps for the larger cancers, holds out hope for greater palliation and control.

2. Better-trained rehabilitation teams for improved restoration of speech for laryngectomies will come. Only 40% are successfully taught esophageal speech at present.

3. Cigarette filters that remove 70% of cigarette tars promise to lower carcinogenic exposure in smokers.

## PROGNOSIS

Vocal cord cancer carries an excellent chance for salvage—80% 5-year and 10-year survival.

Supraglottic and pharyngeal cancer has only a fair chance—35% 5-year survival.

### REFERENCES

Ackerman, L. V., and del Regato, J. A.: Cancer, ed. 3, St. Louis, 1962, The C. V. Mosby Co., pp. 385-461.

Ballantyne, A. J.: Principles of surgical management of cancer of the pharyngeal walls, Proceedings of Ninth International Cancer Congress, Tokyo, Oct., 1966, Berlin, 1967, Springer-Verlag. p. 535 (abst.).

Hollinger, P. H., and Rabbit, W. F.: Late development of laryngeal and pharyngeal carcinoma in previously irradiated areas, Laryngoscope **63:**105-112, 1953.

Lederman, M.: Cancer of the pharynx, J. Laryng. **81:**151-172, 1967.

MacComb, W. S.: Cancer of the larynx, Cancer **19:**149-156, 1966.

MacComb, W. S., and Fletcher, G. H.: Cancer of the head and neck, Baltimore, 1967, The Williams & Wilkins Co., pp. 179-292.

Martin, H. E.: Rehabilitation of the laryngectomee, Cancer **16:**823-841, 1963.

Moore, C.: Smoking and cancer of the mouth, pharynx and larynx, J.A.M.A. **191:**283-386, 1965.

Smith, R. R., Frazell, E. L., Caulk, R., Hollinger, P. H., and Russell, W. O.: The American Joint Committee's proposed method of stage classification and end-result reporting applied to 1,320 pharynx cancers, Cancer **16:**1505-1520, 1963.

Smoking and health, report of the Advisory Committee to the Surgeon General, Public Health Service Publication no. 1103, Washington, D. C., 1964, U. S. Department of Health, Education & Welfare, p. 212.

Chapter 9

# Other head and neck tumors

Such a variety of structures and tissues lie in close proximity in the head and neck that their varied tumors form a confusing array defying neat classification. In this chapter we will try to describe those less common tumors, not mentioned earlier, with which the clinician needs at least a nodding acquaintance.

## CANCER OF THE NASOPHARYNX

### Incidence

The Chinese have an outstandingly high incidence of nasopharyngeal cancer; it outnumbers all other cancers in this race, but it is unusual in western countries. It occurs slightly more often in males. Several studies have failed to uncover a special external initiating factor for nasopharyngeal cancer in the Chinese (burning incense was suggested), nor has any predisposing internal factor been uncovered. Smoking remains highly suspect, however, by analogy to its vital role in cancer of other parts of the respiratory tract.

### Pathology

Histologic types of neoplasms resemble closely those in the oropharynx; epidermoid carcinoma and its variants—undifferentiated, transitional, and lymphoepithelioma—constitute the majority. More than half show anaplasticity; in contrast, well-differentiated tumors are less common. Lymphosarcoma, cylindroma (adenoid cystic carcinoma), other salivary gland tumors, and, rarely, chordoma will occur. No peculiar precancerous lesions develop in this region that we know of, except perhaps the papilloma.

### Natural history

Epidermoid cancer grows slowly to moderately fast in the nasopharynx; it gives symptoms when 2 to 3 cm. in diameter because of the small, bony, rigid enclosure in which it grows. At least one fourth of all such growths invades the cranial cavity via the nerve foramina that contain cranial nerves II, III, IV, V, and VI; this results in cranial nerve palsies of one or several of them. The rest of the cancers first produce unilateral deafness by eustachian tube occlusion, or else nasal obstruction on one side.

*Metastases* occur *commonly* to the upper and mid neck nodes, and later in their course spread to distant organs—spine, lungs, and liver.

The terminal sequence begins when pain becomes severe, leading to narcotics, cessation of food intake, and a bedridden state from weakness and overmedication.

### Diagnosis

Often the first suggestion of nasopharyngeal cancer is a *lump in the neck,* especially in a person of Chinese descent. Nosebleeds, partial deafness on one side, diplopia, nasal obstruction, or fifth nerve neuralgia may also herald this tumor. Perhaps then the physician detects a mass in the neck or sees or feels a lump behind the soft palate. Instead of a mass, the cancer may be only a tiny ulcer seen with an oral mirror placed to view behind the soft palate.

*Biopsy* can be performed under topical mouth and nose anesthesia if one has a proper biting forceps; a palate retractor also helps. *X-ray films* often reveal bony erosions in the base of the skull at the foramen lacerum, ovale, or rotundum. Because the primary is sometimes tiny when metastases occur, the neck metastases may be the only diagnosable tumor mass at first. Aspiration biopsy of the neck mass plays the key role in such a case.

*Nasal polyps* (soft, smooth, jellylike), *juvenile angiofibromas* (in adolescent boys), and *enlarged adenoids* (youngsters usually) may be confused occasionally with cancer. Some physicians believe cancer may begin in a nasal polyp. *Papillomas* of the nares are also considered potentially malignant. They tend to recur.

### Treatment principles

Irradiation of the primary and also of the neck metastases constitutes the first and best mode of treatment. The primary site is inaccessible for surgery. Should the neck metastases get out of hand but the primary be definitely controlled, neck dissection may help control the metastases.

### Common errors

One frequent error with this cancer consists in failure to think of nasopharyngeal cancer or to search the nasopharynx properly for tumor when patients present with nasal obstruction, deafness, or a lump in the neck. Also, we tend to forget that all "nasal polyps" need histologic study.

### Prognosis

A fair chance for 5-year survival exists for these patients—*30% to 35%.*

## SALIVARY GLAND TUMORS

We discuss salivary tumors at this point only because of the anatomic proximity to the respiratory and upper digestive tracts. Here the similarity between the two ends. The salivary glands are designed for external secretion; their structure, function, responsiveness to internal factors, and routes by which external influences reach them all ally them with the pattern of other glands of external secretion, such as the pancreas, prostate, and breast. As we will see, their tumor spectrum is unique and totally different from the tumors arising in the respiratory and mucous-squamous epithelium.

The benign and malignant neoplasms of the salivary glands merit consideration together as a group, despite great variety, because the benign tumors occur relatively often, can mimic cancer, and demand complicated surgical approaches much as do the malignant tumors.

## Incidence

Together benign and malignant salivary gland tumors comprise nearly *1%* of cancers, with an equal male to female ratio, except for the always benign Warthin's tumor. No special geographic distribution, external initiating agents, or internal predisposing factors are known.

## Pathology

Tumors arise in the parotid gland ten times more often than in the submaxillary gland. The chance of a tumor being malignant in the parotid is 1 in 4, whereas in the submaxillary gland it is 2 in 5.

Salivary glandular tissue develops four main types of benign neoplasms: (1) *benign mixed* tumors—most common, (2) *Warthin's* tumor—usually in males, (3) *benign lymphoepithelial lesion of Godwin,* and (4) *oxyphil adenoma*—rare.

Malignant tumors also fall into four groups: (1) *malignant mixed* tumors, (2) *mucoepidermoid carcinoma*—of low, moderate, or high grade but most often low grade (the occasional squamous carcinoma belongs in this group), (3) *adenocarcinoma*—subdivided into adenoid-cystic (cylindroma), acinic cell, and plain, and (4) *anaplastic carcinoma.*

All of these types of tumors, benign and malignant, will appear occasionally in the mouth, oropharynx, or nasopharynx, and originate from the minor salivary glands beneath the mucosal lining. Precancerous lesions do not occur as far as our present knowledge goes. Benign mixed tumors may have a high local recurrence rate unless a rim of a normal gland is taken out with the tumor. Their capsule consists only of compressed local tissues and they invade locally. Many successive local recurrences of benign mixed tumors sometimes seem to precede transformation to cancer.

## Natural history

Benign neoplasms of these glands grow extremely slowly, as we might expect in a benign growth. Patients may first come to the physician with benign mixed tumors that have been bulky but otherwise asymptomatic for 30 to 40 years or more, with periods of indolent growth alternating with periods of quiescence. In contrast, cancers grow moderately fast, showing enough increase in size in 6 months or so to cause symptoms or to bring the patient to the doctor. Untreated parotid cancers attain great local bulk and invade the facial nerve (causing paralysis) and the muscles of mastication; the less differentiated adenocarcinoma and anaplastic cancers metastasize frequently to both neck nodes and lungs. Base of skull extension results in pain and palsies of cranial nerves V, IX, X, XI, and

XII. Death gradually ensues through a sequence of pain, narcosis, undernourishment, inanition, and pneumonia.

### Diagnosis

A *painless lump* in front of, or below, the earlobe, or one in the submaxillary space may be mistaken for a lymph node or a sebaceous cyst. Mixed tumors feel stony hard, movable, bosselated, and sharply defined; cancers feel firm to hard, but with indistinct borders merging into surrounding tissue, and they are relatively immovable. Warthin's tumors and benign epithelial lesions are softer. Slight discomfort and facial weakness constitute frequent presenting complaints in the case of cancer. Diagnosis usually results, after the clinical suspicion of salivary gland tumor, from a formal gland-removal operation, without biopsy. This usually amounts to a superficial parotidectomy or complete submaxillary gland removal. Frozen section study may follow removal. If open biopsy is chosen, the entire wound, including skin, needs excision at the time of definitive removal. X-ray sialograms can only support suspicions, but generally yield no information that alters the operative approach.

Considered in the differential diagnosis of these tumors are the following: *sebaceous cyst, lipoma, myxoma, lymphoma* (occurring rarely in the substance of the salivary glands), *sialadenitis* (firm, tender submaxillary inflammation from stone obstruction), *lymphadenitis, metastatic lymph node* from a primary in the mouth, lip, or scalp, and the *Mikulicz syndrome* (a chronic, recurring, parotid gland swelling with mild, periodic pain).

### Treatment principles

Curative treatment is usually *surgical:* the removal of the entire submaxillary gland, plus all attached muscles in the case of both benign and malignant tumors; superficial parotidectomy (above the facial nerve), or total parotidectomy with sacrifice of the nerve and immediate nerve graft, depending on the size of the growth, symptoms and signs, and the histology. (Salivary tumors, thyroid nodules, and colon cancers constitute three exceptions to the rule that we must secure a biopsy diagnosis before planning treatment.) Cylindromas, or those growths that cannot be cleanly removed, may benefit from x-ray therapy. Neck dissection follows for clinically positive nodes or for anaplastic and plain adenocarcinomas.

### Common errors

A common error in managing salivary gland tumors, happily infrequent today, consists of a mistaken diagnosis of sebaceous cyst near the ear, followed by a minor surgical procedure under local anesthesia in the physician's office. This often results in incomplete removal and sometimes a hopeless scattering of tumor implants, even though the tumors are histologically "benign."

### Prognosis

Patients should never succumb to benign tumors; proper surgery can achieve a local recurrence rate as low as 1%. Cancers that are anaplastic show at best a

30% 5-year survival, but low-grade, differentiated types have a good prognosis —50% to 70% 5-year survivals. Parotid cancers seem somewhat more favorable than submaxillary cancers.

## CANCER OF THE PARANASAL SINUSES (ANTRUM, ETHMOID, SPHENOID, AND FRONTAL SINUSES)

### Incidence

Tumors in these structures develop infrequently, without preference for race, geography, or sex. Chronic sinus infection for many years often seems to precede cancer formation. Reports exist of an increased risk among persons overexposed to radioactive substances deposited in bone, and one report cites a high incidence among wood-finishing workers. If carcinogenic particles present in inhaled air should gain access to these spaces they would be trapped there and in prolonged contact with the mucosa. Thus one can easily imagine external chemical agents playing a role, since they do in other parts of the respiratory tract.

### Pathology

The range of pathologic types resembles that in the nasopharynx and oropharynx; *epidermoid carcinoma* predominates and is thought to arise from squamous metaplasia of the cylindrical respiratory mucosa lining the sinuses. Occasionally salivary gland tumor types or lymphoma occur.

Cancer originates from the nasal cavity even more rarely than from the sinuses. Most malignant neoplasms giving nasal obstruction have invaded the thin bones separating sinuses from the nasal cavity by the time of diagnosis and are considered to be of sinus origin. No identifiable precancerous lesions occur.

### Natural history

A slow to moderate growth rate leads to invasion and destruction of the thin sinus bony walls and then to expansion in the nasal cavity, in the soft tissues of the cheek, or else into the orbit of the eye. Extension also occurs in the pyterygomaxillary space, base of skull, or downward through the hard palate into the mouth.

Sphenoid and ethmoid growths metastasize to the retropharyngeal nodes and then to palpable locations in the neck; antral cancers often embolize first to submaxillary nodes. Venous emboli take root later in lungs or spinal bones.

Local invasion by tumor produces the following ugly and obvious signs: facial deformity, visual defects leading to ophthalmoplegia, nasal obstruction and bleeding, and fifth nerve pain. Death approaches when pain necessitates narcotics and lowered food intake.

### Diagnosis

*Symptoms* of sinus cancer develop relatively late in its course from invasive growth breaking out of the bony confines. A patient gives a long history of sinusitis and nasal discharge. Then he notices a small amount of blood when blowing the nose, increasing blockage of one side of the nose, or a loose upper molar tooth that results from downgrowth of an antral cancer. One or several of the following may occur: swollen cheek, diplopia, facial pain, loose upper molar teeth, and tearing of one eye. Signs correspond to the symptoms. A mass may present in the nose.

*X-ray* films of the facial and nasal bones are essential in assessing the extent of the tumor. *Biopsy* of the most accessible piece of tumor, but not of the neck nodes, follows (neck nodes are assumed to be positive if enlarged and firm, a rule we usually follow in other head and neck cancers). The safest course is to biopsy the tumor in the hospital, since one can encounter uncontrollable hemorrhage or the need for special technical maneuvers in the less accessible masses in the nose or antrum.

*Nasal polyps, fibroosteomas, giant cell tumors,* or other bone tumors of the facial bones may produce some of the above cancer symptoms or signs.

### Treatment principles

*Treatment* consists of some *combination* of *irradiation* and *surgery.* Both modalities are generally needed because these cancers have advanced moderately far when first seen. The fitting of a special dental plate or facial prosthesis in the immediate postoperative period constitutes an essential part of treatment for these patients; the slowly increasing number of dentists trained in maxillofacial prosthetics will soon make possible comprehensive, modern rehabilitation in all of these disfiguring situations.

### Prognosis

Because of late diagnosis, prognosis has generally been poor—10% to 20% 5-year survivals. More recent reports from some centers show survivals around 40% in Stages I and II (localized or confined to the anatomic region). Somewhat earlier diagnosis, more widespread use of radical surgery, and megavoltage radiation techniques all probably can combine to increase the salvage rates.

## TUMORS IN THE NECK

A lump in the neck, if not thyroid and if the patient is an adult, is more likely to be metastatic cancer than any other entity. Martin and Morfit first emphasized this fact. The variety of possible diagnoses of abnormal masses in the neck nevertheless forms a wide spectrum. The great frequency of metastatic disease in the neck is due to the large number of lymph nodes relative to the size of the space. Primary tumors in blood and lymph vessels and nerves rarely occur. Therefore, as we have noted before, since the character of the normal structures in the area determines the frequency and types of its tumors, most neck tumors will be lymph node related, primary, or metastatic.

### Diagnosis

The problem of the lump in the neck presents us with this first decision—is it metastatic, or is it primary? If a negative, complete examination of head and neck, mouth and throat, and nose makes metastatic disease unlikely, or in the case of a supraclavicular node, if a complete chest and gastrointestinal tract survey is negative, then primary tumor possibilities come uppermost in mind. At this stage

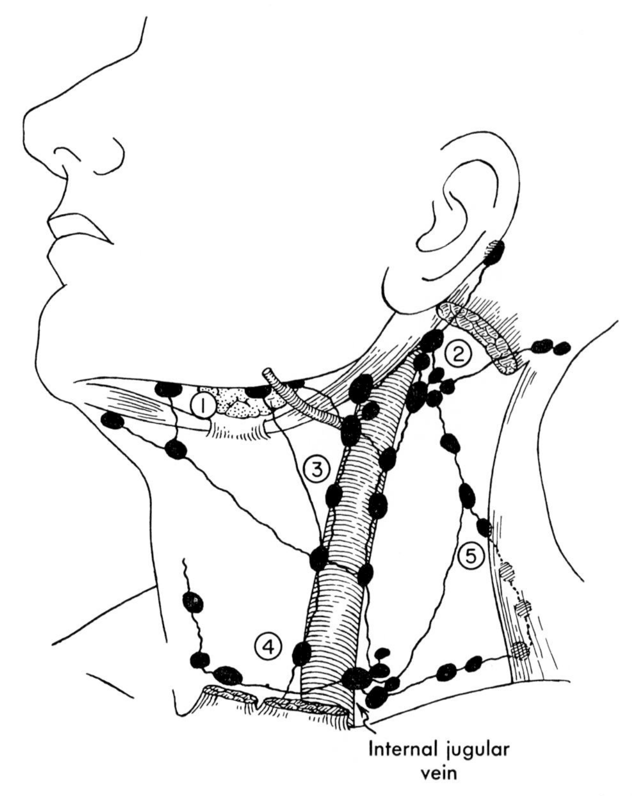


**Fig. 6.** Five main groups, or levels, of neck nodes that drain the mouth, laryngopharynx, nasopharynx, sinuses, and skin. **1,** Submaxillary group; **2,** upper jugular group; **3,** midjugular group; **4,** lower jugular group; **5,** posterior (spinal accessory) chain group.

in the clinician's diagnostic thinking an acquaintance with the many primary neck tumors becomes necessary, especially the neoplasms arising in the lymph tissues themselves.

**Lymphoma.** The various types of lymphoma all may frequently present *first* as neck *masses.* (More detailed data regarding lymphomatous disease appear in Chapter 29.)

*Hodgkin's disease* appears initially in the neck in two thirds of the cases; it usually strikes much younger persons, predominantly males, than do most cancers. Nodes or groups of adjacent nodes present as discrete, rubbery, movable masses.

*Lymphocytic lymphoma* (lymphosarcoma) occurs about as frequently as Hodgkin's disease in the neck nodes. However, it strikes middle-aged or older persons, and the nodes coalesce and become fixed in contrast to Hodgkin's disease.

The *reticulum cell sarcoma* group is a less common lymphoma that can be distinguished from the other two only by histologic study.

Diagnosis of lymphoma demands whole node removal for biopsy; aspiration biopsy and small wedge removal do not give the pathologist enough tissue for accurate classification.

**Leukemia.** The enlarged neck lymph nodes of leukemia are generally smaller and more discrete than the lymphomas.

**Miscellaneous node enlargements.** Other lymph node *enlargements* occur from *tuberculous adenitis* in children, less common than formerly, and from *nonspecific lymphadenitis* that persists longer than usual after nasal or pharyngeal infections. As a rule, these various chronic lymphadenopathies cause no tenderness or other symptoms unless the enlargements have been quick or occur in childhood.

**Developmental anomalies.** Developmental *anomalies,* usually cysts, persist in the occasional growing infant and youngster and yield an interesting variety of tumorous neck masses. These reach the physician at varying ages from childhood to young adulthood, depending upon size and consequent symptomatology.

*Branchiogenic cysts* receive more than their deserved share of attention in view of their rarity. Lateral in the upper neck, they show a squamous epithelial lining and sometimes a partially obliterated but attached branchiogenic fistulous tract to the pharynx.

A *cystic lymphangioma* (cystic hygroma) in an infant, or its remnant at older ages, also causes a neck cyst.

A true *dermoid cyst* on rare occasions will be found in the neck, often containing hair.

The *thyroglossal duct cyst* is the most common neck cyst, occurring in or near the midline anteriorly, with a tract or attachment through the hyoid bone to the base of the tongue.

**Carotid body tumors.** Now and then carotid body tumors arise from the tiny carotid body at, or near, the bifurcation of the common carotid artery. This body consists of chemoreceptor cells that help to control respiration. Its tumors, usually benign, cause pain after several years of slow growth. Removal is difficult and hazardous. Diagnosis is suggested by history, by location in the neck, and by arteriography.

**Miscellaneous tumors.** Except for thyroid gland tumors, covered in Chapter 10, the remaining primary neck neoplasms occur rarely indeed. *Lipomas* are subcutaneous. Cavernous hemangiomas suggest a bunch of compressible small grapes, showing the characteristic bluish tinge if superficial enough. *Parathyroid adenomas* present similar to thyroid masses; only careful complete medical work-up on all patients with cystic bone lesions, renal calculi, or abnormal serum calcium levels can detect the total number of these fascinating, metabolically crucial neoplasms.

## Treatment principles

1. Treatment depends first on whether or not the tumor is primary or metastatic; the decision stems from the clinical work-up and the acuity and wisdom of the physician.

2. If the tumor is primary, most of the above mentioned lesions are *surgical* problems; the main exception is the *lymphoma* group. Here *radiotherapy* and sometimes *chemotherapy* play the main role.

3. If the mass is metastatic, one must find the primary and treat it first. The metastases come second in considerations of treatment. However, if the primary

cancer eludes all search efforts, and if the location of the metastatic node in the neck suggests a mouth or throat primary, radical neck dissection and repeated periodic, continued searches for the primary for the rest of the patient's life proves a worthwhile plan. In other words, one should treat rather than give up when the primary escapes detection.

4. If an abnormal node in the neck is suspicious of metastasis, we treat it as such without node biopsy as long as the primary tumor is proved by biopsy. Node biopsy, often resorted to as a critical diagnostic step, really adds little to the planning of treatment, except in the case of lymphoma.

**REFERENCES**

Ackerman, L. V., and del Regato, J. A.: Cancer, ed. 3, St. Louis, 1962, The C. V. Mosby Co., pp. 228-257, 357-385, 706-736.

Dalley, V. M.: The influence of lymph node metastasis on the prognosis of nasopharyngeal cancer, Proceedings of the Ninth International Cancer Congress, Tokyo, Oct., 1966, Berlin, 1967, Springer-Verlag, p. 532 (abst.).

Foote, F. W., Jr., and Frazell, E. L.: Tumors of the major salivary glands. In Atlas tumor pathology, Sect. IV, Fasc. 11, Washington, D. C., 1954, Armed Forces Institute of Pathology.

Helsper, J. T.: Salivary gland tumors, Med. Sci., pp. 44-53, July, 1965.

MacComb, W. S., and Fletcher, C. H.: Cancer of the head and neck, Baltimore, 1967, The Williams & Wilkins Co., pp. 152-178, 329-389, 488-506.

Martin, H., and Morfit, H. M.: Cervical lymph node metastasis as the first symptom of cancer, Surg. Gynec. Obstet. **78:**133-159, 1944.

Martin, H., and Quan, S.: The racial incidence (Chinese) of nasopharyngeal cancer, Ann. Otol. **60:**168-174, 1951.

Rosenfeld, L., Sessions, D. G., McSwain, B., and Graves, H.: Malignant tumors of salivary gland origin, Ann. Surg. **163:**726-735, 1966.

Sakai, S., and Hamazaki, Y.: On our classification and treatment of the maxillary cancer, Proceedings of the Ninth International Cancer Congress, Tokyo, Oct., 1966, Berlin, 1967, Springer-Verlag, p. 557 (abst.).

Ward, G. E., and Hendrick, J. W.: Tumors of the head and neck, Baltimore, 1950, The Williams & Wilkins Co., pp. 618-755.

Chapter 10

# Cancer of the thyroid

Tumors arising in glands of internal secretion (thyroid, ovary, adrenal, etc.) form a totally different pattern and picture from tumors arising on "lining" surfaces (mouth, stomach, colon, bladder, etc.). The responsiveness of secreting cells to other hormones, the different routes by which external carcinogens may reach these cells, and functional and structural differences of secreting cells from "lining" cells all help to account for the fundamental tumor differences between the two classes of ectodermal tissue.

## INCIDENCE AND DISTRIBUTION

Thyroid cancer develops uncommonly, far less than 1% of all cancers. Females predominate over males by a ratio of 2:1; the average age is much younger than with other cancers. Conflicting reports appear of the relative frequency of thyroid cancer in endemic goiter areas as compared to other geographic locations. In this regard the critical study of Winship and Rosvoll seems the most informative. They conclude that thyroid cancer turns up most often where pathologists and others look hardest for it. Older publications express its occurrence as a percentage of nodular goiters coming to surgery, but the large variation in selection factors negates the permanent value of these figures. Fewer goiters now occur or will be surgically treated than was true 20 years ago. Cancer of the thyroid in children, although rare, seems to be on the increase.

## ETIOLOGY

### External initiating factors

Iodine deficiency probably produces goiter; it may result in cancer in animals as well. Its role in human cancer is less clear, but it may be an indirect contributor to the carcinogenic sequence. (The widespread use of iodized salt will probably continue to reduce the incidence of endemic goiter.)

X-ray therapy given in infancy and childhood for various benign conditions precedes thyroid cancer by an average of 8 years in 80% of Winship and Rosvoll's collected series of over 600 thyroid cancers of youth. We consider this, and other corroborating studies, sufficient evidence to indict as directly carcinogenic x-ray therapy (and also radioactive iodine in diagnostic studies) when given to infants and children. The young gland seems highly susceptible to x-rays. In adults the relation of cancer to x-ray therapy is a weak one.

Thiouracil derivatives contribute to the tumorigenic complex in animals, but no evidence exists that they do so in man.

### Predisposing factors

Excess thyroid-stimulating hormone (TSH) from the pituitary apparently sets the stage for thyroid cancer; it results from an underproduction of thyroxine by the gland or may theoretically arise from other mechanisms. Once cancer has developed, excess TSH often keeps the papillary and follicular tumors growing—a variable, dependent relationship in these highly differentiated types.

## PATHOLOGY

An understanding of thyroid cancer depends upon knowledge of the two major groups, the *differentiated* and the *undifferentiated* cancers. Behavior and prognosis differ between these two groups as widely as between any two in the entire spectrum of human cancer. The differentiated group is happily the common one, often follows a more indolent, benign course than any other cancer; the undifferentiated ones are aggressive, hard to cure, and sometimes rapidly fatal.

Warren and Meissner's *classification* is as follows:

*Differentiated*—80% of all

1. *Papillary*—most common, 50% to 60% of all, least malignant (80% of childhood cancers are papillary)
2. *Follicular*—10% of all (older name was "benign metastasizing goiter"), indolent growth rate
3. *Hurthle cell*—2%, indolent

*Undifferentiated*—20% of all

1. *Small cell* (simplex or solid adenocarcinoma), fast growing, rapidly invasive
2. *Giant and spindle cell*—rare, very fast growing, invariably fatal

A number of unique features of thyroid cancer make it one of the most studied of tumors. First, it requires unusual experience and judgment on the part of the pathologist to distinguish true neoplasms from the hyperplastic nodules of endemic goiters, or to distinguish follicular cancers from the histology presented by variations in the essentially normal gland. Second, although multiple microscopic foci of cancer or widespread intraglandular metastases may be found in whole gland studies, removal of only one lobe for cancer results only rarely in a clinical recurrence in the remaining lobe, so indolent is the growth pattern of the differentiated types. Third, occult thyroid cancer turns up at autopsy as often as clinical cancer does in the living. Fourth, no correlation exists between the size of the thyroid primary cancer and the extent of the metastatic spread, a correlation we find commonly among other cell cancers.

Most differentiated growths (papillary, follicular) show a mixture of histologic patterns; classification is by predominant type.

Benign adenomas are encapsulated and mimic cancers clinically, but the common *fetal* and *embryonal* types are easily distinguishable histologically. Adenomatous nodules of endemic goiter also resemble cancer in the patient, but the gross pathologic appearance is characteristic; they are not true neoplasms.

### Precancerous lesions

Benign thyroid nodules in the experimental animal apparently become malignant. No evidence exists that this happens often in man. Prevailing opinion holds that sometimes cancer and benign nodules and adenomas arise from similar influences, but separately. Cancer develops among adults in the clinically normal gland as often as in the goitrous one, but among children it develops more often in a previously normal gland. However, in young children nearly half of nodular glands have cancer in them.

## NATURAL HISTORY

As indicated above, *papillary* and *follicular* types have a *very slow growth pattern,* both in the enlargement of the primary and in the metastases. A nearly stationary clinical course can occur for 10 or more years. However, eventually these types will invade the larynx and trachea locally, involving the recurrent laryngeal nerve and prethyroid muscles. Most such highly differentiated tumors have on diagnosis metastasized to regional neck nodes (often paratracheal and superior mediastinal nodes first). Follicular cancers invade blood vessels and tend to spread to lungs and bones quicker and more often than papillary types. Sooner or later these indolent types will cause death by laryngeal or tracheal obstruction. They do not seem to parasitize the patient's metabolic and nutritive substances, as do most cancers, because of their slow growth rate. Papillary is the characteristic thyroid cancer of youth—80%. Sloan believes that papillary tumors tend to become anaplastic over the years because of the greater growth rate of anaplastic elements; he thinks we may diagnose an anaplastic cancer of the thyroid 20, 30, 40 years after it began as a predominantly papillary type.

In contrast, the undifferentiated varieties grow fairly rapidly, invade the larynx, trachea, and esophagus in a few months, soon metastasize to regional nodes and lungs, and cause death by inanition and starvation.

Thyroid cancers that metastasize distantly *frequently involve bone,* with consequent bone pain.

## DIAGNOSIS

**History.** Even moderately early symptoms are absent in thyroid cancer. The patient may feel a painless neck lump in the thyroid region. The following signs suggest thyroid cancer: (1) abnormal lateral and posterior neck nodes (metastasis), (2) a single nodule appearing in the gland, (3) marked increase in size of a goiter, (4) extreme hardness of a thyroid nodule, (5) fixation to prethyroid muscles, (6) any thyroid mass in childhood, and (7) hoarseness with a goiter.

**Laboratory studies.** *Radioactive iodine ($I^{131}$) uptake* and *scintiscan* of the thyroid gland and adjacent neck areas form the first definite diagnostic step in all goiters or thyroid masses. "Cold" areas are suspicious of cancer; "hot" ones rarely represent cancer. The gland as a whole usually falls into the euthyroid range, unless cancer coexists with thyroiditis or an overactive nodule is cancerous.

Serum protein-bound iodine determinations and red cell iodine uptake will help decide about other differential diagnostic possibilities such as thyroiditis of various kinds.

**X-ray studies.** X-ray films of the neck sometimes reveal tiny characteristic calcifications (psammoma bodies) in papillary cancer, but their absence means little. Larger calcifications are frequent in adenomatous nodules. Films of flat and long bones complete a work-up for thyroid cancer, since 10% or so have bone metastases; when this tumor does metastasize, it has a predilection for bone sites after first going to neck nodes.

**Biopsy.** Biopsy is *not* the recommended method of diagnosis. *Extracapsular lobectomy* as a formal operation provides the most satisfactory definitive diagnosis; aspiration needle biopsies and wedge biopsies may leave the pathologist short of tissue without a full picture of the tumor in the gland. Biopsy of an abnormal neck node serves as a last resort.

### Differential diagnosis

*Benign adenomatous nodule*—usually present without change for years

Benign *fetal* or *embryonal adenoma*—very discrete

*Hashimoto's thyroiditis*—diffuse, symmetrical, hard enlargement of the whole gland, nearly always in women, often a high titer of antithyroid tissue antibodies

*De Quervains' thyroiditis* (subacute)—a recent, tender, diffuse, enlargement of one lobe with neck pain, generally a self-limiting disease

Healed *chronic thyroiditis* (Riedel's)—very hard; only by histology can one differentiate this from cancer

*Thyroglossal duct cyst*—at or near the midline, cystic, smooth

The differential diagnostic points among various neck masses have been covered before. In children, however, anatomic landmarks remain obscure and lesions such as cystic hygromas, branchial cleft cysts, nonspecific adenitis, and leukemia may be confused with thyroid neoplasms.

## PREVENTIVE MEASURES

1. X-ray therapy to the head and neck areas of infants has virtually ceased in modern medicine; physicians must remember it is carcinogenic to the young thyroid gland, lest the practice revive or $I^{131}$ studies be applied indiscriminately.
2. The increasing reliance on thyroid hormone medication for various thyroid conditions and imbalances tends to reduce TSH stimulation and thus to lower the main background-preparation factor in thyroid cancer.

## TREATMENT PRINCIPLES

Patients with the common papillary type of cancer, and many with follicular cancer also, live so long in normal health, regardless of treatment, that various surgical, medical, and radiologic measures often credited with success have no reliable basis for claims of superiority. In moderately advanced cases with metastases, combinations of modalities are needed; in all differentiated types, medication with thyroid hormone follows initial treatment.

1. *Surgery* stands as the favored form of initial therapy.
   a. *Papillary type*—for this we usually perform an extracapsular lobectomy, removal of the isthmus, unilateral neck dissection, plus careful paratra-

cheal and superior mediastinal dissection. Then thyroid medication to tolerance levels follows surgery. There is more disagreement over this surgical plan than is warranted by the uncommon occurrence of the neoplasm. (The M. D. Anderson Hospital recommends only paratracheal and juxtathyroid dissection routinely, with total thyroidectomy; Crile advocates local node removals, but only when they are suspiciously involved. Memorial Hospital, New York City, finds, despite high incidence of multicentric foci and intraglandular spread of cancer, that lobectomy and neck dissection serve best; they find that only rarely does the remaining lobe develop a palpable tumor.)

b. *Follicular type*—total thyroidectomy plus node dissections where nodes are clinically suspicious of metastases. Thyroid extract to tolerance follows surgery.

c. *Undifferentiated types*—surgery as indicated by the suspected extent of disease.

2. *X-ray therapy* helps control tumor in cases of totally irremovable cancer and single distant metastases, especially in bone or neck areas where surgery has no margin.

3. *$I^{131}$ therapy* is worth a trial for multiple recurrent or metastatic disease in differentiated types. Total thyroid ablation must precede this; tumors can be stimulated to pick up $I^{131}$ by giving a goitrogen or TSH for 10 days, then $I^{131}$ in the period of tissue "rebound."

## COMMON ERRORS

1. As Winship and Rosvoll show, the course of papillary cancer in children is relatively benign so that the performance of mutilating surgery in these patients constitutes an error. Sacrifice of the recurrent nerve, the larynx, and parathyroids is seldom necessary.

2. *Overreliance on $I^{131}$* therapy for metastases in long-term planning can be a mistake. This measure seldom yields satisfactory control.

3. An assumption that massive local and regional papillary cancer means surgery would necessarily mutilate is not warranted. This tumor invades normal tissues later than any other, allowing successful dissections even in the face of bulky, local tumor masses.

## PROMISING DEVELOPMENTS FOR THE FUTURE

1. Complete cessation of x-ray therapy and $I^{131}$ diagnostic tests for benign conditions in infants and children will interrupt one etiologic pathway.

2. Coming widespread understanding of the peculiar, benign behavior of the differentiated types of thyroid cancer will certainly lead to more enlightened management.

## PROGNOSIS

1. Pemberton reported a series of untreated, mixed types of thyroid cancer; 71% lived 3 years and 35% lived 10 years.

2. *Papillary type*—80% live 5 years and 60% to 70% live 10 years and

more. The outlook depends upon age almost as much as upon treatment; the younger the patient at diagnosis, the longer he lives.

3. *Follicular type*—not as good an outlook as with papillary, 30% to 50% live 5 years. Bone metastases are frequent.

4. *Undifferentiated types*—30% have a 5-year survival.

**REFERENCES**

Crile, G., Jr.: Late results of treatment for papillary cancer of the thyroid, Amer. Surg. **160:** 178-182, 1964.

Frazell, E. L., and Foote, F. W., Jr.: The natural history of thyroid cancer, J. Clin. Endocr. **9:**1023-1030, 1949.

Frazell, E. L., and Foote, F. W., Jr.: Papillary cancer of the thyroid, Cancer **11:**895-922, 1958.

Lindsay, S., and Chaikoff, I. L.: The effects of irradiation on the thyroid gland with particular reference to the induction of thyroid neoplasms, Cancer Res. **24:**1099-1107, 1964.

Pemberton, J. deJ.: Malignant tumors of the thyroid gland, Surg. Gynec. Obstet. **69:**417-430, 1939.

Root, A. W.: Cancer of the thyroid in childhood and adolescence, Amer. J. Med. Sci. **246:** 735-749, 1963.

Rose, R. G., Kelsey, M. P., Russell, W. O., Ebanez, M. L., White, E. C., and Clark, R. L.: Management of unilateral thyroid cancer, Amer. J. Surg. **106:**494-500, 1963.

Sloan, L. W.: Of the origin, characteristics and behavior of thyroid cancer, J. Clin. Endocr. **14:**1309-1335, 1954.

Tollefson, H. R., and De Cosse, J. J.: Papillary carcinoma of the thyroid: recurrence in thyroid gland after initial surgical treatment, Amer. J. Surg. **106:**728-734, 1963.

Warren, S., and Meissner, W. A.: Tumors of the thyroid gland. In Atlas of tumor pathology, Sect. IV, Fasc. 14, Washington, D. C., 1953, Armed Forces Institute of Pathology.

Winship, T., and Rosvoll, R. V.: Childhood thyroid carcinoma, Cancer **14:**734-743, 1961.

Chapter 11

# Cancer of the breast

The breast is a gland; like the thyroid, it differs markedly from the conductive, absorptive gastrointestinal, and respiratory organs. It secretes large amounts of nutritive material for relatively short periods (lactation). To make this enormous periodic transformation its tissues possess great sensitivity to hormones, perhaps more reactivity than any other tissue except the uterus. As we would expect, breast cancer reflects the characteristics of its tissue of origin and shows a close and important relationship to endocrines.

## INCIDENCE AND DISTRIBUTION

Cancer of the breast is the most frequent cancer in women—22%. It occurs in men occasionally, about once for every 100 women victims, approximately the same ratio as the amount of breast tissue in the two sexes. It seems more prevalent in white, nulliparous, unmarried, well-to-do women. An artificial menopause exerts some protective influence against breast cancer development. A strong family history of breast cancer increases the risk of developing it by about 10%. This cancer occurs ten times *less often in Japanese* women than in the Americans, English, Danish, or Dutch, in whom it occurs commonly.

## ETIOLOGY

### External initiating agents

No external agents correlate with human breast cancer up to this date, although certain viruses markedly increase the incidence of breast cancer in mice, possibly by altering the endocrine balance.

### Predisposing factors

Many internal factors influence the risk of a woman getting cancer of the breast, all of them linked to endocrines and endocrine balance. A strong family incidence of breast cancer, absence of pregnancies, a first pregnancy late in the childbearing years, delayed menopause, and excess mammotropic hormone of the pituitary all relate to an abnormal hormonal balance, excess estrogen, and/or excess stimulation to ductal and acinar breast tissue. Each increases the risk in women to a slight extent. Sex hormones acting on the substrate breast tissue seems

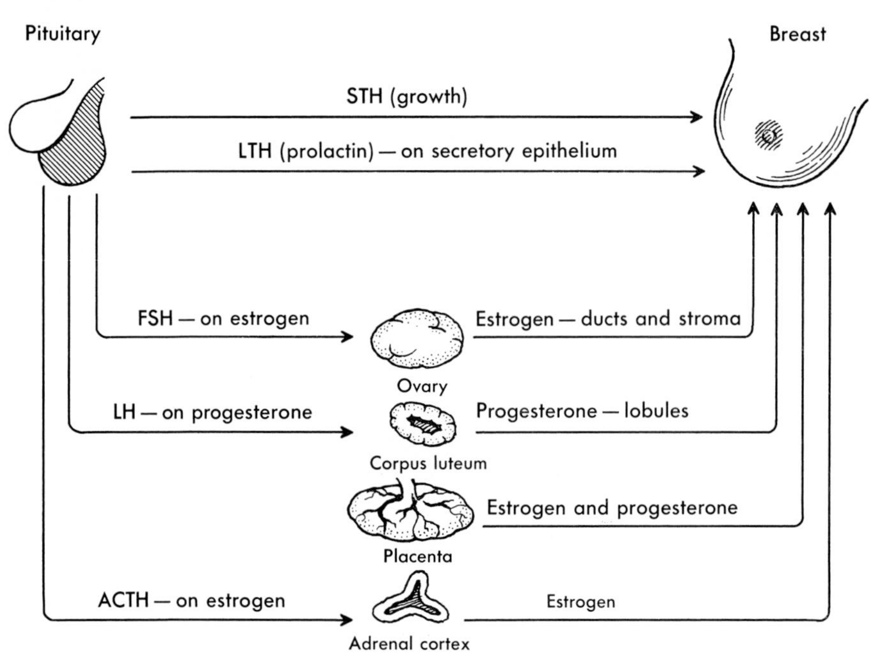


**Fig. 7.** Direct and indirect hormonal stimulation of the breast. (Modified from Kark, W.: Synopsis of cancer, Baltimore, 1966, The Williams & Wilkins Co.)

a necessary stage setting for cancer in both animals and humans. Oophorectomy performed for other reasons reduces the cancer risk if done before the age of 40.

## PATHOLOGY

Benign tumors and breast nodules imitating early cancer abound in the female breast. In women coming to physicians with abnormal breast masses, nearly four masses are benign for every one malignant. Seven benign conditions deserve our attention: (1) fibrocystic mastopathy, (2) fibroadenoma, (3) sclerosing adenosis, (4) periductal mastitis, (5) fat necrosis, (6) eczema of the nipple, and (7) intraductal papilloma and papillomatosis. Only the last of these shows epithelial (ductal) hyperplasia that could presage cancer.

Of the cancers, 80% arise from ductal epithelium; the rest develop from acinar tissue or nonsecretory elements of the breast. Thus all but a few are adenocarcinomas.

A useful classification is one adapted from Stewart:

| | | | |
|---|---|---|---|
| Infiltrating duct | 80% | Paget's disease | 2% |
| Medullary with lymphoid stroma | 5% | Papillary, mucinous, epidermoid | Rare |
| Lobular of acinar origin | 5% | Cystosarcoma phyllodes malignant | Rare |
| Intraductal (comedo) | 4% | Fibrosarcoma, lymphosarcoma, lymphangiosarcoma | Rare |

Occasionally, *inflammatory cancer* of the breast occurs in which a diffuse, pink-red blush colors the skin, which is hot to touch. This fast-growing type invariably causes death in 1 or 2 years despite treatment. Because of the

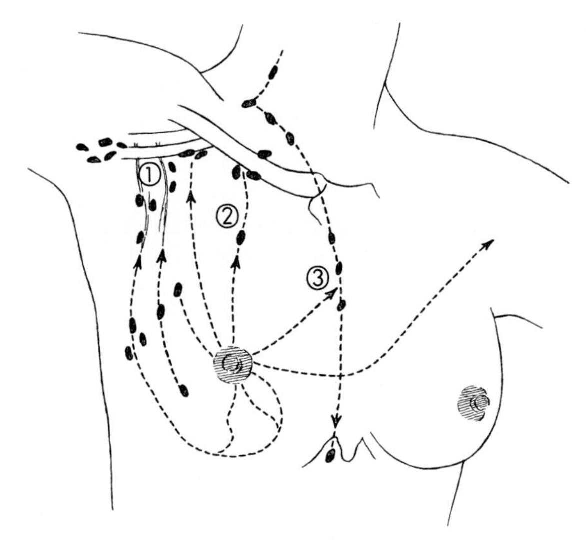


1. Main axillary group
2. Interpectoral node leading to apex of axilla
3. Internal mammary group

**Fig. 8.** Node groups and lymphatic drainage routes of the breast available for cancer cell embolization. (Modified from Ackerman, L. V., and del Regato, J. A.: Cancer, ed. 3, St. Louis, 1962, The C. V. Mosby Co.)

poor outlook, it must be distinguished clinically from the patchy skin redness accompanying many large, less aggressive cancers. Grace and Dao have demonstrated that hypersensitivity of the patient to her own tumor accounts for the peculiar inflammation.

*Paget's disease of the nipple* is an infiltrating duct, or intraductal, cancer beginning in a duct close to the nipple; the cancer invades the skin of the nipple and areola so early that often the primary has not yet developed a palpable nodule.

Medullary cancer has a good prognosis because it grows slowly, often near the tail of the breast, and attains great bulk at times without having metastasized. It spreads to nodes less often and at a later time than infiltrating duct cancers. Comedo or intraductal carcinoma is usually considered a nonmetastizing type that reaches large size and may ulcerate. Malignant cystosarcoma phyllodes, the rare malignant giant fibroadenoma, likewise seldom metastasizes to lymph nodes.

Most of the common infiltrating duct cancers invade breast tissue, fat, skin, and fascia and cause varying degrees of fibrous reaction and lymphatic obstruction, which account for the classic signs of breast cancer—"orange peel" skin and nipple retraction. These cancers embolize in lymphatics, generally to axillary nodes first, proceeding successively from low lateral nodes to high medial nodes beneath the clavicle. Subareolar and medial quadrant cancers travel to internal mammary (intercostal space) nodes as readily or more quickly than to the axilla; sometimes they go directly to the high infraclavicular nodes. Many lymphatics along the internal mammary vessels proliferate into the parietal pleura and mediastinum so that these locations often harbor breast cancer metastases. Vascular connections are profuse in the breast in all directions; cancers invade veins often and blood-borne emboli cause distant metastases in lungs, pleura, bones of the spine, pelvis, and ribs, as well as in the adrenals, ovaries, liver, and brain. Some cancers are multifocal and a few are simultaneously bilateral.

Urban has demonstrated by large routine biopsies of the opposite breast that patients with cancer in one breast have nearly a 20% chance of harboring atypical, precancerous changes, carcinoma in situ, or cancer in the other breast.

### Precancerous lesions

Foote and Stewart first described carcinoma in situ of the breast. Pathologists have been identifying such a stage of preinvasive cancer more and more in recent years—in 10% of opposite breasts where cancer was present on one side and in 30% of opposite breasts where an in situ lobular carcinoma exists on one side. The two following varieties appear: (1) *in situ lobular* carcinoma, which is usually multifocal and carries a 35% risk of developing into invasive cancer in a 20-year period and a 30% chance of cancer developing in the opposite breast (McDivitt and associates); and (2) *noninfiltrating intraductal* carcinoma with lower but definite risks. So well have these precursor lesions been described and documented that we can now devise appropriate cancer preventive treatment.

## NATURAL HISTORY

Like melanomas and thyroid cancers, malignant tumors of the breast exhibit a wide range of behavior; some are quickly lethal despite all treatment, but most grow slowly to moderately fast over a period of some years. Perhaps 10% demonstrate a highly aggressive, uncontrollable character.

Bloom studied the behavior of over 1000 untreated cancers in four series and found close agreement between patients in England and in the United States. Average survival time was over 3 years from onset of symptoms; 20% lived 5 years and 4% 10 years, but life for the untreated patient was miserable with pain and tumor ulceration. He concluded from a comparison with several treated series followed 5 to 15 years that patients benefit considerably from treatment of breast cancer and that the greatest benefit accrues in the more malignant types. No spontaneous regressions occurred in the untreated.

Typically, a 55-year-old woman finds an asymptomatic breast lump; it is usually 1 to 3 cm. in diameter, hard or firm, with indistinct edges, often only a thickening, but definitely an area different from the surrounding breast. Two thirds of tumors present in the outer quadrants and one third are central or in the inner quadrants. In 4 to 6 months the tumor doubles in size and may cause slight skin retraction over it. In another 6 months a low axillary node feels abnormally large and hard; the mass has caused edema ("orange peel" effect) of the overlying skin, slight redness, and some deep fixation to the chest wall. After a few more months ulceration of the skin occurs with larger, higher axillary nodal enlargement; then a cough or dyspnea indicates pulmonary or pleural spread. Back pain may even be the first real symptom when blood-borne emboli reach the

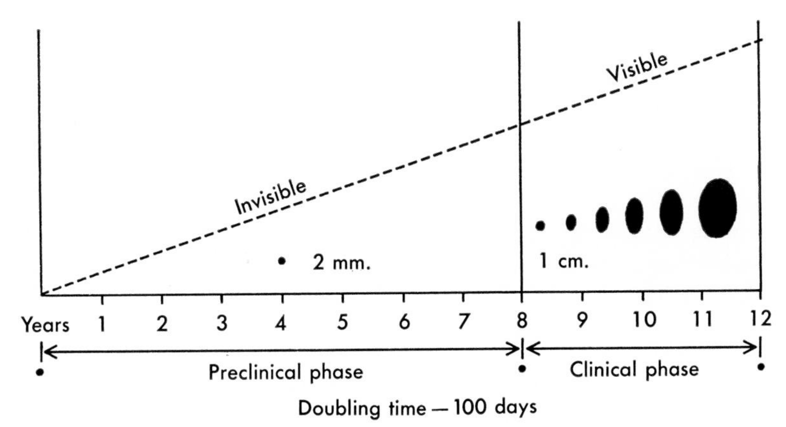


**Fig. 9.** Typical life cycle of breast cancer. Relatively long periods during which a breast cancer exists only in microscopic dimensions are indicated. (Modified from MacDonald, I.: In Nealon, T. F., Jr., editor: Management of the patient with cancer, Philadelphia, 1965, W. B. Saunders Co.)

vertebral bodies via Batson's vertebral venous plexus. Nodal involvement may now be present in the supraclavicular space.

Usually widespread bone, liver, and lung metastases develop, but single distant metastases may sometimes give the major symptoms for long periods, such as a brain metastasis. Death approaches gradually from anorexia, narcosis, inanition, loss of activity, and a terminal pneumonia.

Characteristic of advanced breast cancer are the signs and symptoms of bone metastases present in about one half the patients. Multiple long and flat bones show both osteolytic and occasionally osteoblastic foci, with constantly changing pain patterns that jump from one involved bone to another. Hypercalcemia from bone destruction commonly develops, occasionally without x-ray evidence of bony metastasis, and pathologic fractures often occur. The latter hasten terminal pneumonia if the patient is not kept mobile during management of the fractures.

## DIAGNOSIS

**History and physical examination.** As a rule the patient experiences no early symptoms. Occasionally a nipple discharge (clear, brown, or bloody) may come from a cancer in a large collecting duct. More often this sign comes from a benign intraductal papilloma. The painless lump is the symptom and the sign. Skin dimpling, edema, redness, and nipple retraction seldom accompany a small mass of tumor that has not metastasized. The earliest signs we can detect are slight skin blush, dilated veins, raised nipple level, or skin dimpling with changes in position. Careful, unhurried, and systematic palpation of breasts in both supine and sitting positions can result in great benefit to the woman who has an unsuspected 1 cm. cancer, as the 91% salvage rate in this highly select group demonstrates.

**Mammography.** Mammography can help (1) by deciding about changes that do not feel like definite lumps, (2) by finding suspicious areas we cannot feel at all, (3) by finding suspicious changes in the high-risk opposite breast of a breast cancer patient, and (4) by screening very bulky breasts that are hard to palpate thoroughly. It succeeds most often in older women with fatty breasts, and fails most in young women with scant fatty tissue. In average hands mammography yields an 80% accurate opinion, which is 10% better than clinical judgment. A negative mammogram does not rule out the possibility of cancer. We must still biopsy all faintly suspicious lesions; mammography should not be allowed to replace biopsy, but rather it should be used as a method to show the need for biopsy in additional cases where clinical appraisal fails. This method, unfortunately, cannot qualify as a true screening procedure because of the cost and time needed for it. Ten percent to 15% of mammograms cannot be interpreted because of technical problems.

**Biopsy.** The basic decision in breast diseases is whether or not to biopsy a given lump. The decision rests on the estimated degree of risk that the lump is cancer. The clinician cannot err greatly if he follows the rule of thumb: *when in doubt, biopsy.*

Most patients benefit from having the surgeon do the biopsy because he can (1) best avoid seeding cancer cells in the wound by using proper techniques; (2) best choose among various treatment plans on the basis of a total preoperative study plus biopsy findings; and (3) marshal expert frozen section, pathologic opinion, and radiotherapeutic consultation for an immediate treatment decision without delay and a second anesthetic.

Always done with the patient under general anesthesia in the hospital, open breast biopsy needs only a few minutes to perform and causes no major discomfort or expense to the patient. A small wedge of the true tumor, not the pseudocapsule, serves best if the mass is large—3 cm. or more. Small masses can be excised. The surgeon can lose a tiny cancer after the incision in large, fatty breasts. Excision of an entire pie-shaped segment of breast tissue, down to the fascia, obviates this error. Hemostasis must be meticulous in these biopsies because, if the diagnosis is cancer and uncontrollable circumstances cause delay between biopsy and definitive surgery, considerable blood, containing cancer cells, may extravasate from the biopsy wound and potentially seed cancer cells at some distance. Frozen section study has proved to be 95% accurate. Delay of 3 to 4 days between biopsy and surgery does not worsen the prognosis.

*Aspiration biopsy* with a needle helps save the time of a biopsy when done just before definitive surgery in larger, clinically malignant lesions by those experienced in its performance and interpretation.

Double biopsy is a procedure to determine suitability for curative operation. Here the surgeon takes samples of tissue from (1) primary tumor and (2) infraclavicular axillary nodes. In borderline cases we find it useful to determine suitability for radical mastectomy.

We properly worry about spreading cancer by biopsy. Gentleness, careful hemostasis, and the cutting of the smallest adequate specimen reduce this risk. Misdiagnosis and mistreatment constitute greater risks than potential cancer spread at biopsy.

**Other procedures.** Chest and bone x-ray films, blood chemistry studies, and other laboratory studies, such as cytologic examination of breast discharges, play an adjunctive role in the diagnosis of the primary breast tumor.

**Differential diagnosis**

Faced with the decision about whether or not to biopsy, we gain help from some features of the seven classes of benign breast lesions mentioned before:

*Fibrocystic mastopathy*—a common, mixed lesion composed of duct stasis, multiple cysts, solid fibrous areas, and perhaps intraductal epithelial proliferations. Three types occur: (1) *diffuse*—painful, granular, or coarsely nodular to palpation, (2) *gross cysts*—age 40 to 50, multiple, often bilateral, containing clear yellow or cloudy green fluid, and (3) *localized*—asymptomatic thickening.

*Fibroadenoma*—age 15 to 30, "slippable," discrete, and sometimes multiple; these are mixed tumors. When they grow rapidly, they may be diagnosed as cystosarcoma phyllodes, benign.

*Sclerosing adenosis*—a poorly defined, hard, unilateral nodule that causes no symptoms and has been confused histologically with cancer.

*Periductal mastitis*—arises from erosion and perforation of a major duct under the areola, producing the most common type of inflammatory reaction in the nonlactating, young-to-middle-aged breast. Secondary infection with sinus and abscess formation and an inverted nipple result.

*Fat necrosis*—develops from injury and extrusion of stagnant duct contents into surrounding fat; this results in a mass, often with skin adherence and dimpling.

*Intraductal papilloma and papillomatosis*—these often occur together between 30 and 50 years of age; a yellowish or bloody nipple discharge, usually produced from pressure on an oblong subareolar mass, brings the patient to the doctor. The associated florid papillomatosis may be regarded as a premalignant change.

*Eczema* of the nipple—may mimic Paget's disease and demand a biopsy; it is usually bilateral, however, in contrast to cancer.

## PREVENTIVE MEASURES

One preventive maneuver might reduce the breast cancer incidence slightly—women could be encouraged to have their first child early in the childbearing period—for example, before the age of 25. MacMahon finds evidence that this could reduce the risk somewhat. Universal oophorectomy before the age of 40 is obviously absurd. The most hopeful measures for the future involve earlier diagnosis in all communities. However, we can definitely prevent second primary breast cancers in the opposite breast. Wider and better use of mammography and prompt surgery for any suspicious finding plus careful periodic follow-up examinations should eliminate this small proportion of breast cancer deaths.

## TREATMENT PRINCIPLES

Few substitutes exist today for the adequate regional removal or destruction of cancer. The therapist or surgeon undertaking treatment must accept responsibility for local or regional recurrence because recurrence always raises the possibility that later distant metastases came from the recurrence *after* initial treatment rather than from the primary tumor before treatment.

1. *Radical mastectomy* remains the cornerstone of treatment. By most valid comparisons this very wide local and regional removal benefits more patients with less total suffering than other treatment plans. It requires skill and experience in selection of patients; detailed indications for this operation appear in many references. Some physicians believe node dissection harms patients by removing valuable defense factors against cancer. If this is true, we find it hard to explain why the first metastases of breast cancer occur in the middle of the defense manufactories—the lymph nodes. Nodes should be the last place to find metastases if they actually produce cancerostatic factors during the clinical stages of cancer.

2. *Internal mammary node removals* in continuity with radical mastectomy (the extended radical) have a place in skilled hands for inner quadrant tumors. Such a procedure achieves a 5% to 7% increase in survivals for this group (Urban).

3. Ultraradical surgery (neck and mediastinal dissections) has not improved results.

4. As with most other cancers, the surgeon needs the radiotherapist and vice versa.

5. Radiotherapy alone can often sterilize lymph nodes containing cancer and can achieve an acceptable 5-year control in a selected group of patients (Guttman).

6. The discomfort and disability after radiotherapy to tolerance levels can be considerable; patients do not necessarily prefer it to the sequelae of surgery.

7. *Simple mastectomy and x-ray therapy* (McWhirter's plan) amounts to a partial mastectomy with principal reliance upon irradiation for control. Survivals run 10% lower than in comparable patients who can be treated by radical mastectomy. This plan suits communities in which the quality of radiotherapy exceeds the quality of surgery.

8. Postoperative radiotherapy to the operative field has added disappointingly little to survivals. Therapy seems beneficial to the internal mammary node area in selected cases. Preoperative irradiation also seems to offer little advantage, although on-going studies of this point have not yet been completed.

9. Irradiation constitutes the treatment of choice for isolated metastases.

10. Advocates of no treatment at all, local excision only, or simple mastectomy seem to believe that most breast cancer is essentially incurable by the time it is diagnosed. (Actually only about 10% of cases have the biologic aggressiveness to deserve this hopeless attitude.) Survivals with these weak local efforts run a poor third behind adequate surgery and good irradiation. "Early" diagnosis makes a real difference in end results in cancer of the breast (and in most cancers) up to a certain point, a point that is far from reached in most communities. Diagnosis of smaller and smaller cancers increases at the community level every year, and improvements in community end results due to this factor may be undeservedly credited to conservative rather than radical treatment. Minor operations for cancer will achieve an increasing number of successes because of earlier case finding; but universally applied minor surgery does not achieve an overall optimum salvage.

11. When recurrence occurs, or when the patient presents with distant metastases, the proper sequence of palliative measures follows their degree of effective-

ness in descending order: oophorectomy, hormones, adrenalectomy or hypophysectomy, and chemotherapy.

12. Oophorectomy brings remission to half of the women suitable for it, premenopausal and menopausal. It delays recurrence but does not prolong life.

13. If castration fails, or when relapse occurs, androgens followed by estrogens (or vice versa) may induce remission. The principle of hormone therapy is merely to *change* the hormone environment of the cancer.

14. Operative excision of the adrenals or the pituitary gland secures remissions of about 1 year in one fourth to one third of premenopausal and menopausal patients by removing extragenital sources of sex hormones.

15. Systemic chemotherapy with mustard derivatives or antimetabolites sometimes helps prevent tumor progression. The use of anticancer drugs as adjuvants to surgery may delay recurrences in a special group—premenopausal women with positive axillary nodes (Noer).

## COMMON ERRORS

1. Application of radical mastectomy to incurable patients, such as those with cancerous nodes at the apex of the axilla, obviously achieves little and probably harms the patient.

2. In suitable candidates, however, an inadequate axillary dissection may jeopardize survival chances; a fair number of individuals whose original disease involved multiple midaxillary nodes live for 10 to 15 years after *adequate* radical mastectomy.

3. The withdrawal of serious efforts at control when the first distant metastasis appears may prevent some women from enjoying the best possible palliation via x-ray and hormonal therapy.

4. The application of one treatment plan for all patients never secures optimum results.

## PROMISING DEVELOPMENTS FOR THE FUTURE

1. Increasing exposure of young women to education, such as in the American Cancer Society's program on self-examination of the breast, promises to improve early case finding.

2. Refinement of techniques and reduction of the cost of mammography to make it practical as a screening device would no doubt reduce deaths from cancer of the breast. Another technique, xerography, may offer even greater promise when simplified and refined.

3. The pursuance of epidemiologic studies of breast cancer, such as finding an explanation for the low incidence among Japanese women, would probably add much to control of the disease. Some external agent may play a role, although we know of none as yet, since external carcinogens constitute major factors in so many other cancers.

4. Electron beam x-ray therapy promises better results in the various situations where irradiation works.

5. Improved radioisotopic-scanning techniques offer hope of earlier detection of metastases.

## PROGNOSIS

1. Approximately half of patients not categorically incurable should live 5 years with acceptable treatment. The best clinics report this. Lower overall figures merely indicate late diagnosis, if treatment plans are standard.

2. The results of *radical mastectomy* vary directly with the size of the cancer; 75% achieve 5-year survival with tumors less than 2 cm., whereas only 30% reach 5-year survival with 5 cm. masses. Commenting on this relation between size and prognosis, Stewart says: "No further proof is needed to show the importance of early recognition of mammary cancer."*

3. Radical mastectomy survivals also depend directly on the degree of axillary node involvement; with nodes negative, 80% live 5 years, but with all three levels involved the rate drops to 25% (scarcely more than the untreated series).

4. Cancer diagnosed during pregnancy carries a worse than average outlook, but interruption of pregnancy does not seem to improve the patient's chances. Also, avoiding pregnancy does not lengthen the life of the breast cancer patient.

5. Up to 65 years, age has little effect on prognosis, but old women survive more often than those under 65.

6. Survival percentages drop 10 to 15 percentage points from 5 to 10 years after treatment.

7. Medullary and the rare papillary types of carcinoma generally carry a good prognosis. The histologic finding of nerve sheath or blood vessel invasion augurs a poor outlook.

---

*From Stewart, F. W.: Tumors of the breast. In Atlas of tumor pathology, Sect. IX, Fasc. 34, Washington, D. C., 1950, Armed Forces Institute of Pathology, p. 14.

### REFERENCES

Ackerman, L. V., and del Regato, J. A.: Cancer, ed. 3, St. Louis, 1962, The C. V. Mosby Co., pp. 1060-1132.

Bloom, H. J. G.: The natural history of untreated breast cancer, Ann. N. Y. Acad. Sci. **114:** 747-754, 1964.

Butcher, H. R., Jr.: Radical mastectomy as therapy for mammary cancer. In Ellison, E. H., Friesen, S. R., and Mulholland, J. H., editors: Current surgical management, vol. 3, Philadelphia, 1965, W. B. Saunders Co., pp. 45-52.

Chu, F. C. H.: Radiation therapy of breast cancer, Clin. Obstet. Gynec. **9:**221-234, 1966.

Clemmesen, J.: Statistical studies in malignant neoplasms, vol. 1, Copenhagen, 1965, Danish Cancer Registry, pp. 249-276.

Farrow, J. H.: Common benign lesions of the adult female breast, Clin. Obstet. Gynec. **9:** 170-185, 1966.

Foote, F. W., Jr., and Stewart, F. W.: Lobular carcinoma in situ: a rare form of mammary cancer, Amer. J. Path. **17:**491-495, 1941.

Grace, J. T., and Dao, T. L.: Etiology of inflammatory reaction in breast carcinoma, Surg. Forum **9:**661, 1958.

Guttman, R.: Survival and results after 2-million volt irradiation in the treatment of primary operable carcinoma of the breast with proved positive internal mammary and/or highest axillary nodes, Cancer **15:**383-386, 1962.

Haagensen, C. D.: Tumors of the breast. In Field, J. B., editor: Cancer; diagnosis and treatment, Boston, 1959, Little, Brown & Co., Chapter 4.

James, A. G.: Cancer prognosis manual, New York, 1961, American Cancer Society, Inc.

Macklin, M. T.: Comparison of the number of breast-cancer deaths observed in relations of breast-cancer patients, and the number expected on the basis of mortality rates, J. Nat. Cancer Inst. **22:**927-951, 1959.

MacMahon, B.: Paper on epidemiology of breast cancer, symposium on cancer of the breast, Louisville, Ky., May 12, 1969.

McDivitt, R. W., Hutter, R. V. P., Foote, F. W., Jr., and Stewart, F. W.: In situ lobular carcinoma, J.A.M.A. **201:**82-86, 1967

McWhirter, R.: Should more radical treatment be attempted in breast cancer? Amer. J. Roentgen. **92:**3-13, 1964.

Moore, C., and Shaw, H.: Carcinoma of the breast, Arch. Surg. **75:**598-604, 1957.

Noer, R. J.: Personal communication, 1967.

Segaloff, A.: Endocrine background of breast cancer, Clin. Obstet. Gynec. **9:**186-194, 1966.

Snyder, R. E.: Mammography: contributions and limitations in the management of cancer of the breast, Clin. Obstet. Gynec. **9:**207-220, 1966.

Stewart, F. W.: Tumors of the breast. In Atlas of tumor pathology, Sect. IX, Fasc. 34, Washington, D. C., 1950, Armed Forces Institute of Pathology.

Urban, J. A.: Evaluation of newer techniques of treatment for breast cancer, Clin. Obstet. Gynec. **9:**235-251, 1966.

Chapter 12

# Cancer of the lung

## INCIDENCE AND DISTRIBUTION

Most neoplasms of the lung are cancers; they are frequent and comprise 10% of all malignant neoplasms. More common than any other male cancers, lung cancers cause 15% to 16% of male cancer deaths, 3% of female cancer deaths, giving about a five to one male to female ratio. Lung cancer is increasing faster than any other cancer, both in males and females; it killed twice as many men in 1965 as in 1950.

Scotland, England, Wales, and Finland lead other countries in lung cancer death rates; their rates run twice as high as those in the United States. Rates are lowest in Japan, Norway, and Sweden for reasons unknown.

## ETIOLOGY

### External initiating agents

Most authorities indict cigarette smoking as a necessary factor in the sequence of events leading to the majority of lung cancers. The President's Advisory Committee on Smoking and Health brands cigarettes a definite causative factor. Cigarette smoke condensate (tar) contains various carcinogenic polycyclic hydrocarbons, and has produced cancer in several species of laboratory animals and in various animal organs—skin, mouth, bladder, and cervix. Squamous and undifferentiated lung cancers, together comprising over half of the human cancers, are rarely found in noncigarette users.

Because urban death rates exceed rural death rates from lung cancer, with equal cigarette inhaling habits in both groups, more recent critical work on other possible factors in polluted urban air have broadened the etiologic possibilities. Some investigators believe that, despite unmistakable association with cigarette smoking, multiple factors have been operative in the increasing incidence of lung cancer. Some of the other suspected external agents that are often inhaled in polluted city and industrial air are as follows: oil and gasoline engine exhaust fumes, road tar fumes, dust in cobalt and uranium mines, and chromate and asbestos dust.

Since we increasingly suspect multiple external factors as causative, we cannot expect the elimination of one factor from the environment to reduce the attack rate of lung cancer by the percentages of cancers correlated with that particular factor (Kotin and associates).

Average length of exposure and average dosage for cigarettes in lung cancer patients have been estimated; they amount to one package per day for 30 years.

### Predisposing factors

No hormonal, genetic, or metabolic predisposing factors are known. The common pulmonary diseases (pneumonia, tuberculosis, and histoplasmosis) often coexist with cancer and may act as cancer promoters.

## PATHOLOGY

Classifications vary, but in a general way lung cancers fit into the following six groups, the three commonest not unlike the types that occur in the upper respiratory tract:

|  |  |
|---|---|
| Squamous or epidermoid | 50%-60% of all |
| Undifferentiated (anaplastic) | 15%-20% of all |
| Adenocarcinoma | 10%-20% of all |
| Oat cell (small, round cell) | 10%-15% of all |
| Terminal bronchiolar ("alveolar cell") | 3%- 5% of all |
| Bronchial adenoma (Grade 1 carcinoma) | 1%- 2% of all |

The common squamous and undifferentiated cancers compose a group linked statistically with cigarettes; they arise in the bronchi from the columnar, ciliated bronchial epithelium, which first probably undergoes squamous metaplasia. Often they occur in smaller subsegmental bronchi, grow centrally, and cause symptoms when they invade a large bronchus. Adenocarcinomas and bronchiolar tumors grow from mucous gland epithelium, predominantly in peripheral locations. Upper lobes harbor cancer more often than lower lobes. Bronchial adenomas arise from mucous glands, always in the major bronchi, and resemble carcinoids of the intestines histologically and in their low malignant potential and infrequent metastases.

The less common type of terminal bronchiolar cancer appears as diffuse or focally distributed clumps of tumor in the walls of the alveoli; it is usually bilateral, probably multicentric in origin, grows slowly, and metastasizes very late, if at all, outside the lungs. Of interest is a benign variant of bronchiolar cancer, pulmonary adenomatosis, which is similar to the weakly contagious disease of sheep, *jaagsiekte*.

The common cancers can proliferate into the bronchial lumen as a bulky growth or grow peribronchially. They often invade blood vessels early, embolizing to other sites in the lung, then distantly to liver, bones, adrenals, kidneys, and brain. They spread as well by lymphatics to segmental, interlobar, and then to subcarinal, paratracheal, and mediastinal lymph nodes. Proceeding out of the chest, the lymph pathways from the right and lower left lungs carry emboli to the right supraclavicular nodes and from upper left lung to the left supraclavicular nodes. Direct extension to the pleura produces effusions with tumor cells or adhesions, and new lymphatics in adhesions carry tumor emboli across the pleural space. In this manner metastases occur in the chest wall, axilla, and diaphragm. Superior sulcus tumors and peripheral cancers may produce rib and spine invasion and erosion. Direct invasion of structures contiguous to lungs commonly develops, such as in the pericardium, diaphragm, or aortic wall.

Two syndromes produced by lung cancer show distinctive features: (1) *superior sulcus tumor*—an apical lung cancer causing pressure on the brachial plexus with arm and hand pain and neurologic changes; sometimes a Horner's syndrome develops; and (2) *superior vena caval compression syndrome*—a picture of chest, neck, and upper extremity edema, with blueness and venous distention, caused by a lung tumor or metastasis obstructing the superior vena cava.

Most symptoms and signs of lung cancer arise from bronchial obstruction by tumor that either develops endobronchially or compresses the bronchus from growth outside in the lung parenchyma. Partial obstruction leads to infection and pneumonitis distally, then further obstruction to atelectasis, abscess formation, or bronchiectasis. The infectious process often masks the underlying tumor.

### Precancerous lesions

At autopsy Auerbach and associates have found atypias and carcinoma in situ at multiple bronchial sites more often in lung cancer patients than in others. The bronchial epithelium has its cancer precursors, in all likelihood, just as other lining tissues do, although we cannot see them easily in the living patient.

## NATURAL HISTORY

Typically, a heavy-smoking male, between 40 and 60 years old, notes a cough that is persistent, at first nonproductive but later productive, and occasionally slight hemoptysis. Half of the patients will present with this symptomatology. The other half begin with symptoms of lung infection, cough, fever, and sweats. As the cancer progressively occludes a major bronchus, organizing pneumonitis, atelectasis, and abscesses of varying degrees may result with consequent increasing cough, malaise, fever, dyspnea, and weight loss. Occasionally hoarseness develops from left recurrent nerve involvement at the arch of the aorta, or pleural effusion develops from visceral pleural tumor extension or metastases.

Oat cell and undifferentiated types grow relatively fast, causing a terminal state in 1 to 2 years from first symptoms; epidermoid and squamous cancers and adenocarcinomas grow at a more moderate rate, remaining silent without symptoms for several years in some cases, especially if located peripherally. Bronchial adenomas grow very slowly as a rule. Rigler has brought to our attention the prolonged existence of lung cancers—90% show x-ray findings before symptoms—and in half the silent interval is 2 to 3 years and more; in some growths the interval is 3 to 5 years.

Lung cancers kill patients rapidly once the irremediable progression of lung infection and destruction begins behind the obstructing tumors. Rapid deterioration of all vital functions occurs, especially the respiratory function.

## DIAGNOSIS

**History.** As indicated in previous sections, lung cancers give symptoms only when large enough or so located in the bronchus as to give partial obstruction. Cough and slight hemoptysis occur commonly; localized wheeze, chest discomfort, dyspnea, low-grade fever, sweats, and anorexia occur less often as initial symptoms. Seldom do any "early" symptoms occur. Peripheral lesions may grow silently to moderate size. Physical signs are those produced by bronchial obstruction, secondary pneumonitis, and consolidation.

**X-ray studies.** On a chest film, which is the first laboratory measure used in diagnosis after the history and physical, a small "coin" lesion in the peripheral lung may be picked up before symptoms develop, or an area of localized emphysema may indicate a tiny silent obstructing tumor that casts no shadow itself. Chest films can be used for screening large groups of healthy persons for lung cancer; Guiss estimates that about 70 possible curable tumors will result from x-ray films of 2 million chests. One third of "coin" lesions are "early" cancers. Most positive x-ray films reveal a hilar mass or a segmental pneumonitis or atelectasis, representing moderately advanced cancer.

**Cytology.** Cytology plays a large role in lung cancer diagnosis; five deep-cough sputum specimens collected and processed carefully will yield malignant or suggestive cells in 70% to 80% of lung cancers. This is as productive as one bronchial washing for cell study, twice as often positive as bronchial biopsy. As in other cancers, cytology leads us to proceed to formal biopsy, which has to be performed at bronchoscopy or at exploratory thoracotomy.

**Bronchoscopy.** The third step in the lung cancer work-up is bronchoscopy. It not only can secure a diagnosis by visualization and biopsy of the cancer in one of the main bronchi in 30% to 40% of cases, but it gives one a chance to obtain bronchial washings for cytologic study if the lesion cannot be seen. By bronchoscopy one can evaluate the patient for operability by obseravtion of cords, trachea, carina, etc.

**Biopsy.** Many chest surgeons advocate routine *scalene node* biopsy, even though nodes are not enlarged, to help estimate curability and to secure a tissue diagnosis when previous methods fail. Our clinic finds this a relatively unrewarding maneuver.

*Needle biopsy* through the chest can be done safely by experienced physicians and can yield a tissue diagnosis in large tumors.

**Thoracotomy.** Exploratory thoracotomy completes the sequence of diagnostic steps. We may be forced to this step if all other methods fail and suspicion of lung cancer is high. Thoracotomy may also be the only way to determine operability.

## Differential diagnosis

Distinctions among three classes of lesions need consideration here—primary infections versus secondary infections accompanying neoplasms, benign tumors versus malignant tumors, and metastatic neoplasms versus primary growths. Masses in the lung present many diagnostic possibilities. With the tremendous increase in lung cancers, differential diagnostic procedures in the lung are of increasing frequency and importance.

**Infections.** Infections that can mimic cancer comprise the usual list of common lung diseases—lung abscess, organizing pneumonia, tuberculosis, tuberculoma, silicosis, histoplasmosis, coccidiomycosis, and sarcoidosis. X-ray films, sputum examinations and cultures, and skin tests all help differentiate; often one must rely on educated guesses, the passage of time, and response to antibiotic therapy to distinguish infection from cancer.

**Benign tumors.** Tumorlike lesions and benign tumors occur in some variety in the lung: (1) hamartomas simulate peripheral silent cancers; they cast a well-defined, nonchanging, peripheral shadow, and show complex, unorganized tissues under the microscope; (2) cavernous vascular lesions (arteriovenous fistulas) are usually multiple and associated with compensatory polycythemia; (3) intrabronchial fibromas and chondromas are usually pedunculated; and (4) mesotheliomas of the pleura occur rarely.

**Metastases.** With a rich network of blood vessels in two separate circulations supplying the lung, it is small wonder that so many cancers growing elsewhere embolize to the lung. Cells stop and grow to form lung metastases largely because the lung capillaries of the pulmonary circuit constitute the first small vessel filtering bed for the systemic venous blood. Embolizing cells from cancers of the rectum, kidneys, testicles, ovaries, breast, and soft part sarcomas, as well as many others, frequently stop and grow in the lungs. As we would expect, they are usually multiple. Multiple tumor masses in the lungs must be considered metastatic rather than primary until proved otherwise. Primary lung cancer may metastasize via the rich peribronchial and peripulmonary vessel lymphatics to other sites in the lung, but does not do so very often. Breast cancer frequently reaches the lungs by way of the intercostal lymphatics that then travel along the substernal vein to the parietal pleura. In a few cases we can see at bronchoscopy a metastatic lesion obstructing a bronchus and then we can secure positive biopsy. Differential diagnostic examinations and procedures in other parts of the body to eliminate extrapulmonary primary neoplasms sometimes need to be thorough and extensive to determine whether a lesion is primary or metastatic. Here we rely heavily on gastrointestinal and genitourinary tract x-ray films.

**Lymphomas.** These tumors may arise primarily in lung parenchyma; they commonly occur in the mediastinal lymph nodes and thus can resemble lung cancer metastases to nodes on an x-ray film. These diseases are covered in Chapter 29.

## PREVENTIVE MEASURES

All studies point to the vital role of polluted air in the etiology of lung cancer, be it pollution from industrial wastes, transport vehicle exhausts, or tobacco smoke. Any burned, volatilized organic material may be a threat. The problem for preventive medicine appears obvious—cleaning our air constitutes a major health objective. Many maneuvers will help, not the least of which is eliminating or effectively filtering the chemical carcinogens from tobacco smoke. Possibly, also, we must actively teach young children never to smoke; such advice may have a greater effect the younger the child.

## TREATMENT PRINCIPLES

1. Surgery in the form of lobectomy, or sometimes pneumonectomy, plus regional node removal, constitutes the most reliable curative type of treatment.

2. Careful pulmonary function studies preoperatively ensure against our creating a pulmonary cripple by surgery.

3. Preoperative x-ray therapy—megavoltage—appears worthwhile.
4. Radiotherapy helps relieve symptoms of pain, infection, fever, and cough and may sometimes arrest lesions to prolong life.
5. Chemotherapy with nitrogen mustard or other drugs may palliate patients for short intervals.
6. X-ray therapy achieves some 5-year survivals in superior sulcus tumors and marked palliation of the superior vena caval syndrome.

## COMMON ERRORS

1. Misdiagnosis—false negative x-ray or sputum reports—allows unnecessary tumor progression before treatment.
2. Failure to carry out wide "radical" surgery, when the tumor is well differentiated and the patient is in good condition, may jeopardize survival.

## PROMISING DEVELOPMENTS FOR THE FUTURE

1. Cigarette smoke filters that remove carcinogens.
2. Strict industrial worker safeguards.
3. Automotive exhaust purifiers.
4. Replacement of coal- and oil-burning sources of energy with "clean air" sources.
5. Annual or semiannual health check-ups with chest films and sputum cytology, especially in high-risk individuals, will salvage some slow and moderate growth-rate cancer victims. The practicing physician would do well to insist on this regimen with all his male patients who smoke.

## PROGNOSIS

1. Although only 7% to 10% of all lung cancer patients live 5 years because of the large proportion of late diagnoses and aggressive, fast-spreading tumors, the survival rates of those patients who can be resected with cure in mind amounts to approximately one third. Lung cancer outlook is not good, but not hopeless.
2. Interestingly, the best prognosis obtains in a group who delayed in seeking medical attention the shortest time after symptoms and also in another group delaying the longest—a year or more. Evidently, a short delay helps treatment succeed in some tumors before they spread to incurable stages, whereas a long delay constitutes a selection process of the least biologically malignant neoplasms in which salvage is high with all sorts of irregular management.
3. Invasion of organs and tissues outside the lung proper nearly always constitutes a fatal sign.
4. Cancers confined to lung and intersegmental or interlobar nodes yield 40% 5-year survivals; mediastinal node metastases makes a big difference—the rate drops to 7%.
5. The average length of life amounts to 10 to 16 months; 85% of patients are dead within 2 years of diagnosis.
6. Prognosis for resectable tumors runs highest with squamous cancer—30% 5-year survivals. Resectable adenocarcinomas and resectable undifferentiated types permit 5-year survivals in 20% of patients.

**REFERENCES**

Ackerman, L. V., and del Regato, J. A.: Cancer, ed. 3, St. Louis, 1962, The C. V. Mosby Co., pp. 461-511.

Auerbach, O., Stout, A. P., Hammond, E. C., and Garfinkel, L.: Changes in bronchial epithelium in relation to cigarette smoking and in relation to lung cancer, New Eng. J. Med. **265:**253-267, 1961.

Auerbach, D., Stout, A. P., Hammond, E. C., and Garfinkel, L.: Bronchial epithelium in former smokers, New Eng. J. Med. **267:**119-125, 1962.

Bloedorn, F. G., and Cowley, R. A.: Irradiation and surgery in the treatment of bronchogenic carcinoma, Surg. Gynec. Obstet. **111:**141, 1960.

Extent of cancer illness in the United States, Public Health Service Pub. 547, U. S. Department of Health, Education and Welfare, Washington, D. C.

Fletcher, C. M.: Cigarette smoking and the prevention of lung cancer. In Wagner, G., editor: Proceedings of Symposium on Cancer Facts and Statistics (Krebs-Dokumentation und Statistik maligner Tumoren), Berlin, Oct., 1965, Stuttgart, 1966, F. K. Schattauer-Verlag, pp. 183-192.

Guiss, L. W.: Dividends and defects of the mass-survey method in detecting lung cancer, Ca. Bull. **4:**56, 1954.

James, A. G.: Cancer prognosis manual, New York, 1961, American Cancer Society, Inc.

Kotin, P., Mitchell, I. A., and Falk, H. I.: The role of polluted urban air and associated factors in the pathogenesis of respiratory tract cancer. In Wagner, G., editor: Proceedings of Symposium on Cancer Facts and Statistics (Krebs-Dokumentation und Statistik maligner Tumoren), Berlin, Oct., 1965, Stuttgart, 1966, F. K. Schattauer-Verlag, pp. 171-182.

Liebow, A. A.: Tumors of the lower respiratory tract. In Atlas of tumor pathology, Sect. V., Fasc. 17, Washington, D. C., 1952, Armed Forces Institute of Pathology.

Lombard, H. L., and Snegireff, L. S.: An epidemiological study of lung cancer, Cancer **12:**406, 1959.

Ochsner, A., Jr., and Ochsner, A.: Cancer of the lung: recognition and management, Surg. Clin. N. Amer. **46:**1411-1425, 1966.

Review of Bronchogenic Carcinoma, Acta Chir. Scand. **347** (supp.):6-42, 1965.

Rigler, L. G.: The natural history of lung cancer, In Ariel, I. M., editor: Progress in clinical cancer, vol. 1, New York, 1965, Grune & Stratton, Inc., pp. 571-594.

Smoking and Health. Public Health Service Pub. 1103, report of the Advisory Committee to the Surgeon General, Washington, D. C., 1964, U. S. Department of Health, Education and Welfare.

Wynder, E. L., and Hoffman, D.: Experimental aspects of tobacco carcinogenesis, Dis. Chest **44:**337-346, 1963.

Chapter 13

# Cancer of the esophagus

An organ like the esophagus, which only conducts and propels food along its stratified squamous epithelial lining, should develop cancers in the same general way and of the same types as we have seen in the mouth and throat with similar lining. And so it does. The basic neoplastic developmental and growth process is the same in both areas. Only the gross location differs to produce different symptoms and different problems of diagnosis and treatment.

## INCIDENCE AND DISTRIBUTION

This cancer comprises only 2% of all cancers and possesses roughly the same male to female ratio as in the upper digestive tract, 4:1. Pockets of unusually high incidence of esophageal cancer occur all over the world (at random)—in parts of South Africa, southern Russia, Honan Province of China, Puerto Rico, Japan, France, Finland, and in the Negro population of eastern South Carolina. For example, it occurs oftener in the indigent population of Louisville, Kentucky, than does stomach cancer. Many authors report an increasing incidence of this neoplasm in recent years.

## ETIOLOGY

### External initiating agents

As in the oral and laryngopharyngeal epithelium, *tobacco* and *alcohol* are highly suspect carcinogenic factors. Many dietary components also have come under suspicion regarding esophageal cancer—for example, smoked and spicy foods. The very spotty epidemiologic distribution suggests external factors rather than genetic or metabolic internal derangements. Interestingly, history of a *previous mouth* or *throat cancer* emerges in these patients far more frequently than chance would allow, pointing toward a common etiology for both mouth-throat and esophageal cancer. Auerbach and associates find possibly precancerous changes in the esophageal epithelium of smokers that are seldom present in nonsmokers, although such changes and differences are not as pronounced as in his similar study of bronchial mucosa.

The fact that most cancers occur at points of narrowing in the esophagus, namely, at the level of the bifurcation of the trachea (middle esophagus) and at the lower end where it enters the stomach, means that swallowed substances could maintain more prolonged contact at these sites. Chronic irritation may similarly be concentrated there. A higher incidence of cancer in abnormally strictured areas of the esophagus reinforces the concept that stasis helps cancer develop.

### Predisposing factors

Deficiencies in vitamins and other essential food constituents probably contribute, since cancer in the cervical esophagus arises so commonly in Swedish women with an iron and vitamin deficiency syndrome (Plummer-Vinson syndrome). As we have mentioned before, *dietary deficiency* is linked so closely with overuse of alcohol, *liver disease,* and heavy smoking that the four have been hard to separate for accurate analysis; all four associate statistically with cancer of the esophagus and probably predispose to it.

## PATHOLOGY

Nearly all the cancers are squamous or epidermoid; some may be differentiated squamous cancers, but most are relatively anaplastic. Adenocarcinomas account for only 10%, usually arising from the cardia of the stomach and invading the esophagus, or else coming from misplaced gastric mucosa at the lower end of the esophagus. Rarely a true adenocarcinoma develops from "cardiac glands" that may lie at any part of the esophageal lining.

Located most often in the middle third, next most frequently in the lower third of the organ, esophageal cancers grow as ulcerating, infiltrating, or proliferating masses that quickly penetrate all muscular layers of the thin esophageal wall with varying degrees of fibroplastic reaction and surrounding inflammation. Obstruction to passage of food occurs in 90% of these tumors and causes the first symptoms. Tumors seed themselves submucosally by the rich intramural lymphatic network to such an extent that surgeons have come to regard the whole length of the esophagus as potentially cancer-involved when the tumor is 5 cm. or more in diameter. Lymph node metastasis occurs commonly, long before blood-borne distant spread, to nodal groups at the hilar and subcarinal areas, then in one half of cases downward to the subdiaphragmatic nodes around the origin of the left gastric artery. Direct invasion of contiguous structures develops soon because of the lack of an outer serosal coat on the esophagus, so that aortic wall, left mainstem bronchus, trachea, left recurrent laryngeal nerve, pleura, phrenic nerve, and pericardium often become involved. Upper third and cervical esophageal tumors spread to supraclavicular, paratracheal nodes and can invade the carotid sheath and other adjacent structures.

We seldom can find evidence for the multicentric origin of esophageal cancer; also we cannot very well correlate the degree of differentiation of the cancer with the extent of spread. So rapid is the downhill course once esophageal stenosis occurs that 30% to 40% of patients have no lymph node metastases at death.

### Precancerous lesions

Although leukoplakia often occurs in the esophagus, its incidence and proximity to cancer do not connect well in studies (mainly autopsies) that are available at present. The inaccessibility of the organ and the large size of the cancers when recognized probably obscure most precancerous changes. We find carcinoma in situ at the edges of invasive cancers on occasion.

## NATURAL HISTORY

The garden variety of esophageal cancer grows at a moderately fast rate. A male smoker-drinker of about 55 years of age typically first experiences a few episodes where food sticks in his throat or midchest area when eating a heavy meal with large chunks of meat. He finally washes down the food or vomits and forgets the incident. But then solid food hesitates regularly in passage, and slight discomfort occurs on swallowing, which comes from esophageal spasm. After 4 to 5 months of insidiously increasing dysphagia he begins living on liquids and rapidly loses weight. After a few more months liquids will not go down except with great effort and he begins to spit out his accumulating saliva. He becomes thin, emaciated, weak, and hungry and has pain on swallowing. Only a small nasogastric feeding tube or a feeding gastrostomy will now prevent him from dying of dehydration. Even with restored feedings, inanition and terminal pneumonia overtake him from aspiration of the saliva he cannot swallow. Shortly before death, he may develop a productive cough from tumor erosion into the left mainstem bronchus or trachea with a tracheoesophageal fistula, which leads to pneumonia. Hoarseness may indicate recurrent nerve involvement. Patients seldom live long enough to experience symptoms from distant metastases to lungs and liver.

## DIAGNOSIS

**History.** Dysphagia always means esophageal cancer until proved otherwise, just as hoarseness of the voice should suggest laryngeal cancer. Dysphagia is really the only symptom of cancer of the esophagus, coming on gradually as described above. Occasionally a patient feels substernal fullness or a pressing pain from esophageal spasm. Since a 3 mm. opening will allow most food to pass on through the esophagus, the degree of circumferential invasion and stenosis, or the total bulk of the tumor mass, must be considerable before any swallowing difficulty at all occurs. Whereas dysphagia constitutes a late symptom usually, cough, hoarseness, and extreme weight loss occur even later in the course of the disease. Signs of esophageal cancer are absent unless advanced cancer causes palpable cervical nodes, drooling, emaciation, or dehydration.

**X-ray studies.** Nearly all diagnoses result from the *barium swallow* x-ray studies, which can pinpoint the level of obstruction and describe characteristic deformities caused by the cancer.

**Esophagoscopy.** Then esophagoscopy must be done to secure a confirming biopsy, which succeeds in 85% of cases. A few patients need repeat attempts and gentle dilatations, even at the risk of perforation, to visualize pure tumor for biopsy.

**Cytology.** Cytology on esophageal washings, taken either from a nasogastric tube passed to the point of obstruction or to the cardiac end of the esophagus, or taken at esophagoscopy, has proved a valuable adjunct to diagnosis. It yields accurate reports in 90% of instances.

**Additional studies.** *Bronchoscopy* and *laryngoscopy* also produce needed information about the extent of cancer involvement, such as bronchial invasion or cord paralysis.

### Differential diagnosis

Nine of ten tumorous lesions of the esophagus are cancer. The others make up an assortment of uncommon conditions:

*Achalasia* produces symptoms similar to cancer but involves younger ages, is always the terminal esophagus, and has a somewhat different x-ray picture. Similarly differentiated from cancer is *peptic esophagitis* with *hiatus hernia.* We depend upon careful x-ray study and esophagoscopy for delineation.

*Cysts*—bronchial cysts or cystic duplication of the esophagus can occur. Gastric gland cysts develop at the lower end.

*Benign tumors* arise rarely in the esophageal muscle wall, but are principally leiomyomas, which may be polypoid. Benign fibrovascular polyps may also develop, but even more rarely. Fibromas, angiomas, etc. occur. These unusual neoplasms all tend to cluster at the two narrow points in the lumen, as do the cancers.

*Diverticula,* either pharyngeal or at the midesophagus, can be distinguished, since they fill with barium.

*Chest tumors extrinsic* to the esophagus may compress the organ and produce luminal narrowing, such as intrathoracic goiter, mediastinal lymphoma, or aortic aneurysms. Signs unrelated to esophageal cancer will point to these conditions.

*Strictures* of the esophagus can mimic cancer. A history of lye ingestion, negative biopsies and cytology, plus careful x-ray study help to clarify the diagnosis.

## PREVENTIVE MEASURES

Esophageal cancer occurs infrequently in most locales, and conviction about etiology is too spotty for us to advocate elimination of possible external initiating agents (tobacco and alcohol). However, its occurrence constitutes another piece of evidence favoring the importance of balanced, vitamin-adequate dietary intake because this cancer obviously has intimate connections with diet.

## TREATMENT PRINCIPLES

1. Only 10% to 15% of patients exhibit potentially curable lesions on diagnosis; for these may experts now favor preoperative megavoltage x-ray followed in 4 to 6 weeks by surgical resection of the esophagus and reconstruction of a swallowing passage with stomach or a segment of colon.

2. A number of palliative measures relieve symptoms and delay starvation but do not significantly prolong life: (a) x-ray therapy, (b) nasogastric feeding tube passed through the tumor when possible, (c) a feeding gastrostomy, and (d) bypass operation with mobilized stomach or colon.

3. Dilatations of the tumor site and prosthetic devices passed through the tumor to establish a passage help only the occasional patient.

4. Chemotherapy offers little or nothing.
5. The occasional tumor of the cervical esophagus demands extensive surgery, often including laryngectomy and neck dissection after preoperative irradiation.

## COMMON ERRORS

1. Many errors can occur in diagnostic procedures, of course. Failure to esophagoscope all patients with dysphagia, false confidence that temporary subsidence of dysphagia means benign disease, reliance on a false negative biopsy report, or failure to utilize fully modern cytologic techniques on esophageal washings, all may delay diagnosis and prolong suffering.
2. Failure to pursue vigorously curative x-ray therapy and surgery in the more favorable cervical and lower segment cancers may deny salvage to an occasional patient.
3. Esophageal perforation often occurs at esophagoscopy because cancer has destroyed the esophageal wall—more a complication of diagnosis than an error.

## PROMISING DEVELOPMENTS FOR THE FUTURE

Identification of etiologic factors and prevention of esophageal cancer seems our only hope in this neoplastically dismal segment of the anatomy. Preoperative irradiation is being widely employed more and more with increasing resectability rates, and many surgical specimens now show sterilization of the cancers. This may improve results. At the present time we cannot evaluate this improvement.

## PROGNOSIS

Prognosis relates to location of the cancer in the esophagus more than to other factors because incurability results from involvement of irremovable vital structures. Most cancers develop in the middle segment of the esophagus adjacent to the trachea, major bronchi, and aorta; here salvage approximates zero. Ten percent to 20% of patients with cancers located in the neck survive 5 years and 20% to 30% of those with lower segment tumors survive. However, overall esophageal cancer salvage runs only 5% to 10% at best. Life expectancy from first symptom averages 9 months without treatment; one quarter will live slightly more than 1 year. Palliative treatment may extend life 4 to 6 months in some cases.

### REFERENCES

Ackerman, L. V., and del Regato, J. A.: Cancer, ed. 3, St. Louis, 1962, The C. V. Mosby Co., pp. 553-578.

Auerbach, O., Stout, A. P., Hammond, E. C., and Garfinkel, L.: Histologic changes in the esophagus in relation to smoking habits, Arch. Environ. Health **11:**4-15, 1965.

Burge, J. P., and Ochsner, J. S.: Management of esophageal tumors, Surg. Clin. N. Amer. **46:**1457-1467, 1966.

Parker, E. F., and Gregorie, H. B., Jr.: Carcinoma of the esophagus, Curr. Probl. Surg., April, 1967.

Prolla, J. C., Taebel, D. W., and Kirsner, J. B.: Current status of exfoliative cytology in diagnosis of malignant neoplasms of the esophagus, Surg. Gynec. Obstet. **121:**743-752, 1965.

Raphael, H. A., Ellis, H. F., and Dockerty, M. B.: Primary adenocarcinoma of the esophagus, Ann. Surg. **164:**785-796, 1966.

Sherman, C. D.: The surgical treatment of cancer of the esophagus. In Ariel, I. M., editor: Progress in clinical cancer, New York, 1965, Grune & Stratton, Inc., pp. 605-619.

Stout, A. P., and Lattes, R.: Tumors of the esophagus. In Atlas of tumor pathology, Sect. V, Fasc. 20., Washington, D. C., 1957, Armed Forces Institute of Pathology.

Chapter 14

# Cancer of the stomach

In our progress down the digestive tract we now reach an organ in which the lining tissue abruptly changes from relatively inactive squamous epithelium of the structures above to a digestive mucosa. Gastric mucosa actively secretes acid, pepsin, but mainly mucus, as well as at least one hormone; it also absorbs. Its tumors likewise become different in a number of respects; the commonest adenocarcinoma shows a general biologic pattern that will be repeated throughout the rest of the intestinal tract.

## INCIDENCE AND DISTRIBUTION

The only change in incidence of a cancer as dramatic as the recent rise in lung cancer is the dramatic fall in cancer of the stomach among Caucasians. Current incidence rates amount to one half of those 30 years ago for both males and females. The decline may be more apparent than real (Barclay), but most authorities accept it as real. We cannot account for this marked reduction, but certainly the meager recent improvement in diagnosis and treatment cannot be given the credit. As of the year 1967, 4% to 5% of all cancers in the United States occurred in the stomach. Men fall victim twice as often as women.

Stomach cancer is still the commonest male cancer in Japan, Finland, Chile, Austria, Iceland, and many parts of the Soviet Union in contrast to its relatively low rate in the United States, Australia, and Canada. Over half of the male cancer deaths in Japan result from gastric cancer. Most countries with a high incidence show a high frequency of cancer of the esophagus also.

## ETIOLOGY

### External initiating agents

Cancers of the stomach do not correlate closely with tobacco and alcohol usage. The feeding of carcinogenic polycyclic hydrocarbons produces stomach cancer in mice and rats (and cancers in other organs too), but the only definitive human studies involving external carcinogens consist in the finding of benzpyrene in the smoked fish that Icelanders consume in such quantity. Evidence for an external carcinogen is mainly epidemiologic; a dietary factor best accounts for the trends and distribution of stomach cancer. Haenszel lists the following possibilities: (1) a natural carcinogen in food, (2) a carcinogen introduced in the preparation of food, and (3) the absence of some protective factor in food.

### Predisposing factors

A great deal of work has been done that has unearthed a number of factors associated with higher gastric cancer occurrence: (1) *group A blood* correlates significantly with this cancer; (2) a strong *family history* increases the risk; (3) *achlorhydria* similarly raises the chance that a person will develop stomach cancer; and (4) *intrinsic factor deficiency,* linked to pernicious anemia and also associated with chronic gastritis and achlorhydria, predisposes to gastric cancer. (See also precancerous lesions.)

## PATHOLOGY

**Adenocarcinomas.** Ninety-five percent of stomach cancers are adenocarcinomas; some cancers are well differentiated but most are poorly differentiated or anaplastic. They arise from the common mucosal cell, the mucus-producing cell, and at least a trace of mucin may be seen in all adenocarcinomas from the colloid to the scirrhus types. They grow in five different gross patterns that relate importantly to prognosis: (1) the *superficial spreading*—uncommon, extensive, least aggressive, (2) the *ulcerating infiltrative*—commonest of all, usually in the distal part of the stomach and at the lesser curvature, (3) the *polypoid*—uncommon, well circumscribed, late to metastasize, and relatively curable, (4) the *diffuse* ("linitis plastica")—10% of all stomach cancers with an insidious submucosal and intramuscular spreading pattern that converts the whole stomach into a stiff leatherlike reservoir, seldom cured, and (5) *carcinoma arising in a gastric ulcer*—a type that develops occasionally at an ulcer edge.

Degrees of histologic differentiation of these cancers correlate inversely with lymphatic spread and thus with prognosis. Most cancers arise in the antrum and lesser curvature, but a few occur in the fundus and at the greater curvature.

Spread of the superficial and the diffuse types occurs via intramural lymphatics, as in the esophagus, and the occasional cancers of the cardia penetrate the esophagus to cause obstruction. Direct penetration through the muscular wall takes place in the common infiltrative type to involve the serosa and contiguous organs (liver, pancreas, spleen, transverse colon), or to cause peritoneal seeding. The "colloid," mucus-producing type sometimes seeds transperitoneally to both ovaries, giving the "Krukenberg tumor" syndrome (Chapter 21).

Lymphatic metastases develop early and often to the following groups of regional nodes on all sides of the stomach: (1) the proximal gastric segment involves first the fundal, superior pancreaticosplenic and greater curvature nodes; (2) the middle segment involves mainly the fundal, superior lesser curvature nodes and infrapyloric and retropyloric nodes; (3) cancers of the lower segment embolize mainly to the peripyloric and lesser curvature groups of nodes (Fig. 10). Size and location of the primary does not affect the degree of nodal involvement; 60% to 70% of resected stomachs show nodal spread. Blood-borne distant metastases develop late in liver, lungs, and bones.

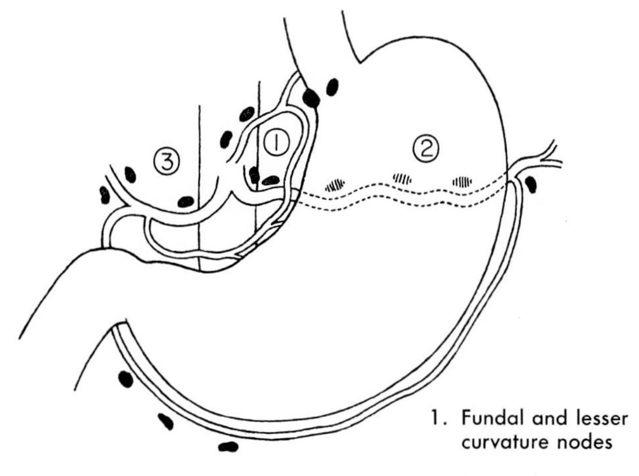


**Fig. 10.** Locations of principal lymph nodes through which lymphatics draining the stomach pass. (Modified from Ackerman, L. V., and del Regato, J. A.: Cancer, ed. 3, St. Louis, 1962, The C. V. Mosby Co.)

**Other gastric neoplasms.** The remaining 5% of malignant gastric neoplasms consist principally of two kinds. (1) *Lymphomas* (any one of the main types, except Hodgkin's disease) may arise de novo as a localized initial growth from the lymphoid elements in the stomach wall, or they may appear in the stomach as a secondary manifestation of systemic disease. These tumors may grow as a soft projecting mass, a disklike whitish plaque on the mucosa, or a diffuse proliferation making giant rugae. (2) *Leiomyomas or leiomyosarcomas* are silent, slow-growing muscle tumors that tend to attain great bulk, ulcerate centrally, and may bleed profusely but carry a fairly good prognosis.

## Precancerous lesions

*Chronic gastritis* and *intestinal metaplasia* of the mucosa occur so commonly with cancer, as does epithelial hyperplasia, that suspicion of an etiologic relationship naturally arises. Achlorhydria is also a concomitant of these processes.

*Pernicious anemia* will give rise to stomach cancer in 10% of the cases. It features atrophic mucosal changes, intrinsic factor deficiency, macrocytic anemia, and achlorhydria.

*Gastric polyps* (adenomatous polyps) develop infrequently in the stomach as compared to the colon, but 5% to 10% of stomachs will show cancer when they are single, and 15% to 30% will develop cancer when polyps are multiple. Polyps smaller than 2 cm. are generally benign, but those larger are often malignant. Here, too, a link may exist with polyps, atrophic gastritis, and achlorhydria. Rather than become embroiled in inconclusive controversy over the malignant potential of a polyp, the reader would profit more from considering that polyps and cancer probably arise from the same basic causative complex, whatever that may be. The rare villous adenoma in the stomach carries a high cancer potential, as it does in the rectum.

*Gastric ulcer* develops a cancer in its edge to account perhaps for one out of every twenty stomach cancers. Gastric ulcer and cancer may occur together. Mason states that stomachs liable to gastric ulcer are also liable to gastric cancer.

## NATURAL HISTORY

Gastric cancer grows at a moderate rate, and silently reaches 5 cm. or larger in size without interfering with the function of this large distensible organ. After 4 to 6 months of gross enlargement, vague symptoms begin, such as weight loss, fatigability, anorexia, and epigastric uneasiness. By this time the tumor has metastasized to regional lymph nodes at the various peripheries of the stomach in half of the cases, or perhaps a tumor at the pylorus or cardia will begin to obstruct at a smaller size with consequent pain and vomiting. Further progression leads to emaciation, anemia, epigastric pain after eating, and a palpable upper abdominal mass representing the primary tumor, or liver or omental metastasis. Occasionally extensive peritoneal seeding produces a "shelf" of tumor felt rectally in the cul-de-sac of the peritoneum. Lung metastases may develop, as well as a supraclavicular nodal mass. Pulmonary embolism causes death in many terminal patients because of the blood clotting disturbance that often accompanies abdominal carcinomatosis. The liver shows metastases in 70% at death, the peritoneum in 40%, and the lungs in 30% of the cases. Two years after first symptoms 80% to 90% of patients will be dead.

## DIAGNOSIS

**History.** Early symptoms seldom appear in cancer of the stomach; most tumors are silent until sizable. One patient in ten, however, will have had ulcerlike pain relieved by antacids much of his adult life; then he will note a change in the symptoms as the first indication of cancer. Occasionally the cancer itself causes symptoms suggesting peptic ulcer from the first. Usually the patient notes symptoms only of a moderately advanced neoplasm, such as weight loss, distaste for food, especially meat, epigastric distress after meals, or vomiting from an obstructing mass. Any vague change in digestive pattern deserves investigation. *Signs* of gastric cancer are those produced by advanced disease such as a palpable epigastric tumor, a fluid wave, jaundice, and a left supraclavicular metastasis. Seldom do gastric cancers bleed in large amounts.

**X-ray studies.** The main technique we rely on for diagnosis is x-ray study (gastrointestinal barium series) of the stomach. It maintains a 90% accuracy rate in pinpointing frankly cancerous or highly suspicious abnormalities. No method substitutes for the absolute proof of a biopsy, but x-ray film approximates definite diagnosis in most stomach lesions. Gastric ulcers give x-ray diagnosticians some trouble; 10% to 20% that appear benign turn out to be malignant. X-ray study has been disappointing as a screening method for stomach cancer.

**Cytology.** Gastric cytology has now developed to a point at which, with a careful technique of stomach irrigation without mucus-digesting enzymes, cancer cells can usually be found and a definitive diagnosis made as often as with x-ray

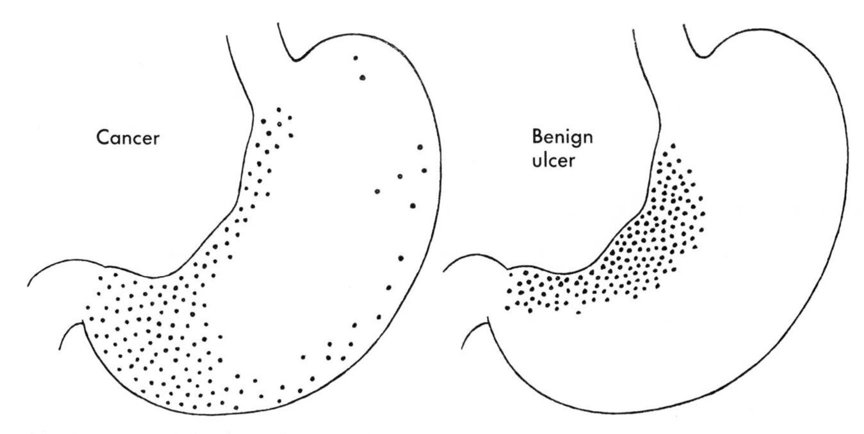


**Fig. 11.** Cancer and benign ulcer of the stomach do not differ very much in their general anatomic locations within the organ. (Modified from Stout, A. P.: Bull. N. Y. Acad. Med. **23:**106, 1947.)

films. Cytology fails when lesions do not exfoliate cells, as in lymphomas and leiomyosarcomas, but exceeds the accuracy of x-ray films in recurrent cancer, in lesions of the cardia, and in equivocal gastric ulcers. This method yields only a rare false positive report.

**Laboratory studies.** Laboratory studies contribute suggestive or supporting evidence for cancer. *Achlorhydria* after histamine occurs in 70% of gastric cancers, but this obtains in some healthy persons over the age of 55 also. Macrocytic anemia that is refractive suggests gastric cancer. *Occult blood in the stool* also alerts us to a cancer somewhere in the gastrointestinal tract. Other less localizing changes may be found with gastric cancer—elevation of serum bilirubin and mean red cell corpuscular volume, and depression of serum proteins and plasma prothrombin levels.

**Biopsy.** *Laparotomy* and biopsy must be done in many cases to make a diagnosis or to verify an x-ray opinion. A portion of an extragastric mass such as a hard regional lymph node is easiest to secure. If a gastrotomy opening becomes necessary, several biopsies from inside the stomach ensure diagnosis of the true lesion. A small doubtful ulcer needs complete excision and frozen section study.

**Miscellaneous studies.** *Gastroscopy* with the new Fiberoptic gastroscope often yields helpful information for the clinician, but it is seldom the decisive diagnostic tool.

*Peritoneoscopy* helps some clinicians avoid laparotomy by discovering conclusive evidence of incurability in the form of peritoneal implants or liver metastases.

## Differential diagnosis

In addition to the confusion aroused by gastric polypoid lesions and gastric ulcers, a number of other pathologic conditions must be distinguished from cancer by characteristic symptoms and x-ray findings. *Prolapse* of gastric *mucosa* through the pyloric ring, *pyloric hypertrophy, pylorospasm, achalasia, foreign bodies* (phyto- and trichobezoars), and *extrinsic tumor masses* pressing on the stomach, all have their distinctive findings to help the clinician decide about further diagnostic efforts. Giant gastric rugae may appear with hypertrophic gastritis or with lymphoma. Rare benign neoplasms may give trouble, such as *leiomyomas,* a carcinoid tumor, or eosinophilic granuloma. As mentioned above, villous adenomas are equivalent to low-grade cancers.

## PREVENTIVE MEASURES

Only the identification and elimination of essential extrinsic carcinogens for stomach cancer can conceivably prevent the disease from occurring. It is vitally important for us to find whatever change in our habits (probably dietary habits) has caused this cancer to decrease in incidence. If we do not know what the beneficial change is, we may reverse it in our ignorance, and cause the cancer to increase again.

## TREATMENT PRINCIPLES

1. *Surgery* constitutes the only curative treatment at present. This usually implies a subtotal gastrectomy, since most cancers arise in the distal part, but a total gastrectomy may be needed at times. Complete removal of adjacent lymph node groups pays dividends because 10% of theoretically curable patients with positive nodes survive 5 years. The additional excision of omentum and spleen is common practice. Extirpation of the distal pancreas and transverse colon when these structures are directly invaded also benefits some patients.
2. *X-ray therapy* does not cure gastric cancer; it seldom even palliates the primary tumor because of its location, but it may relieve symptoms from isolated metastases. Lymphomas comprise a special exception to this rule. If a gastric lymphosarcoma seems the only focus in the body, surgical removal followed by irradiation should be used. If it is one of several foci—generalized disease—x-ray therapy alone may be best. Leiomyosarcoma responds only to surgery.
3. A gastric ulcer generally needs a surgical procedure if it fails to heal with subsidence of symptoms after 3 to 6 weeks of strict medical management in the hospital.
4. Stomach polyps less than 2 cm. in diameter may be observed; if larger or multiple, the risk of cancer rises and requires prompt surgical attention.
5. A careful search for evidence of incurability should always precede surgery to spare the hopeless patient an operation. A purely palliative resection helps only the patient with obstruction or one with the rare severe hemorrhage.
6. Chemotherapy with 5-fluorouracil or methotrexate may relieve symptoms for short intervals but is generally without benefit. Regional infusion of these drugs via the hepatic artery palliates a few patients with liver metastases.

## COMMON ERRORS

1. Physicians who have never seen stomach cancer cured may make the mistake of giving up as soon as the diagnosis is made. Others may persist in unsuccessful medical management of gastric ulcer for many months because they believe that the patient is inevitably doomed if the ulcer proves to be malignant. Fair numbers of 5-year survivals reported from the best clinics give the lie to

these attitudes. Differences in survival between rural community hospitals and large urban clinics exist; they depend on the diagnostic acumen of the primary physician who finds the curable lesion, not so much on the skill of the surgeon.

2. Another frequent error lies in assuming that long-standing symptoms mean incurable cancer. They can mean the opposite; biologically slow-progressing tumors produce a long period of symptomatology without spreading beyond hope of cure. Conversely, a short symptomatic period may correlate with a fast-growing, aggressive tumor.

3. Finally, the physician needs always to remember that a bulky tumor may represent the 5% that are leiomyosarcomas or lymphomas, where therapy is always rewarding, rather than representing an incurably large adenocarcinoma.

## PROMISING DEVELOPMENTS FOR THE FUTURE

*Enzymatic differences* between the normal and precancerous stomach may eventually lead to successful screening tests for gastric cancer. Promising alterations have been found in the lactic dehydrogenase in the gastric juice of normal and abnormal stomachs, and in the aminopeptidase content of normal mucosa versus mucosa undergoing intestinal metaplasia.

## PROGNOSIS

Because of its inaccessibility and relative lack of sensitivity to minor stimuli, the stomach tolerates the ravages of cancer to an advanced degree before demanding attention. Most patients are incurable when first seen; even though a majority of them can be resected, most resections are palliative only. Including all patients, only 7% survive 5 years.

Five-year survivals when the cancer has not penetrated all layers, or when nodes are negative, approximate survivals in other organs—35% to 40%. The presence of metastases in nodes alone cuts survival rates to one third of this—12%. Therefore, in the stomach we are dealing with cancer that behaves very much as cancer in other locations, spreading mainly by direct infiltration and lymphatic emboli. Curability remains dependent upon the local extent of the primary and the presence or absence of nodal metastasis. As we would expect, also, the more anaplastic the tumor the worse the outlook. Patients with ulcerlike symptoms from their cancers have a better than average prognosis.

### REFERENCES

Ackerman, L. V., and del Regato, J. A.: Cancer, ed. 3, St. Louis, 1962, The C. V. Mosby Co., pp. 579-626.

Barclay, T. H. C.: The current status of cancer of the stomach in Saskatchewan, Canada, Prog. Clin. Cancer **2:**209-221, 1966.

Eisenberg, M. M., and Woodward, E. R.: Gastric cancer: a midcentury look, Arch. Surg. **87:**810-824, 1963.

Haenzel, W.: Variation in incidence of and mortality from stomach cancer, with particular reference to the United States, J. Nat. Cancer Inst. **21:**213, 1958.

Harkins, H. N.: Stomach and duodenum. In Harkins, H. N., Moyer, C. A., Rhoads, J. E., and Allen, J. G., editors: Surgery, principles and practice, ed. 2, Philadelphia, 1961, J. B. Lippincott Co., pp. 687-695.

Hoerr, S. O., Hazard, J. B., and Bailey, D.: Prognosis in carcinoma of the stomach in relation to microscopic type, Surg. Gynec. Obstet. **122:**485-494, 1966.
Hoerr, S. O., and Hodgman, R. W.: Carcinoma of the stomach, Amer. J. Surg. **107:**620-636, 1964.
James, A. G.: Cancer prognosis manual, New York, 1961, Amer. Cancer Society, Inc.
Lumpkin, W. M., Crow, R. L., Jr., Hernandez, C. M., and Cohn, I., Jr.: Carcinoma of the stomach, Ann. Surg. **159:**919-931, 1964.
Marshak, R. H., and Feldman, F.: Gastric polyps, Amer. J. Dig. Dis. **10:**909-931, 1965.
Mason, M. K.: Surface carcinoma of the stomach, Gut **6:**185-193, 1965.
McNeer, G.: The stomach, In Nealon, T. F., Jr., editor: Management of the patient with cancer, Philadelphia, 1966, W. B. Saunders Co., pp. 561-603.
Pack, G. T.: Tumors of the stomach, Texas J. Med. **61:**811-816, 1965.
Stout, A. P.: Tumors of the stomach. In Atlas of tumor pathology, Sect. VI, Fasc. 21., Washington, D. C., 1953, Armed Forces Institute of Pathology.
Taebel, W., Prolla, J. C., and Kirsner, J. B.: Exfoliative cytology in the diagnosis of stomach cancer, Ann. Intern. Med. **63:**1018-1026, 1965.

Chapter 15

# Cancer of the small intestine

The small intestine comprises 85% of the lining area of the entire gut, but strangely develops only 2% to 3% of the gastrointestinal neoplasms. Relative mobility of the food column in the small intestine compared to the relative stasis that obtains in the stomach and colon seems to us the significant physiologic difference that may explain this disparity of tumor incidence (see Etiology). Types of tumors exhibit more diversity than those in the stomach; the otherwise rare carcinoids emerge as relatively common in the distal small gut and appendix. Small bowel tumors provide an interesting study in comparative neoplasia.

## INCIDENCE AND DISTRIBUTION

Small bowel neoplasms are so uncommon that they can only be counted as a proportion of all gastrointestinal tumors—approximately 2% to 3%. Rochlin and Longmire found only 650 cases in reviewing 40 years of cancer publications. They occur more or less equally in men and women and show no racial predilection. The disparity in incidence between small bowel and stomach-colon cancers applies only to adenocarcinomas and carcinoids; the sarcomas of nonepithelial origin occur here with about the same frequency as in the stomach.

## ETIOLOGY

### External initiating agents

There is every reason to suspect chemical carcinogens of being active in the causative mechanism of small bowel tumors, since they seem to be in some higher areas of the digestive tract. In addition to ingested foodstuffs, various substances excreted by the liver in the bile impinge on the intestinal mucosa. Some studies suggest that bile contains carcinogenic chemicals, but their specific nature is still obscure. We may surmise that whatever the substances are, they simply have less time to impinge on the mucosal cell in the extremely mobile small bowel than in the other parts of the tract. The food solution also exists in a more dilute form in the small intestines. Dosage of carcinogens delivered to the cell depends somewhat on the length of time a solution has contact with mucosa. We have already seen the importance of "mucus reservoirs" in relation to mouth and throat cancers and of areas of narrowing in the esophagus related to the location of its tumors. In a similar way the concept of relative mobility or stasis of food solutions fits very well with tumor distribution in the various segments of the lower digestive tract.

### Predisposing factors

None are known.

## PATHOLOGY

With increasing variety of function of normal cells, tumors from these cells also increase in variety. The small bowel, a most active secreting and absorbing organ, exhibits four main types of cancer:

1. *Adenocarcinomas*—50% of the group. This is the same garden variety of cancer of mucus-producing cells found in the stomach and colon. Duodenal cancers are nearly all adenocarcinomas. Some adenocarcinomas develop in the jejunum as well, but a few develop in the ileum. Generally they constrict, stenose, and so obstruct the lumen of the bowel, metastasize to regional nodes in the mesentery, and penetrate the gut wall to involve adjacent organs. They may embolize via the portal vein system to the liver.

2. *Carcinoid tumors*—15% of the group. These tumors constitute a unique type of low-grade malignant tumor, often multiple, arising from the argentaffin, Kultschitsky, cells of the small bowel mucosa. The firm, yellow, submucosal growths may produce serotonin and occur most often in the appendix and occasionally in the ileum. They grow very slowly, metastasize to regional nodes, and

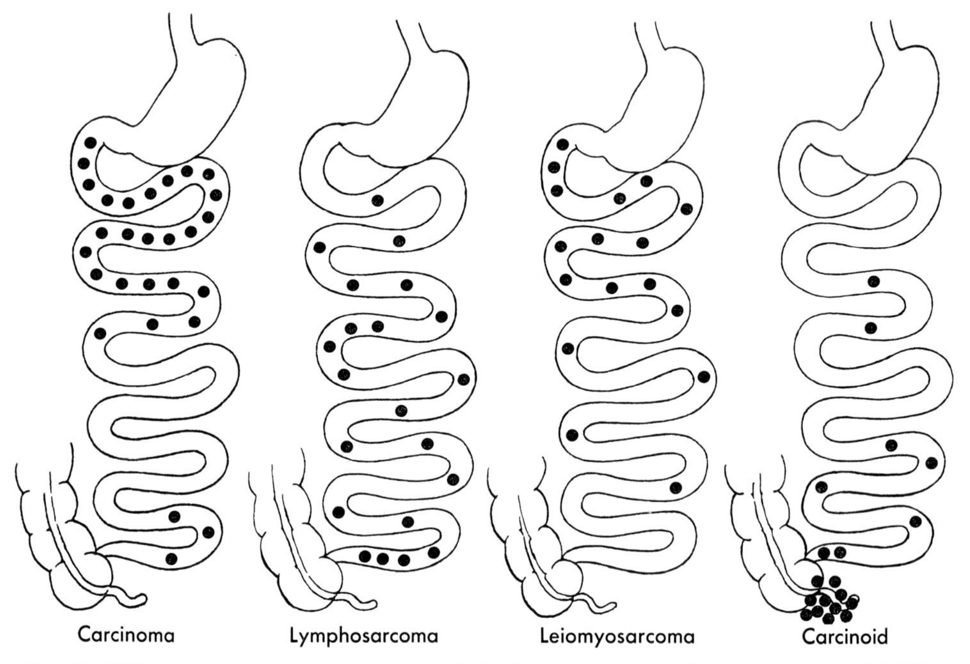


**Fig. 12.** Different anatomic concentrations of the four types of small bowel tumors. (Modified from McPeak, C. J.: In Nealon, T. F., Jr., editor: Management of the patient with cancer, Philadelphia, 1965, W. B. Saunders Co.)

may produce symptoms after many years of development. One in ten will cause a carcinoid syndrome from extensive functioning liver metastases. Histologically, similar tumors arise in the bronchi, pancreas, testicle, and ovary.

3. *Lymphomas*—15% of the group. As in the stomach, lymphocytic lymphoma (lymphosarcoma) and the reticulum cell sarcoma group may develop from intramural lymphoid collections in jejunum and ileum, producing tumors that obstruct the lumen and produce the typical symptoms of pain, nausea, and vomiting.

4. *Leiomyosarcomas*—10% of the group. These tumors develop in all three segments of the small bowel (duodenum, jejunum, and ileum) from smooth muscle about as often as they do in the stomach. They usually bleed profusely, seldom involve nodes, grow slowly, and metastasize late to liver and lungs.

Benign tumors occasionally originate in the small bowel and are mainly of two types—adenomatous polyps and benign leiomyomas. Hemangiomas, lipomas, or neurofibromas rarely develop.

The appendix rarely exhibits a neoplasm. When it does so, the type is usually that of a carcinoid, which occurs here more frequently than in the entire small bowel. Mucoceles of the appendix may sometimes rupture or may be ruptured, resulting in an essentially malignant syndrome from the seeding of myxoid material throughout the peritoneal cavity—the troublesome condition called *pseudomyxoma peritonei.*

### Precancerous lesions

The malignant potential of an adenomatous polyp anywhere in the gastrointestinal tract engenders much argument. Certainly the rare small bowel polyps over 2 cm. in size or the sessile ones deserve suspicion of being precancerous or frankly malignant. They are probably best considered a result of the same basic abnormal conditions that produce cancers such as those in the stomach.

## NATURAL HISTORY

Abdominal symptoms of several different kinds begin the clinical course in these various tumor types. With adenocarcinoma the patient first feels crampy pain after meals, then distention and vomiting, all the signs of intestinal obstruction; this may proceed to perforation and to peritonitis and death, if untreated. Carcinoids grow silently and metastasize to regional nodes years before symptoms occur. Some are found incidentally on x-ray study. They may occasionally enlarge enough to obstruct the gut, although the great distensibility of the distal small bowel means that a circumscribed, noninfiltrative tumor like this must attain considerable size before obstructing. The carcinoid syndrome from excess circulating serotonin (flushing, cyanosis, diarrhea, weakness, etc.) occurs only rarely when the tumor has been spreading for some years and liver metastases themselves secrete large amounts of serotonin. Carcinoids eventually cause death after prolonged enlargement in numerous abdominal sites.

Leiomyosarcomas grow slower than carcinomas and show the same tendency to bleed as their stomach counterparts. In fact, all of these four types bleed in half of the instances, resulting in anemia, occult blood in the stools, or melena.

These sarcomas bulge away from the lumen at first but may also obstruct. Death results from the complications of obstruction or bleeding.

Lymphomas can cause all of the clinical signs mentioned above, but death usually ensues from generalized lymphomatous disease and emaciation from large multiple foci of catabolically active tumor.

## DIAGNOSIS

**History.** Symptoms and signs develop late in the course of these neoplasms and are not specific, as shown by the fact that only 20% of cases are diagnosed before operation. Often the patients' vague complaints lead to calculated guessing on the physician's part, and he diagnoses all of the more common abdominal ailments before thinking of small bowel tumor. Some of these commoner conditions are peptic ulcer, biliary tract disease, and bowel obstruction from adhesions or inflammatory diseases. Abdominal pain and localized tenderness commonly occur first, then a syndrome of intestinal obstruction from stenosis or intussusception, or a bleeding triad that may be acute or chronic—hematemesis, melena or occult blood in the stool, and weakness and anemia. Perforation from a tumor with the signs of acute abdominal catastrophe develops in a few patients. Periampullary growths in the duodenum may obstruct the common duct and lead to jaundice (a syndrome common with cancer of the pancreas, described in Chapter 16). Occasionally one can feel an abdominal mass, which may occur anywhere in the abdomen since the small gut is so mobile. Two thirds of patients commonly have symptoms of pain, weight loss, and vomiting for over 6 months before treatment.

**X-ray studies.** A barium x-ray study of the small bowel gives more definitive information than any other diagnostic maneuver. It is quite efficient in the fixed duodenum, but less so in the "floating" jejunum and ileum. Diagnostic accuracy at best is poor—25%. Injection of barium through an intestinal tube passed to the point of obstruction gives best delineation of the tumor.

**Laboratory studies.** Laboratory studies help us with a definitive diagnosis of carcinoid tumors where one in four produces elevated serotonin breakdown product levels (5-hydroxyindolacetic acid) in the urine.

**Biopsy.** Most diagnoses must be made at *laparotomy* where biopsy of a suspiciously metastatic lymph node or a "blind" small bowel resection with immediate frozen section study finally yields the answer. Opening the small bowel lumen for a direct biopsy of the primary risks peritoneal contamination by bacteria and tumor cells.

**Clinical syndromes.** Two rare clinical syndromes aid us now and then to suspect unusual intestinal tumors: (1) the *Peutz-Jeghers syndrome*—melanosis of lips and buccal mucosa often associated with intestinal polyposis and (2) *malignant acanthosis nigricans*—hyperpigmentation and papillary hypertrophy of skin folds that seem congenitally linked to occurrence of bowel cancer, both large and small.

### Differential diagnosis

Almost any affliction of abdominal organs that can produce acute or chronic obstruction to gut or bile tract, bleeding, or pain must be considered in differentiating small bowel tumors from other ailments. Gallstones, cysts and tumors of the pancreas, volvulus, internal hernia, adhesions, intussusception from other conditions, regional enteritis, peptic ulcer, acute appendicitis, tumors of the stomach and colon, and ovarian cysts can all simulate some of the varied presenting pictures of small bowel tumors. Metastases to the small bowel develop on occasion from widely disseminated cancers of other sites such as melanoma.

## PREVENTIVE MEASURES

Unless we find external carcinogens or viruses that trigger these neoplasms or discover that they result from the same carcinogenic complex that applies to other gastrointestinal tumors, hope of prevention remains small.

## TREATMENT PRINCIPLES

1. *Surgery* constitutes the best treatment, since it is generally needed to make a diagnosis and since the area of anatomy involved tolerates x-ray therapy poorly. One can use either a resection of the small bowel segment involved along with mesentery and regional nodes or a bypass operation in cases where palliative relief of obstruction is required. Cancers of the duodenum, if curable, may require pancreatoduodenectomy; those in the terminal ileum may require a right hemicolectomy.

2. X-ray therapy plays a key role in managing lymphomas; we use x-ray therapy usually *after* surgery because profound diagnostic difficulty in the small bowel prevents preoperative use.

3. Palliative surgery for carcinoids differs from that ordinarily employed for incurable cancer because these tumors grow so slowly and sometimes cause symptoms by excessive serotonin production. Surgical excision of as much gross tumor as possible helps the patient even though some tumor remains.

## COMMON ERRORS

Many surgeons faced suddenly with an incurable carcinoid tumor do not remember its indolent growth pattern and troublesome functioning ability. They often omit the careful dissection and removal of most of the tumor, which may mean real palliation even though not a cure.

## PROMISING DEVELOPMENTS FOR THE FUTURE

None are foreseen.

## PROGNOSIS

Survivals with the commonest cancers, the adenocarcinomas, fall well below those obtained from the same type in the colon because of difficulties of diagnosis in the small bowel and the advanced stages of the tumors when treated. Approximately 20% survive 5 years, although nearly half of the patients survive when the cancer has not metastasized.

The outlook brightens considerably with the other less common varieties of small bowel cancer—carcinoids, 50% 5-year survival; lymphomas, 40% 5-year survival; and leiomyosarcomas, 50% 5-year survival.

**REFERENCES**

Diffenbaugh, W. G., and Anderson, R. E.: Carcinoid (argentaffin) tumors of the gastrointestinal tract, Arch. Surg. **73:**21-37, 1956.

Dorman, J. E., Floyd, C. E., and Cohn, I., Jr.: Malignant neoplasms of the small bowel, Amer. J. Surg. **113:**131-135, 1967.

Ebert, P. A., and Zuidema, G. D.: Primary tumors of the small intestine, Arch. Surg. **91:** 452-455, 1965.

Fortner, J. G.: An appraisal of the pathogenesis of primary carcinoma of the extrahepatic biliary tract, Surgery **43:**563-571, 1958.

Mattingly, T. W., Andrus, E. C., Biorck, G., and Manion, W. C.: The functioning carcinoid tumor: a serendipity in diagnosis, Trans. Amer. Clin. Climat. Ass. **77:**190-203, 1965.

McPeak, C. J.: The small bowel. In Nealon, T. F., Jr., editor: Management of the patient with cancer, Philadelphia, 1966, W. B. Saunders Co., pp. 634-656.

Ostermiller, W., Joergenson, E. F., and Weibel, L.: A clinical review of tumors of the small bowel, Amer. J. Surg. **111:**403-410, 1966.

Pagtalunan, R. J. G., Mayo, C. W., and Dockerty, M. B.: Primary malignant tumors of the small intestine, Amer. J. Surg. **108:**13-18, 1964.

Rochlin, D. B., and Longmire, W. P., Jr.: Primary tumors of the small intestine, Surgery **50:**586-592, 1961.

Smith, F. H., and Murphy, R.: Cutaneous melanosis associated with gastrointestinal disease, Med. Clin. N. Amer. **50:**349-359, 1966.

Chapter 16

# Cancer of the pancreas

The pancreas is a complex exocrine and endocrine gland that secretes diverse substances from many types of cells. Several varieties of tumors arise within it. Grossly it resembles the parotid gland, a purely digestive exocrine gland, in which mixed tumors predominate, but no such tumors appear in the pancreas.

## INCIDENCE AND DISTRIBUTION

Pancreatic cancer comprises 1% to 2% of all cancers, occurs twice as often in men as in women, and is the fifth leading cause of cancer deaths among males. It has increased in the last two decades, especially in men, and now equals stomach cancer in this country, since the latter has been dropping in incidence. No one has described significant geographic variations in incidence.

## ETIOLOGY

### External initiating agents

No real clues exist here. Most cancers are of ductal cell origin and two thirds occur in the head of the gland. We tend to agree with Fortner that a reasonable chance exists that carcinogens in bile can regurgitate into the major pancreatic ducts and remain there for an adequate time to begin the carcinogenic process.

### Predisposing factors

No common factors have emerged as yet. A tiny group of tumors, cystadenomas of the pancreas, occur in women with profound hormonal imbalances and a peculiar tendency toward malignant tumors at various other sites.

## PATHOLOGY

Pancreatic tumors develop mainly from two of the many types of cells—ductal cells that perform a lining function and beta islet cells in the islets of Langerhans. Ninety percent of tumors are *adenocarcinomas* of duct cell origin. The latter grow at a moderate rate, produce much fibrosis and often a surrounding zone of pancreatitis, and compress and block nearby pancreatic ducts leading to cystic dilatation of the blocked ducts and to atrophy of the sensitive defunctionated acini. Islets seem tough and persist in the face of advancing tumor and fibrosis. One can find focal areas of squamous metaplasia in some blocked ducts. In addition to these scirrhous adenocarcinomas, benign cystadenomas may arise from ductal cells; these are rare, small, multilocular tumors of the tail that resemble serous cystadenomas of the ovary.

Tumors of acinar origin rarely occur.

*Islet cell growths* usually develop from the beta (insulin) cell of the islet and 90% are benign; two thirds of the neoplasms produce insulin with the expected clinical result of episodes of hypoglycemia. The tumor causing the *Zollinger-Ellison ulcerogenic syndrome* comes from a "nonbeta" cell that secretes a gastrinlike hormone. This hormone can produce a fulminating peptic ulcer disease by stimulating gastric hypersecretion. No tumors of the alpha, glucagon-secreting cell of the islet have been described.

Grossly we find most of the adenocarcinomas in the *head of the gland,* where the hard, whitish nodular neoplasm grows silently, replacing normal gland; then it begins to involve the surrounding duodenum or the colonic mesentery, or posteriorly the portal and mesenteric veins. Symptoms generally only appear when the tumor obstructs the duct of Wirsung or the common bile duct by direct invasion or compression, or when metastatic nodes at the porta hepatis shut off bile flow. Common duct obstruction results in an enlarged, dark green liver with dilated bile radicles, fibrosis and, if no previous inflammation has scarred it, a dilated gallbladder containing thick dark bile that later turns pale and thin. The same changes occur when tumors of the periampullary duodenum or of the ampulla of Vater proper obstruct the common duct (Chapter 17).

Carcinomas of the *body* and *tail* of the pancreas can enlarge to great size without characteristic symptomatology; no vital structures lie easily available for invasion. The cancers in this location do eventually fuse to the vertebral bodies, obstruct splenic vessels and mesenteric veins with consequent venous thromboses or splenic infarction, and invade the celiac plexus of nerves with resulting intractable pain.

*Tumors of islet cells* usually arise in the body and tail of the gland because islets are more numerous there. They develop as small, vascular, reddish nodules, never over 5 cm., and can be multiple. Islet cell hyperplasia, rather than full-blown neoplasia, can also produce symptoms of hypoglycemia. Insulinomas and ulcerogenic tumors often are associated with other endocrine gland tumors in thyroid, parathyroid, or adrenal glands.

Direct *spread* by cancers of the pancreatic head occurs into duodenum, colon, and stomach, but not easily into the free peritoneum. Hepatoduodenal nodes at the liver hilum usually show metastases, and later deposits appear in the para-aortic and posterior mediastinal nodes. Virchow's node at the left base of the neck becomes clinically involved in only 3% of instances. Blood-borne metastases then produce small nodules, first in the liver and then in the lungs or bones. Cancers of the body and tail spread more widely, gain easier access to the peritoneal cavity as they grow, and often result in abdominal carcinomatosis, widespread involvement of the liver, lung, and other distant blood-borne sites in addition to multiple regional node metastases.

## Precancerous lesions

We know of none.

## NATURAL HISTORY

Cancers of the head of the gland may produce insidious, vague indigestion, anorexia, and bulky fatty stools from blockage of pancreatic digestive enzymes (lipase, amylase), but usually *jaundice* from common duct obstruction occurs first, with marked weight loss and often pain in the right upper quadrant. Emaciation develops within weeks from poor absorption of food, liver dysfunction, low food intake, anorexia, and narcotic use. The average patient dies of cachexia and liver failure in 6 to 9 months after the onset of symptoms.

*Body* and *tail* pancreatic cancers may grow to great size with only vague symptoms. The principal abnormality is steady epigastric pain, which radiates to the back and is relieved by forward bending. The physician often can feel an epigastric mass behind the stomach when these patients finally come in. Increasing pain, narcotic addiction, anorexia, marked weight loss, emaciation, and signs of widespread abdominal metastases progress rapidly.

By contrast the small, usually benign islet cell tumors do not obstruct or invade, but only produce physiologic imbalances from oversecretion of insulin or a gastrinlike hormone. The size of the tumor makes no difference in the amount of hormone produced. Three degrees of hypoglycemia can occur with insulinomas: (1) mild fatigue and restlessness, (2) pallor, sweating, fear, tachycardia, and tremor from adrenalin overcompensation, and (3) staggering, confusion, diplopia, and violence simulating epilepsy or drunkenness. Ulcerogenic tumors may cause marked gastric hypersecretion with an episodic fulminating illness due to gastric ulcers that can be fatal from ulcer complications. Refractory diarrhea and a low potassium syndrome may also accompany the illness.

## DIAGNOSIS

As with other digestive and respiratory tract tumors, obstruction of a major passage is the event that leads to symptoms that lead to diagnosis.

**History and physical examination.** Findings in the inaccessible pancreatic cancer occur late in the course of its growth, and patients delay an average of 6 months or more after the start of symptoms. When common duct occlusion develops in cancers of the head, *jaundice, clay-colored stools,* weight loss, an enlarged gallbladder, and pain all demand investigation. More elusive signs come from pancreatic duct occlusion and disturbed functions, such as vague indigestion, steatorrhea, thirst, and urinary frequency associated with beginning diabetes. Cancers in the body and tail of the pancreas, lacking vital passages to obstruct, engender the following quite late symptoms and signs: epigastric pain, a mass with transmitted pulsation from the underlying aorta, and peripheral thrombophlebitis. Functioning islet cell tumors yield hypoglycemic attacks, often identified by Whipple's triad—central nervous system abnormalities with convulsions, a fasting blood sugar below 45, and relief by the administration of sugar. Refractory, recurrent gastric ulcers must suggest an ulcerogenic pancreatic tumor as part of the differential diagnosis.

**X-ray studies.** Changes in the normal contour of duodenum and stomach by encroaching pancreatic cancer show up in barium x-ray studies and help considerably in the diagnosis of tumor and in determining its extent, but such changes come only from advanced cancer (exception—ampullary area tumors). Newer techniques defining more subtle changes are being developed, such as celiac and mesenteric arteriography, percutaneous hepatic cholangiography (just prior to operation), and splenoportography. Pancreatic calcification, if found, is not associated causally with cancer, nor does the 20% concurrence of gallstones and pancreatic cancer help clarify a difficult differential problem.

**Laboratory tests.** The laboratory offers many helpful tests, although some tests are surprisingly little used, especially various analyses of *duodenal drainages.* When we analyze duodenal aspirates, particularly for amylase and lipase activity, especially after secretin (plus pancreozymin) stimulation, any reduction in pancreatic exocrine function can usually be detected. *Oral radioactive fat absorption tests* also give fairly reliable information about pancreatic lipase production in the absence of clinical symptoms. In obstructive jaundice serum bilirubin and *alkaline phosphatase* levels run high, cephalin flocculation and thymol turbidity remain normal, whereas transaminase determinations are moderately elevated. Occult blood occurs in the stool only with ampullary cancers, and stools show no bile or urobilinogen in complete common duct obstruction. Urine urobilinogen is absent, but urine bilirubin is high in obstructive jaundice. Glycosuria and a high blood sugar may mean diabetes from tumor destruction of islets, whereas low fasting blood sugar or a typical *tolbutamide* response curve may indicate an insulinoma.

**Cytology.** Because histologic diagnosis in pancreatic cancer can present formidable problems, the pursuance of cytologic study of duodenal drainages after secretin stimulation needs encouragement. By this study one may sometimes differentiate chronic pancreatitis and gallstone obstruction from cancer.

**Exploratory laparotomy.** Nine of ten pancreatic cancers coming to exploration are nonresectable for cure; thus the definitive histologic diagnosis usually comes from an easy biopsy of a metastasis (node or nodule). For the patients presenting an undiagnosed mass in the substance of the gland, without metastasis, we can only suggest a mobilization of the duodenum and pancreatic head, with fingers above and below, and careful exploration with a needle followed by "knife-core" of tumor tissue under good vision. The risk of hemorrhage and fistula seems preferable to a blind resection of an unknown mass that may not be cancer. Second biopsies may be needed. Accuracy of direct biopsy is still only 90%, so often do surrounding pancreatitis and bleeding obscure the true tumor.

## Differential diagnosis

The first problem in cases of jaundice constitutes elimination of *hepatocellular jaundice;* cephalin flocculation and thymol turbidity should be negative or only weakly positive with obstructive jaundice of short duration. Once obstructive jaundice seems certain, the field of possibilities narrows to three—*common duct stone, chronic pancreatitis,* and *cancer.* Proper x-ray investigation should be able to define the occasional confusing aortic aneurysm or traumatic pseudocyst of the pancreas.

To distinguish stone in the common duct from cancer of the head of the pancreas may be impossible clinically, but generally stone patients are female with a history of previous attacks of colicky, right upper quadrant pain, vomiting, and often chills, whereas cancer patients are generally male and show a weight loss and an enlarged gallbladder and liver.

Attempts to differentiate clinically between the *four cancers* that cause obstructive jaundice (cancers of common duct, ampulla of Vater, periampullary duodenum, and head of the pancreas), although important, do not lend themselves to any useful generalizations.

*Chronic pancreatitis* usually shows calcifications, a history of typical attacks of vomiting and pain, a diffusely enlarged gland, an absence of malignant cells on cytology, and negative biopsies.

## PREVENTIVE MEASURES

None are known.

## TREATMENT PRINCIPLES

1. Surgery alone can cure these cancers, but few diagnoses are made with the growth localized and operable. Surgery carries a high operative mortality—12% to 30%.
2. Patients with cancers of the head of the pancreas survive for 5 years so seldom that the experts use the standard operation of pancreatoduodenectomy only for the occasional small tumor, reserving it mainly for the more favorable cancers of the ampulla, common duct, and duodenum.
3. Operative removal of distal pancreas, spleen, and appropriate adjacent organs is worth trial in the rare operable cancer of the body and tail.
4. Conservative segmental excision of the usually benign functioning islet cell tumors suffices, if accompanied by a thorough search for multiple tumors. Local tumor removal plus total gastrectomy is needed in the ulcerogenic tumors.
5. Radiotherapy usually gives little help to patients with these cancers.
6. Palliative relief of jaundice often results from cholecystojejunostomy, choledochoduodenostomy or, preferably, choledochojejunostomy.
7. Chemotherapy seldom causes tumor regression or symptomatic relief.

## COMMON ERRORS

1. Some physicians may assume that obstructive jaundice comes from cancer when gallstones really cause it.
2. Surgeons may occasionally perform unjustified pancreatoduodenectomies because of inexpert knowledge of what constitutes incurability in these cancers, or because of poor clinical judgment, when biopsies are negative, in cases of chronic pancreatitis.
3. Multiple islet cell tumors can easily be missed.

## PROMISING DEVELOPMENTS FOR THE FUTURE

1. A radioactive scanning technique for the pancreas with selenium 75–tagged methonium shows promise, as do refinements in methods to do quick, total body scans.
2. Methods of obtaining angiograms in and around the pancreas, alone or in combination, promise to help delineate neoplasms better in the future.

## PROGNOSIS

Five-year survivals in adenocarcinoma of the pancreas are so rare that Child and Frey speak of the achievements of pancreatoduodenectomy in terms of palliation only. Of 366 resections in sixteen reported series, twenty-six lived 5 years (7%). Published operative mortality rates vary from 12% to as high as 50%.

### REFERENCES

Ackerman, L. V., and del Regato, J. A.: Cancer, ed. 3, St. Louis, 1962, The C. V. Mosby Co., pp. 736-759.

Buckwalter, J. A., and Raterman, L.: Recent developments in the diagnosis of pancreatic and alimentary and biliary tract neoplasms, Iowa Med. Soc. J. **54:**172-177, 1964.

Chey, W. Y., Shay, H., and Nielsen, O. F.: Diagnosis of diseases of the pancreas and biliary tract, J.A.M.A. **198:**257-262, 1966.

Child, C. G., and Frey, C. F.: Pancreatoduodenectomy, Surg. Clin. N. Amer. **46:**1201-1213, 1966.

Fortner, J. G.: An appraisal of the pathogenesis of primary carcinoma of the extrahepatic biliary tract, Surgery **43:**563-571, 1958.

Hermann, R. E.: Current concepts in the surgical management of cancer of the pancreas and peripancreatic region, Med. Times **94:**571-584, 1966.

Monge, J. J., Judd, E. S., and Gage, R. P.: Radical pancreatoduodenectomy, Ann. Surg. **160:**711-722, 1964.

Rhoads, J. E.: Pancreas. In Harkins, H. N., Moyer, C. A., Rhoads, J. E., and Allen, J. G., editors: Surgery, principles and practice, ed. 2, Philadelphia, 1961, J. B. Lippincott Co., Chapter 31.

Soloway, H. B.: Constitutional abnormalities associated with pancreatic cystadenomas, Cancer **18:**1297-1300, 1965.

Winegarner, F. G., Hague, W. H., and Elliott, P. W.: Tissue diagnosis and surgical management in malignant jaundice, Amer. J. Surg. **111:**5-7, 1966.

Chapter 17

# Cancer of the biliary tract and liver

Although some selective absorption takes place in the gallbladder, the extrahepatic biliary tract mainly conducts bile to the intestine. Cancers of this tract are of one fairly uniform type. The liver performs many varied functions—excreting, secreting, detoxifying, and metabolizing—but two kinds of cells, the parenchymal liver cell and the "lining" bile radicle cell, largely compose the functional elements of this huge organ. The basic tumor spectrum of the liver is therefore not large, despite the varied chemical reactions inside the parenchymal cell, and falls into two main groups from the two principal cells of origin.

## INCIDENCE AND DISTRIBUTION

Biliary tract cancers outnumber liver cancers by five to one. Liver tumors are rare in the United States, but very common in parts of Africa, Asia, and Indonesia, where they develop at younger ages and seem to be on the increase. We know of few remarkable differences in biliary tract cancer distribution. Hepatic cell cancers (hepatomas) occur five times more often than duct cell cancers (cholangiocarcinomas). Lumped together, the tumors of this chapter equal over 1% of all cancers, half as frequent as pancreatic neoplasms but much more common than small bowel cancers. Men acquire more liver and common duct cancers than women, but gallbladder cancer shows just the reverse—a five to one preponderance for women.

## ETIOLOGY

### External initiating agents

**Biliary tract.** Fortner has induced animal cancers with bile from patients with cancer of the gallbladder. The insertion of sterile foreign bodies produced gallbladder cancer in guinea pigs. One may recall here again the predilection of cancer for locations of concentration and stasis, which exactly describes the gallbladder. Chemical carcinogens may well be present in bile.

**Liver.** Many chemical compounds induce liver cancer in experimental animals—butter yellow, dimethylnitrosamine, 2-acetylaminofluorene, and aminoazotoluene;

more recently mycotoxins have fallen under suspicion as human liver carcinogens. The aflatoxins (*Aspergillus flavus*) particularly have been closely implicated in the high incidence of hepatomas in certain African tribes who allow molds to contaminate food supplies in areas of high humidity. Liver parasites may possess carcinogenicity; *Clonorchis sinensis* and *Opisthorchis viverrini* infect many South China and Southeast Asian persons, where a relatively high incidence of liver cancer exists.

### Predisposing factors

**Biliary tract.** Much analysis and many published reports concern the predisposing effect of *gallstones* on gall tract cancer; 1% to 4% of gallstone patients develop these cancers, whereas 80% to 90% of gallbladder cancers have concomitant stones, and about half of common duct cancers show them. Fortner's and Petrov's work cited above is pertinent. We personally believe that the concentration of bile plus stasis promote both stones and cancer, and the specific effect of the foreign body (stone) constitutes but one factor in the process.

**Liver.** Many publications direct attention to the high frequency of hepatic cell cancer in cirrhotic livers when compared to normal ones; the implied causal relation fails to bear close scrutiny, however, as Steiner's recent worldwide studies on cirrhosis show. Cirrhosis of certain kinds and cancer may coexist because of basic abnormal stimuli toward both. Malnutrition does not appear to trigger cancer but may act as a promoter.

## PATHOLOGY

**Biliary tract.** Gallbladder cancers grow usually as differentiated adenocarcinomas, with gallstones generally present in the dome or in the neck of the organ; the common scirrhous type scleroses the gallbladder and invades the liver bed at an early stage, but the papillary and mucinous types form slow-growing, bulky, intraluminal masses that become secondarily infected. Epidermoid cancers also appear occasionally. Direct growth into adjacent stomach, colon, duodenum, as well as liver occurs frequently, and half of the patients have positive periportal or peripancreatic nodes when explored. An occasional benign gallbladder polyp or papilloma develops, but these are not necessarily precancerous.

Tumors of the extrahepatic ducts are adenocarcinomas, circumscribed and papillary or diffusely invading, slow-growing, and constricting; most occur at the lower end of the tract—the common duct, the confluence of cystic with common hepatic, or in structures around the ampulla (common pancreatic duct, duodenal mucosa adjacent to ampulla or ampulla of Vater proper). The exact site of origin of these neoplasms is usually obscure because of overgrowth by the time of diagnosis. The microscopic, gross, and clinical picture of obstructive jaundice presents in the duct proximal to tumor and in the liver; one half exhibit regional node metastases at operation.

**Liver.** A single, large tumor mass with small satellite nodules often characterizes hepatomas, although a diffuse type with smaller multiple nodules develops as well, often with cirrhosis. Gall finds liver cancers most commonly with postnecrotic cirrhosis (20%), next with posthepatic, but seldom with nutritional cirrhosis. One in ten cases of hemochromatosis of the liver also shows cancer.

Microscopically hepatomas exhibit a great variety of structure, often with bizarre cells that produce bile, a variety recalling the many functions of the normal hepatic cell. In contradistinction, cholangiocarcinomas produce a rather uniform adenomatous pattern. Both cancers probably begin as a single focus but present as multiple foci because of early intrahepatic vascular metastases.

*Direct extension* constitutes the most common route of spread, followed by hepatic and portal vein seedings, first in the liver itself, then in the lungs. Positive nodes at the hilum of the liver and mesentery of the colon or in the retroperitoneal chain are common. Cancer gains easy access to the chest through lymphatics in the "bare area" of the liver and posteriorly at the origins of the diaphragm.

The liver harbors *metastatic* cancerous nodules from primaries in the stomach, intestines, and pancreas far more often than it develops primary cancers itself because venous blood from these organs drains through the liver via the portal circulation first, before entering the systemic circulation. Thus the liver arrests cancer cells in the venous blood from most abdominal organs. Some embolizing malignant cells reach the liver through its second, hepatic circulation as well. Breast cancers reach the liver via lymphatics and stomach cancers may invade it directly. No reliable gross characteristics of a metastatic nodule exist. The histology of liver nodule biopsy usually suggests either metastatic or primary tumor. The finding of an extrahepatic primary clinches the diagnosis.

### Precancerous lesions

Except for the rare carcinoma in situ in a gallbladder papilloma, no such lesions occur.

## NATURAL HISTORY

**Biliary tract.** Generally a long symptomatology of gallbladder disease from the stones that coexist precedes gallbladder cancer, and with increasing tumor growth the colicky pain becomes steadier and weight loss begins. Jaundice finally develops from metastatic nodes compressing the common duct, and secondary inflammatory complications often precipitate operation or death. By contrast, jaundice usually ushers in the clinical phase of cancers of the extrahepatic bile ducts without previous symptoms. Then pain develops and the full-blown obstructive jaundice syndrome settles in with ascending cholangitis as a frequent late complication.

**Liver.** Symptoms of primary liver cancers are vague and late, such as steady right upper quadrant pain, indigestion, weakness, and weight loss. Later exertional dyspnea may begin from an enlarged liver and ascites. Some reports describe intraperitoneal hemorrhages, febrile illnesses, and even hypoglycemia. Inanition and cachexia come on within a few months after diagnosis. One half of both groups of patients die within 6 months after the onset of symptoms.

## DIAGNOSIS

**History and physical examination.** Cancer of the gallbladder yields no characteristic symptoms or signs; it is a disease of older women with findings typical of recurring cholecystitis and only occasionally do pain, weight loss, and jaundice come on even reasonably early, such as with a small tumor mass in the cystic duct. *Obstructive jaundice* may occur early with small tumors of the common duct or ampullary area, but no easy clues differentiate such tumors from stone or pancreatic cancer. Liver cancer similarly produces vague findings of weight loss, abdominal fullness, upper abdominal pain, weakness, anorexia, plus symptoms and signs of the often accompanying cirrhosis—abdominal fullness and ascites.

**X-ray studies.** The diagnosis in biliary tract cancer may stem from a flat abdominal film rather than from a cystogram in which the gallbladder fails to fill or shows only stones. Barium study of the duodenum may reveal deformity of the papilla in ampullary cancer. Percutaneous *transhepatic cholangiography* done just before surgery may help delineate common duct neoplasms. Plain abdominal films also may reveal liver deformity or diaphragmatic invasion by tumor.

**Liver scan.** Radioisotopic scanning by the production of scintigrams, using $I^{131}$ rose bengal, can achieve nearly 80% accuracy in spotting tumor defects of more than 1.5 cm. in the liver substance. This is an indispensable study when liver tumors, primary or secondary, are suspected. Of course, a scan cannot tell one type from another.

**Laboratory examinations.** Laboratory studies (blood, stool, urine, and liver function), mentioned in the discussion of cancer of the pancreas, will aid the physician in making the distinction between obstructive and hepatocellular jaundice. However, no specific chemical test for tumor exists. Liver function tests may remain quite normal until tumors grow very large. *Alkaline phosphatase* and *Bromsulphalein retention* tests show the earliest changes. Transaminase determinations are less sensitive to neoplastic replacement of liver. Analyses for bile and pancreatic ferments in duodenal drainage may occasionally suggest the location of biliary tract neoplasms by the presence of one and not the other. *Cytology* is worth doing on any duodenal aspirate; it will help when positive, since false positive reports seldom occur, but false negatives abound.

**Biopsy.** Needle biopsy of the liver shows tumor of some type, not always accurately classified, in 85% of large primary and metastatic masses. However, the physician trying to aspirate small masses fails frequently to hit the neoplasm and risks hemorrhage, and may cause delay in diagnosis.

**Exploratory laparotomy.** Usually only direct open biopsy at operation gains histologic proof of these cancers.

## Differential diagnosis

In distinguishing tumors of the four specific locations in the extrahepatic biliary tree from cancer of the *head of the pancreas* and *common duct stone,* our notes under pancreas apply. The following two additional findings may help: (1) occult blood in the stool comes only from ampullary cancers, not from biliary tumors; and (2) the finding of malignant cells in duodenal aspirates with normal pancreatic ferments points more toward common duct cancer than to other tumors.

Liver *cysts* of developmental or parasitic origin occasionally occur.

The long-standing *cirrhotic liver* is usually smaller than normal, not larger as it is with tumor, and a long history of intestinal complaints accompanies cirrhosis. Focal cirrhosis may closely simulate metastatic cancer.

*Metastatic liver tumors* occur often from primaries in stomach, bowel, pancreas, endometrium, breast, esophagus, and lung, and from melanomas of the skin; therefore, by the laws of probability, nearly all liver tumors should be metastatic. It follows that a survey of these major suspect organs constitutes part of a liver tumor work-up. If no extrahepatic primary is found, needle biopsy or laparotomy must follow. Now and then a solitary large tumor mass represents a benign hemangioma. Small (1 to 2 cm.) hemangiomas commonly mimic an isolated metastatic nodule, but the vascular lesions are bluish and compressible, unlike the hard, white metastases.

## PREVENTIVE MEASURES

1. Cholecystectomy for all gallstones to prevent cancer from developing in 1% to 4% of these gallbladders does not make sense statistically. Cholecystectomies for stones are justified, however, to prevent the common inflammatory complications of stones, and so this surgery incidentally interrupts the cancerous process in some cases.

2. We can relatively easily eliminate from our environment substances highly suspected of carcinogenicity, such as the azo dyes in industry and mycotoxins that contaminate stored food *(Aspergillus flavus, Penicillium islandium,* and *P. rubricum).*

3. Measures to develop and enforce proper screening for carcinogenicity of all food additives and preservatives and a stepped-up search for inadvertent carcinogenic food contaminants may be hard to institute. We need an acceptable screening test. The abundance of agents causing experimental liver cancer may make this organ a good candidate for an animal screening test.

## TREATMENT PRINCIPLES

1. As with the pancreas, surgery offers the only curative measure, but it can seldom be used in these advanced cancers.

2. Pancreatoduodenectomy, partial hepatectomy, or a right or left hepatic lobectomy comprise the operative spectrum when cure seems possible.

3. Among liver tumors, the apparently solitary, well-demarcated hepatomas, not the diffusely infiltrative tumors, lend themselves to resection. Gallbladder cancer invades liver just between lobes and so presents an anatomic problem; either a wedge of liver needs removal at the base of the gallbladder, which risks an inadequate margin, or else the right lobe plus the medial segment of the left lobe must be sacrificed, which may leave insufficient viable liver.

4. Pancreatoduodenectomy generally suits only the more favorable cancers—those of the ampulla of Vater, periampullary mucosa, and distal common duct.

5. Radiotherapy can palliate some liver neoplasms.

6. Liver infusion of chemotherapeutic drugs by intravascular catheter may secure an occasional worthwhile remission of both primary and metastatic masses.

7. Choledochojejunostomy may palliate some distal biliary tract cancers. One may also force one limb of a T-tube through a cancer to relieve biliary obstruction temporarily.

## COMMON ERRORS

These complicated tumor situations do not permit generalizations.

## PROMISING DEVELOPMENTS FOR THE FUTURE

1. Refinements and wider availability of *liver scanning* techniques offer hope for better diagnosis.

2. Carefully planned *combinations* of newer diagnostic methods, such as *pancreatic exocrine function* tests, *splenoportography, selective arteriography,* and *transhepatic cholangiography* can pinpoint the exact location and suggest degree of resectability in four of five cases of tumor of the extrahepatic biliary ducts.

## PROGNOSIS

**Biliary tract.** Only an occasional patient survives 5 years, although one in three survives with the more favorable carcinoma of the ampulla of Vater. Most die within 1 year of onset of symptoms.

**Liver.** Now and then a patient will survive long term after removal of a liver tumor; such survivors are rarer than those with cancer of any other organ, and most of the survivors are children with pathologically unusual neoplasms not described above.

### REFERENCES


Ackerman, L. V., and del Regato, J. A.: Cancer, ed. 3, St. Louis, 1962, The C. V. Mosby Co., pp. 759-792.

Buckwalter, J. A., and Raterman, L.: Recent developments in the diagnosis of pancreatic alimentary and biliary tract neoplasms, Iowa Med. Soc. J. **54:**172-177, 1964.

Cattell, R. B., and Prytels, L. J.: An appraisal of pancreatoduodenal resection, Ann. Surg. **129:**840-849, 1949.

Flemma, R. J., and Shingleton, W. W.: Clinical experience with percutaneous transhepatic cholangiography, Amer. J. Surg. **111:**13-22, 1966.

Fortner, J. G.: An appraisal of the pathogenesis of primary carcinoma of the extrahepatic biliary tract, Surgery **43:**563-571, 1958.

Fortner, J. G., and Randall, H. T.: On the carcinogenicity of human gallstones, Surg. Forum **12:**155, 1961.

Hermann, R. E.: Current concepts in the surgical management of cancer of the pancreas and peripancreatic region, Med. Times **94:**571-584, 1966.

Higginson, J.: Geographic considerations in liver disease, Prog. Liver Dis. **2:**211-227, 1965.

Litwin, M. S.: Primary carcinoma of the gallbladder, Arch. Surg. **95:**236-240, 1967.

Nelson, R. S., Elizalde, R., de, and Howe, C. D.: Clinical aspects of primary carcinoma of the liver, Cancer **19:**533-540, 1966.

Pack, G. T., and Islami, A. H.: Surgical treatment of hepatic tumors, Prog. Liver Dis. **2:**499-511, 1965.

Patton, R. B., and Horn, R. C., Jr.: Primary liver carcinoma, Cancer **17:**757-768, 1964.

Sato, T., Kakizaki, G., Saito, Y., Maki, T., and Koyama, K.: A combined method of diagnosis in malignant jaundice, Arch. Surg. **95:**207-216, 1967.

Steiner, P. E.: World problem in the cirrhotic diseases of the liver; their incidence, frequency, types and aetiology, Trop. Geogr. Med. **16:**175, 1964.

Strohl, E. L., Reed, W. H., Diffenbaugh, W. G., and Anderson, R. E.: Carcinoma of the bile ducts, Arch. Surg. **87:**567-577, 1963.

Warren, K., and MacDonald, W. M.: Cancer of the biliary tract. In Nealon, T. F., Jr., editor: Management of the patient with cancer, Philadelphia, 1966, W. B. Saunders Co., Chapter 25.

Whipple, A. O., Parsons, W. B., and Mullens, C. R.: Treatment of carcinoma of the ampulla of Vater, Ann. Surg. **102:**763-779, 1935.

Chapter 18

# Cancer of the colon and rectum

For the purpose of understanding neoplasia, it is misleading to separate the colon and the rectum. The colorectal mucosa is more or less uniform and performs relatively simple functions, absorbing fluid and electrolytes and helping to pass along and excrete unneeded foodstuff by the production of mucus. The tumor spectrum is simple and limits itself mainly to one type and its variants.

## INCIDENCE AND DISTRIBUTION

Colorectal adenocarcinoma is the *commonest visceral cancer* when both sexes are considered together; it constitutes 13% of all cancer, exceeded only by cancer of the skin. The male to female proportion is approximately equal, although one registry reports higher colonic rates in women and higher rectal rates in men. In women breast cancer occurs slightly more often than colorectal cancer, and only lung cancer exceeds it in men. The disease generally manifests itself in the elderly.

Highest rates occur in Europe and the lowest rates occur in Japan, Finland, and Chile, where stomach cancer rates run high. The inverse relation between the incidence of stomach and colorectal cancer in the latter countries merits study. Second colorectal cancers occur in 5% to 6% of patients.

## ETIOLOGY

### External initiating agents

None are known. But some compelling reasons exist to suspect that chemical carcinogens in the feces may trigger the cancerous sequence. For one, the organ concentrates useless or harmful material while at the same time holding it for excretion; stasis obtains here far more than elsewhere in the digestive tract. We would expect, if an ingested agent were active, that it would have its best chance for longest contact at highest dosage in the colorectum, and the nearer the anus the greater the chance. And this is just what we find—most digestive passage cancers occur in the colorectum and two thirds of these occur in the last foot of the 24-foot passage, the rectum, and the sigmoid.

Second, laboratory studies in animals reveal a number of chemical carcinogens that exhibit specific action in the colorectum—cycasin, dimethylnitrosamine, aflatoxins. One investigator suggests that bacterial flora of the gut must convert these compounds before they can initiate cancer.

### Predisposing factors

Following the above theoretical observations we would expect that chronic constipation should predispose to colorectal cancer. Indeed, it has been often indicated as a factor, but the association is difficult to document. We know of no common constitutional defect related to this cancer, although many reports of high incidence in families suggest that genetics may play a part.

A rare hereditary disease, *congenital familial polyposis of the colon,* based on an autosomal dominant gene, afflicts half of the offspring of an affected parent. Cancer inevitably develops in these persons before the age of 40, presumably from one of the thousands of colorectal polyps. Similarly inherited but less common, the *Peutz-Jeghers syndrome,* exhibits colonic polyps in one third of persons with the other stigmata—mucocutaneous pigmentations. By contrast polyps in this condition are fewer and scattered, carrying little threat of cancerous degeneration. An even rarer congenital disease complex, *Gardner's syndrome* (exostoses, benign skin and soft tissue tumors, and colonic polyps) demonstrates a high incidence of colorectal cancer. Interestingly, no inherited disease includes a tendency to colorectal cancer without exhibiting multiple polyposis, but the common isolated adenomatous polyp found so often in older persons carries with it a relatively low cancer potential (see below).

## PATHOLOGY

Developing from the same mucus-producing cell as its counterparts higher in the digestive tract, *adenocarcinoma* of the colorectum dominates the field, comprising 98% of the cancers. Lymphomas, of course, arise sometimes in the colorectum, as they do higher. Squamous carcinomas develop occasionally in the lower rectum and anal canal, and carcinoid tumors will occur in the rectum.

Microscopically most adenocarcinomas show fairly good differentiation (80%), whereas a few are undifferentiated or show a predominantly mucinous picture. Now and then we find one of these cancers growing as a gross polypoid lesion, which augurs for easy curability, but most cancers grow as fungating, ulcerating, or infiltrating tumors that stenose and obstruct the lumen, bleed in small amounts, invade through the bowel wall to involve adjacent structures, and often perforate.

Adenocarcinomas distribute themselves in the colorectum as follows:

|  |  | |
|---|---|---|
| Rectum | 50% | ⅔ of all |
| Sigmoid | 20% | |
| Descending colon | 7% | |
| Transverse colon | 7% | |
| Right colon | 16% | |

Spread occurs by direct extension to neighboring organs, by lymphatic embolization to regional nodes in orderly progression, or by venous channels to liver or lungs (usually later than the establishment of lymphatic metastases), by free peritoneal implant, and by intraluminal implants at points of trauma in the mucosa distal to the tumor. Since most cancers arise in the pelvis, the bladder, vagina, uterus, ovaries, seminal vesicles, sacrum, ureters, and small bowel often become invaded and involved. Nodal spread occurs in sequence from the nearest mesen-

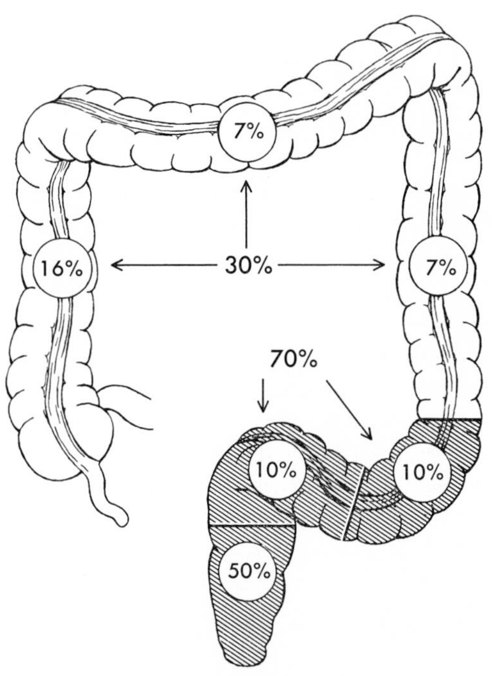


**Fig. 13.** Distribution frequency of colorectal cancer shows high concentration in rectum and sigmoid.

teric node to the next highest, and only in retrograde manner when most nodes in the forward flow path are blocked. Nodal metastasis to pelvic iliac nodes and levator nodes occurs uncommonly in rectal cancer. Sometimes inguinal nodes harbor metastases in low-lying rectal and squamous, anal canal growths.

Unlike many other cancers, size is not related to frequency of positive nodes; many of the well-differentiated tumors grow to great size without metastasizing. Most blood-borne tumor emboli drain into the middle and inferior hemorrhoidal veins and thence to the systemic circulation. Metastases develop in the following structures in descending order of frequency: nodes, peritoneum and omentum, liver, lungs, bones.

A simple, popular pathologic classification based on degree of invasion and nodal spread follows Duke's studies: "Duke's A"—only muscularis involved; "Duke's B"—extension through all layers of bowel wall; and "Duke's C"—presence of positive regional nodes (Fig. 14). These groups directly relate to prognosis.

Microscopic blood vessel invasion in the tumor specimen constitutes another valuable, serious prognostic sign found in one fourth to one third of cases.

Multiple colorectal cancers occur fairly often and some pathologists describe occasional multifocal origin and carcinoma in situ in the mucosa.

## Precancerous lesions

The common small *adenomatous polyps* that develop singly or two or three in scattered patterns in persons after middle age are lesions of small malignant

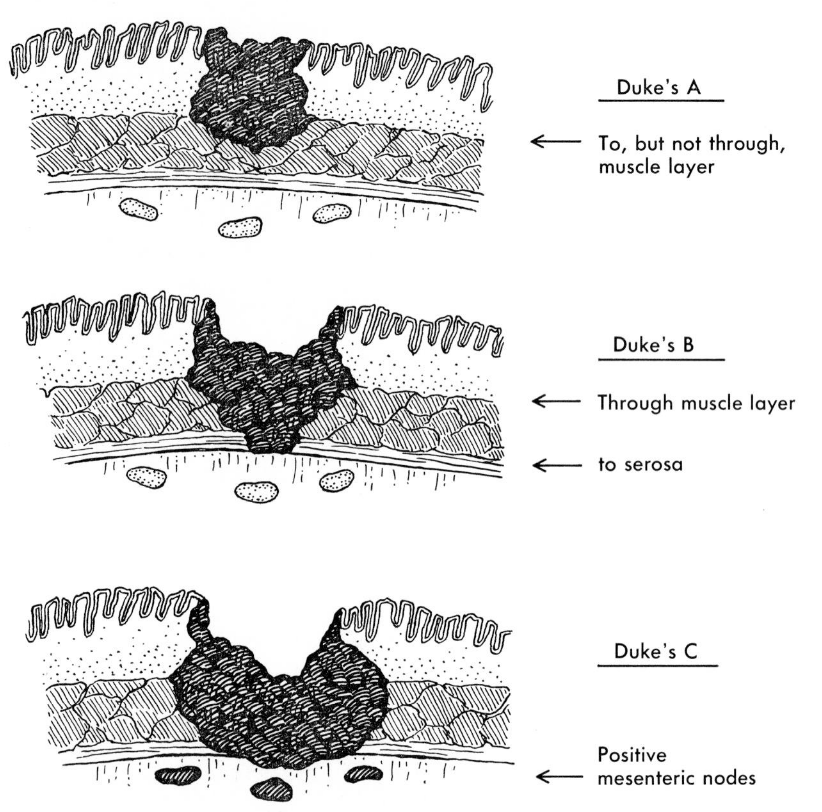


**Fig. 14.** Duke's classification of colorectal cancer, which is often used by pathologists in reporting their studies of resected cancer specimens; this classification relates closely to the prognosis. (Modified from Ackerman, L. V., and del Regato, J. A.: Cancer, ed. 3, St. Louis, 1962, The C. V. Mosby Co.)

potential (Ackerman and del Regato, Spratt and associates, Castleman and Krickstein, Welch and Burker, and Turrell and Haller). We emphasize this point to prevent the delusion that studied eradication of these isolated polyps amounts to a major cancer prevention effort. In all probability it does not. Cancer arises from these polyps rarely when compared to the number of such polyps; it usually develops de novo as a tiny ulcer or plaque that we cannot easily see. If polyps were a common precursor, we should expect a hundred or so cancers from the thousands of polyps in familial polyposis, but generally only one or two cancers occur. Adenomatous polyps, which seldom grow larger than 1 cm., may well result from the same general abnormal influences that generate cancer, so that the colorectum with polyps may be the one that is cancer prone. Polyps are a signal of general mucosal abnormality rather than each one being a potential small cancer. Polyps of the rectum sometimes disappear spontaneously after subtotal colectomy for polyposis, which suggests that stasis no longer obtains to allow luminal contents to produce abnormality. Other kinds of polyps share benignity with adenomatous polyps—the juvenile polyp, the lymphoid polyp, the inflammatory polyp, and the simple mucosal excrescences.

These observations do not imply that cancer can never arise in polyps. Cytologic cancer is sometimes found in the tuft of a polyp, but this early change seldom invades the stalk and seldom metastasizes. Some gross polyps are actually small polypoid cancers from the start (see below).

The following are a number of less common lesions that precede invasive cancer with great regularity:

*Congenital familial polyposis* (described elsewhere).

*Villous (papillary) adenomas* are best considered low-grade cancers, since 25% to 40% show invasive cancer. These are called villous polyps when small.

*Ulcerative colitis* carries a high risk of cancer (30 times that of a normal person) if the process involves the whole colorectum and has been present for over 10 years. Most cases have no so-called pseudopolypi (islands of normal mucosa surrounded by coalescing ulcers); thus cancers do not develop from these "polyps" either.

*Bowen's disease* of anus, *leukoplakia* of the anal area, chronic rectal *fistulae,* and lymphogranuloma venereum may possess premalignant properties as precursors of the occasional squamous cancer of the anal region.

## NATURAL HISTORY

Most colorectal cancers *grow slowly*. A doubling time of over 600 days has been determined by some investigators in contrast to doubling times of 100 days or so in many breast and lung growths. The old story repeats itself—the cancer remains asymptomatic for months or years until large enough to obstruct. The earliest indications are really late in the tumor's course. An insidious change in bowel habit, excess gas, mucus in the stool, a trace of blood in the stool, anemia, and slowly increasing constipation all presage the bulky tumor mass. As size increases further, gas pains and diarrhea develop as well as distention and obstipation from obstruction, tenesmus in the case of rectal masses, or more profuse bleeding. However, massive bleeding from colorectal cancer is rare.

Obstruction comes about easier in the left colon than in the cecum or rectum because (1) the lumen is narrower, (2) the contents are more solid (than in the cecum), and (3) the wall is less distensible, more muscular. The type of growth pattern that obstructs is the common annular, constricting, "napkin ring" variety. Roughly, it requires 1 year for a gross cancer to encircle the lumen completely. Occasionally a polypoid mass may form the head of an intussusception.

Death approaches from the dehydrating effects of unrelieved intestinal obstruction or from free perforation and peritonitis, localized perforation and abscess formation, or inanition from massive catabolic tumor involvement. Sometimes the liver is replaced by metastases and ascites develops from myriad peritoneal implants, or occasionally respiratory failure occurs from lung metastases. Half of untreated patients die within 2 years after the onset of symptoms and all are dead in 4 years.

## DIAGNOSIS

**History.** The following treacherously mild symptoms initiate the clinical phase of colorectal cancer: any change in bowel habit, a trace of blood at stool falsely attributed to hemorrhoids or constipation, excess gas or mild episodes of diarrhea called "something he ate," or an increase in the need for laxatives. Occasionally a hernial weakness becomes worse because of excessive straining at stool due to the rectal mass of tumor. In the same way latent hemorrhoids can enlarge and bleed from increased straining at stool. Later "gas pains" and borborygmi from impending obstruction may come on, or else steady pain from localized perforation and abscess formation may occur. More marked and definite symptoms develop from rectal and sigmoidal tumors than from the late-obstructing right colon lesions. The latter must be quite large to produce any symptoms, and then they cause only vague, cramping discomfort, weakness from anemia, anorexia, or occasionally a palpable mass.

**Physical examination.** A careful *digital rectal* examination, done best in the squatting position, can detect half of colorectal cancers and nearly all of the rectal growths. *Blood* on the examining finger alone indicates the need for a full cancer work-up. Rectal examination should also be done with the patient lying down and the other hand on the abdomen; in women it is combined with a vaginal examination. Abdominal masses, an enlarged or nodular liver, areas of tenderness, spasm, bowel distention indicating bowel obstruction or impending perforation, hernias, and hemorrhoids may all be found as indications of the cancer.

**Sigmoidoscopy and biopsy.** These procedures can be easily performed in the office after a self-administered small enema immediately preceding the "scoping." Sigmoidoscopy surveys the rectum and rectosigmoid segments and will reveal an additional one fourth of all the cancers not felt digitally. All suggestively symptomatic persons, and ideally all persons over 40, need this maneuver as part of a complete work-up. One percent of these asymptomatic persons will exhibit cancers. *Multiple biopsies* often are required to secure an accurate assessment of the true nature of the lesion. Small lesions can be completely removed for biopsy. Sigmoidoscopy always precedes an x-ray study with barium to enhance good vision of the lesion and to detect partially obstructing lesions before barium inserted above them converts them to completely obstructing ones. "Scoping" all persons with symptomatic hemorrhoids and hernias may be wise.

**Barium x-ray examination.** This study always *follows* sigmoidoscopy if the latter failed to show abnormality; it scans the colon above 25 cm. for filling defects suggestive of neoplasia. If sigmoidoscopy has revealed a cancer, barium enema surveys the rest of the large bowel for polyps and second cancers. X-ray study has difficulty in clear delineation of some tumors in the lower sigmoid and in the cecum. It can seldom diagnose rectal lesions or tumors at any location less than 1 cm. in diameter. Care must accompany a barium study in partially obstructing lesions lest they be made completely occlusive by inspissated barium. Post-evacuation and air-contrast films best delineate polyps.

**Laboratory studies.** These studies play an adjunctive role in diagnosis. *Occult blood* appears in the stool in nearly all cancers and alerts the physician to pursue the work-up; blood counts often reveal secondary anemia so common in right colon cancer from faulty hematopoiesis; occasionally a low-potassium syndrome associated with large villous adenomas will be detected by electrolyte studies.

**Cytology.** Cytologic studies and silicone-foam enemas are still experimental. Silicone foam may be injected rectally when liquid; this then solidifies to form a solid cast of the sigmoid and rectum which, when expelled, can be studied for tumor defects and adherent tumor cells.

**Laparotomy.** Exploratory laparotomy will sometimes make the definite diagnosis when other methods fail; excision of a positive mesenteric node, a peritoneal implant, or a metastatic liver nodule constitutes the safest method. Opening into the bowel lumen for biopsy risks peritonitis and cancer spread so that sometimes a lesion must be resected on educated clinical judgment alone, risky as this may be. This situation arises when a cancer perforates into the free peritoneal cavity, necessitating an emergency operation without any of the orderly, sequential studies outlined above.

**Coloscopy.** This procedure involves "scoping" the bowel through bowel-wall incisions at laparotomy to scan the mucosa directly for second primaries. Coloscopy has a limited application because many authorities fear it will risk the spreading of cancer when performed in the presence of a known cancer.

### Differential diagnosis

A myriad of abdominal illnesses mimic colorectal cancer, and *diverticulitis* probably gives more trouble than any other one condition. An x-ray film often cannot differentiate the two; even though diverticulosis has no causal relation to cancer, the two may coexist. Thus the finding of diverticula above or below the lesion does not make the diagnosis. Diverticulitis causes most patients to give a history of previous attacks, a short duration of their present illness, and a feeling of dull, constant pain, with localized abdominal tenderness, whereas cancer causes most patients to show weight loss and blood in the stools with little abdominal pain. Massive bleeding, however, comes more likely from uninflamed diverticulosis.

*Ovarian* and *uterine tumors* and masses can feel on bimanual pelvic examination exactly like a rectosigmoid cancer; sigmoidoscopy and barium enema will clarify the matter. Endometriosis may rarely develop as a discrete mass in the rectal wall in young women, but sigmoidoscopy in this circumstance shows no mucosal change.

In the right colon symptoms and signs of cancer are vague at best; *appendicitis* in the elderly, *gallbladder disease,* ovarian *cysts,* intussusception, small bowel obstruction, regional ileitis, and segmental *ulcerative colitis* may simulate cancer and require appropriate x-ray studies for differentiation.

## PREVENTIVE MEASURES

A signal lack of specific knowledge about etiologic factors keeps us from developing any significant program for colorectal cancer prevention. Only in familial polyposis and in certain cases of ulcerative colitis can we employ colectomies for prevention (see below), but these instances are a tiny proportion of the whole large problem. ("Polyp hunting" may achieve early diagnosis, rather than prevention, by keeping cancer-prone persons under surveillance.)

## TREATMENT PRINCIPLES

### Polyps

1. Observe carefully all colons and rectums with small polyps under 1 cm. (remove and destroy those within endoscopic range); reexamine these persons every 6 months for life.

2. Surgically remove the relatively few polyps over 1 cm. in size, as well as those that are obviously growing, and examine the stalk at frozen section, since the incidence of cancer in these larger polypoid lesions is high. If cancer exists in the stalk, one must perform a standard cancer operation.

### Premalignant conditions

**Familial polyposis.** Total or subtotal colectomy in the late teens to prevent the very virulent cancer these patients will inevitably develop before the age of 40.

**Chronic ulcerative colitis.** Total colectomy for all patients with involvement of the whole colon for more than 10 years; careful observation with periodic x-ray films and individualized selective surgery for those with segmental involvement for over 10 years.

### Cancer

1. Surgery provides the mainstay of curative and much palliative treatment.

2. When the tumor lies approximately 12 cm. or more above the anus, a resection of bowel and mesentery with primary anastomosis to restore continuity constitutes the operation of choice.

3. Below 10 cm. most surgeons elect to perform an abdominoperineal resection with permanent colostomy.

4. Palliative resections help most patients; these apply when the cancer is removable but distant metastases prevent cure.

5. Palliative colostomies help only patients with bowel obstruction.

6. Resections of adherent adjacent organs or parts thereof (bladder, uterus, vagina, and small bowel), in addition to standard cancer curative operations when no distant metastases preclude cure, pay good dividends; survival rates approach those of the overall group. Adherence of tumorous bowel to adjacent organs more often results from inflammation than from cancerous invasion. The same surprising benefit accrues to patients with abscesses, fistulas, and free perforations. Panhysterectomy should be done for margin in all low-lying cancers in females.

7. Careful operative technique yields fewer local recurrences by using maneuvers such as covering the outside of the tumor, ligation of the bowel above and below the cancer, early and high ligation of vessels, and excision of crushed bowel ends before suturing.

8. Surgical removal of villous adenomas is done with a moderately conservative procedure as though they were low-grade, nonmetastasizing cancers.

9. Preoperative radiotherapy for rectal and rectosigmoid cancers improves the survival rate for patients whose cancers have metastasized to regional nodes (Duke's C).

10. Irradiation controls many perineal recurrences and can successfully palliate inoperable patients.

11. When the above measures fail, various chemotherapeutic drugs given by several routes achieve short-term palliation in one patient of every five.

12. Squamous carcinoma of the anal area usually requires an abdominal perineal resection with careful consideration of inguinal node dissections if nodes are at all suspicious of metastases.

13. Surgical exploration must be done for most local recurrences, since "second look" resections yield some cures.

## COMMON ERRORS

1. The assumption that blood at stool comes from hemorrhoids, with omission of sigmoidoscopy and a barium enema.
2. Omission of the digital rectal examination in physical examinations.
3. Excessive zeal for radical additions to standard operations, such as pelvic node dissections, para-aortic node dissections, pelvic exenterations, and subtotal colectomy as a prevention against second cancers in which the rare added survivals do not exceed the added operative mortality.
4. Excessive concern for anal sphincter preservation by "pull-through" operations that, in most surgeons' hands, yield unsatisfactory sphincteric control of defecation.
5. Inadequate, "give-up" surgery for localized cancer that involves adjacent organs or for perforated cancers or fistulized cancers because of ignorance of the fair prognosis in these situations.
6. Failure to follow cancer patients for life, since new primaries are frequent.

## PROMISING DEVELOPMENTS FOR THE FUTURE

1. Identification of chemical agents in feces that activate the cancerous process may give us a controllable factor in the causative complex.
2. We need a cytologic screening method for the early detection of colorectal cancer.
3. Wider use of preoperative irradiation may add somewhat to survivals.
4. Fiberoptic "scopes" and the longer sigmoidoscopes that are under development may promote easier and earlier diagnosis.

## PROGNOSIS

Five-year survivals approximate true cures in colorectal cancer, since few patients die of cancer after 5 years.

Survival rates for all patients diagnosed fall in the 25% to 35% range and rise to around 40% in a few well-organized clinics in high intelligence communities. Survivals show definite improvement over the last several decades because of reduced operative mortality, increased operability and resectability, and possibly from somewhat earlier diagnosis. This improvement of roughly 15% in overall figures is now leveling off. Efforts toward earlier diagnosis seem to reward us in the colorectum because asymptomatic tumors found in detection centers nearly all achieve cure.

Polypoid cancers, Duke's A cancers, and those with negative nodes all have survival rates of 65% or better. One half are cured who have resections for cure. High grade lesions, those showing vein invasion, those with positive nodes or adjacent organ extension, or cancers causing acute bowel obstruction or perforation all have a poorer-than-average outlook. One patient in four survives with adjacent organ attachment, fistula, or perforation.

Approximately 30% of patients are incurable on admission to the hospital primarily because of liver metastases. Operative mortality remains at 5% to 10%.

## REFERENCES


Ackerman, L. V., and del Regato, J. A.: Cancer, ed. 3, St. Louis, 1962, The C. V. Mosby Co., pp. 645-706.

Belleau, R., and Braasch, J. W.: Genetics and polyposis, Med. Clin. N. Amer. **50:**379-392, 1966.

Botsford, R. W., Aliapoulios, M. A., and Curtis, L. E.: Results of treatment of colorectal cancer at the Peter Bent Brigham Hospital, Amer. J. Surg. **109:**566-571, 1965.

Castleman, B., and Krickstein, H. I.: Do adenomatous polyps of the colon become malignant? New Eng. J. Med. **267:**469-474, 1962.

Cole, D. R., Rousselot, L. M., and Grossi, C.: Chemotherapy for colorectal cancer, Surg. Clin. N. Amer. **45:**1075-1086, 1965.

Cole, W. H., Roberts, S. S., and Graham, A. L.: Carcinoma of the colon, Arch. Surg. **91:** 547-557, 1965.

Glenn, F., and McSherry, C. K.: Carcinoma of the distal large bowel, Ann. Surg. **163:**838-845, 1966.

Hinton, J. M.: Risks of malignant change in ulcerative colitis, Gut **7:**427-432, 1966.

James, A. G.: Cancer prognosis manual, New York, 1964, American Cancer Society, Inc.

Miller, L. D., Boruchow, I. B., and Fitts, W. J., Jr.: An analysis of 284 patients with perforative carcinoma of the colon, Surg. Gynec. Obstet. **123:**1212-1218, 1966.

Morton, D. L., and Goldman, L.: Diverticulitis and carcinoma of the sigmoid colon, Amer. J. Surg. **103:**55, 1962.

Moss, N. H.: End results in the treatment of cancer of the colon and rectum, Proceedings of Fifth National Cancer Conference, Philadelphia, 1964, J. B. Lippincott Co., pp. 627-633.

Pagtalunan, R. J. G., Dockerty, M. B., Jackman, R. J., and Anderson, M. J., Jr.: Histopathology of diminutive polyps of the large intestine, Surg. Gynec. Obstet. **120:**1259-1265, 1965.

Polk, H. C., Jr., Spratt, J. S., Jr., Bennett, D., Copher, G. H., and Butcher, H. R., Jr.: Surgical mortality and survival from colonic carcinoma, Arch. Surg. **89:**16-23, 1964.

Ramiriz, R. F., Culp, C. E., Jackman, R. J., and Dockerty, M. B.: Villous tumors of the lower part of the large bowel, J.A.M.A. **194:**863-867, 1965.

Rhoads, J. E., Dudrick, G. J., and Miller, L. D.: Colectomy for cancer: techniques and pitfalls, Surg. Clin. N. Amer. **46:**1163-1177, 1966.

Spratt, J. S., Jr., Ackerman, L. V., and Moyer, C. A.: Relationship of polyps of the colon to colonic cancer, Ann. Surg. **148:**682-690, 1958.

Statistics on cancer, Ca Bulletin—publication of American Cancer Society, Inc. **17:**34-43, 1967.

Stearns, M. W., Jr.: Preoperative radiation in carcinoma of the rectum, Proceedings of Fifth National Cancer Conference, Philadelphia, 1964, J. B. Lippincott Co., pp. 489-493.

Stewart, H. L.: Site variation of alimentary tract cancer in man and experimental animals as an indicator of diverse etiology, Harold Dorn Memorial Lecture. In Proceedings of Ninth International Cancer Conference, Tokyo, Oct., 1966, Berlin, 1967, Springer-Verlag, p. 7 (abst.).

Stewart, H. L.: Personal communication, 1966.

Turrell, R., and Haller, J. D.: Adenomas of the colon and rectum, Surg. Clin. N. Amer. **45:** 1117-1139, 1965.

Welch, C. E.: Carcinoma of the colon and rectum, Med. Sci. **11:**266-275, 1962.

Welch, C. E., and Burke, J. F.: Carcinoma of the colon and rectum, New Eng. J. Med. **266:** 211-219, 1962.

Chapter 19

# Cancer of the cervix

The vaginal portion of the cervix possesses a squamous "lining" epithelium that abruptly changes at the external os to a columnar type. This columnar type lines the crypts and irregularities of the endocervix and produces mucus. Both epithelia, nevertheless, produce a more or less uniform type of tumor; the situation is not unlike that obtaining in the oronasopharynx.

## INCIDENCE AND DISTRIBUTION

Cervical cancer comprises 7% of female cancers, exceeded by breast, colorectal, and skin cancer. Incidence and mortality rates have been declining markedly in the last 30 years. Hammond and Seidman show a 50% improvement in death rates from 1930 to 1963 and attribute this partly to better treatment, partly to earlier diagnosis, but mainly to the prevention of the occurrence of invasive cancer by the detection and eradication of precancerous lesions through *cytologic screening.* The total number of new cases per year increases, however, because more carcinomas in situ come to light as the result of ever wider use of cytology, and these lesions are often lumped in with the total group. The incidence of carcinoma in situ and invasive cancer rise and fall together in different populations, supporting the widespread conviction that one precedes the other.

Chile, Japan, Denmark, Portugal, Puerto Rico, and Austria head the list with high incidence rates, whereas at the bottom of the list come Israel, Iceland, Norway, and Australia. American Negro women develop many more cervical cancers than American white women. (Some reasons for this irregular distribution will be suggested below.)

This cancer strikes women at younger ages than most other major neoplasms; the mean age of diagnosis for invasive cancer is 50 years.

## ETIOLOGY

### External initiating agents

Many authorities have documented the close connection between two factors—sexual activity and childbearing—and cancer of the cervix. Early first intercourse, a large number of children, and sexual promiscuity characterize high-risk women; nulliparity, unmarried status, and late marriage describe the low-risk group. Nuns almost never acquire cervical cancer; many prostitutes do acquire it. Jewish women have the lowest incidence of any racial-social group, suggesting that circumcision of males and consequent lower smegma dosage to the cervix may reduce the risk. The evidence indicting smegma is not completely convincing, but it deserves consideration as a main triggering factor, especially when we recall that smegma in the uncircumcised male constitutes a sine qua non for cancer of the penis. More recently a significantly higher antibody titer against a herpeslike virus has been found in women with cervical cancer than in normal women; thus virus initiation is possible. A high incidence of cervical cancer generally prevails among American Negroes, not because of racial, inherited susceptibility, but owing to socioeconomic and other factors (Lundin and associates). Geographic and racial distributions can very likely be explained by analysis of sexual practices.

### Predisposing factors

No one now believes that internal physiologic imbalances or genetic traits exert much influence on cervical cancer development. Emphasis today rests largely on factors cited above; *age at beginning intercourse* seems the most important single factor, followed by circumcision of partner, number of children, etc. Some of these may act by inducing physiologic disturbances that may then bear on etiology.

## PATHOLOGY

*Epidermoid carcinomas* of moderate differentiation comprise the vast majority of cervical cancers. Squamous metaplasia or epidermidization of the columnar epithelium of the cervical canal can easily explain the occurrence of this type in the endocervix. A few at each end of the histologic spectrum are anaplastic or well differentiated. *Adenocarcinomas* make up only 5% of all, have a tortuous glandular pattern, and produce mucin. Rarely a female infant will develop a third type, sarcoma botryoides, which is nearly always fatal.

Most cancers arise at the junction of squamous and columnar epithelium at the external os *(squamocolumnar junction)*. A few cancers arise on the portio vaginalis and some 10% arise in the endocervix. (Our principle that stasis and concentration generally determine location is harder to apply here than in the intestinal tract; other factors, such as cellular instability and susceptibility where two tissues join or the point of maximum dosage of externally introduced substances, seem more important "localizers" in the cervix.)

Epidermoid or squamous cancer can present three different gross appearances: (1) a cauliflower-like *exophytic growth* that expands into the vagina and may infiltrate only slightly at first—a picture of a favorable type of lesion that characterizes other cancers in other organs as well, (2) a *nodular infiltrating variety* that often begins in the endocervix and remains hidden for some time, and (3) the common *ulcerating tumor* that destroys the cervix and leaves a gaping cavity.

Cervical cancer, like mouth cancer, remains localized to adjacent tissues and regional nodes for relatively long periods of time. Spread by direct invasion takes place in any of six directions. After it traverses the tough fibrous stroma of the cervix, the tumor most often gains momentum and progresses laterally, either to one side or the other, in the loose parametrial tissue that is rich with lymphatics and blood vessels. It may also grow in the subepithelium of the vagina, outward into the fornices and downward along the vaginal walls, or else it can grow upward to the internal os and expand into the endometrial cavity. Progression in anterior-posterior directions is less common; when it occurs, the anterior or posterior vaginal fornices can become involved first, or the bladder, uterosacral ligaments, or rectum itself may be invaded directly. The ureters often suffer compression from the tumor-associated fibrosis around them incident to the cancer's parametrial spread.

Lymphatic metastases generally wait until the tumor attains some size; the risk of positive pelvic nodes is directly related to the size of the primary cancer. External iliac, obturator, internal, and common iliac nodes develop metastases in that order. Late in the course blood-borne distant metastases to lungs and bones occur in about half of uncured patients.

**Precancerous lesions**

Throughout history no other area of the human body has ever been so intently studied in so many persons as has the cervix; carcinoma in situ of the cervix has undergone such extensive investigation that it may stand as a model of a cancer precursor lesion. Ackerman states: "It seems certain that carcinoma in situ [of the cervix] precedes the development of infiltrating carcinoma in a high proportion of instances."*

So closely established is its connection with invasive cancer that carcinoma in situ is actually referred to as cancer. Although advantageous for cancer control, this "overcall" may mislead us into believing the following two falsehoods: (1) that carcinoma in situ is a lethal condition and (2) that it always progresses to invasive cancer. It is not lethal and it can remain stationary or even regress, especially during and after pregnancy. Jeffcoate finds that four of every 1000 women have in situ cancer and that somewhere between 30% and 80% will progress to invasive cancer.

Seldom a grossly discernible lesion, carcinoma in situ of the cervix is discovered frequently today because of a happy coincidence of factors: (1) the development of cytology through the Papanicolaou smear and (2) the fact that it usually develops in one small area—the squamocolumnar junction, the cervical canal, and the portio vaginalis. Also it easily desquamates its abnormal cells. Thus a successful screening method becomes possible. Fortunately, also, most women will submit to examination. The lesion has a mean age of appearance at 35 years—10 years earlier than the mean age of invasive cancer. Erickson and Sprunt find evidence that around the time of the menopause, host resistance breaks down and in situ lesions often rapidly become invasive. All agree that the lesion needs complete eradication when found and that this comprises a highly successful cancer prevention measure.

---

*From Ackerman, L. V., and del Regato, J. A.: Cancer, St. Louis, 1962, The C. V. Mosby Co., p. 993.

## NATURAL HISTORY

Owing to the relatively slow growth rate of most cervical cancers, early symptoms are so innocuous that they are considered within normal limits by many premenopausal women. Slight *spotting of blood after coitus,* a little *watery vaginal discharge, elongation of a menstrual period,* or minimal intermenstrual spotting should, but seldom does, occasion an immediate trip to the doctor. As the tumor breaks into surrounding structures after a year or so, discharge of yellow, foul-smelling, infected, or bloody material commences and increases. Vague lumbar back pain, radiating to one hip and down the thigh, may come from parametrial invasion. Extension into the base of the bladder at first causes slight changes in urinary habit, but pain and frequency come later and may gradually worsen until a vesicovaginal fistula develops. A rectovaginal fistula usually appears only after x-ray treatment has weakened local tissues. Lower extremity edema derives from large amounts of pelvic tumor blocking iliac lymphatic and venous channels. The clinical course follows a prolonged downhill pattern, ending after several years in terminal uremia from bilateral ureteral blockage. Sometimes small bowel loops suffer invasion by the pelvic mass of tumor and cause kinking and intestinal obstruction. A cachectic picture may supervene from repeated vaginal hemorrhages, anemia, secondary infection of the tumor-filled vagina, weight loss, and narcotic overuse. Most untreated patients die within 2 years of onset of symptoms, whereas those treated unsuccessfully live in general about 4 years.

## DIAGNOSIS

**History.** Abnormal vaginal bleeding, however slight and thin, persistent vaginal discharge, plus back or hip pain constitute the main presenting complaints of these patients. Duration and intensity of bleeding and discharge do not correlate with the extensiveness of the cancer; in fact, these so-called "early" symptoms result more often from benign cervical and uterine conditions, so that a history does little more than tell us in what anatomical region to begin our investigation. Carcinoma in situ causes no symptoms; any symptoms with the precancerous state result from a coincident, unrelated condition.

**Physical examination.** A speculum inspection of the cervix precedes bimanual examination in the pelvic routine because the Papanicolaou smear (scraping or swabbing of the cervix) needs to be done before there is any disturbance of the desquamated cell depots (cytology is described below). In inspecting the cervix, one gains help from painting it with an iodine solution *(Schiller test)* to outline areas that do not stain and thus have abnormal mucosa. Unstained areas and lesions need biopsy. After this, vaginal-abdominal and vaginal-rectal-abdominal bimanual examinations are performed to determine the extent of the tumor and assign the clinical stage. One feels for thickening, fixation, and nodules in the various fornices surrounding the cervix, the parametria on either side, and the rectovaginal septum in the lower vaginal tract, and then one palpates each lateral pelvic wall for lumps suggesting metastatic lymph nodes.

Staging of the cervical cancer must be done largely at this same time if the diagnosis is reasonably certain. Staging consists of a clinical estimate of *extent* of the cancer, and one generally follows the international staging system (Fig. 15):

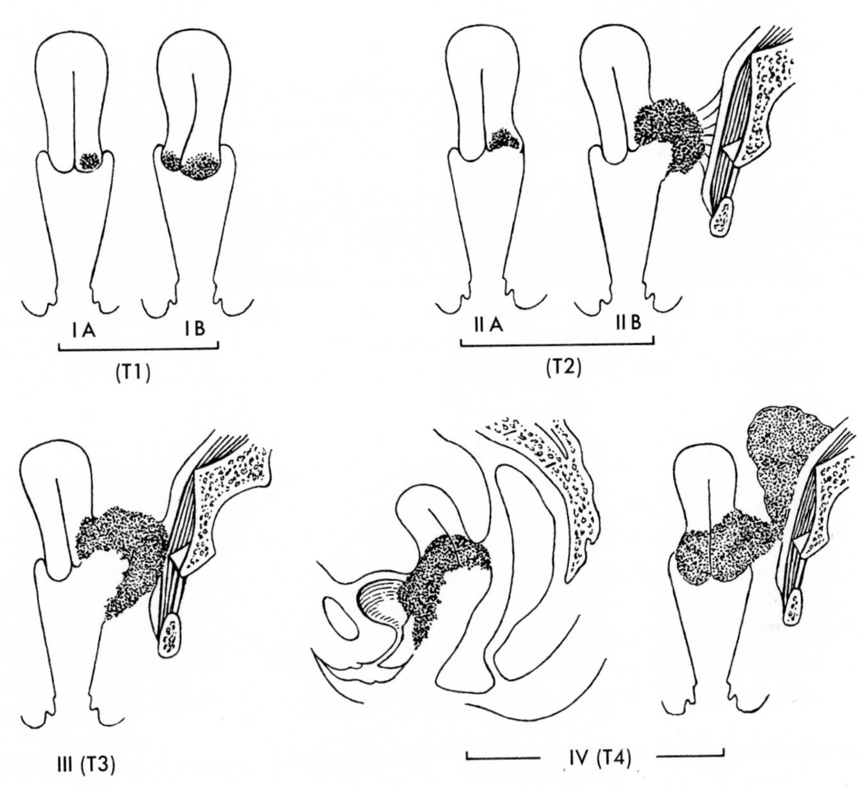


**Fig. 15.** Simplified version of staging for cancer of the cervix, using the international classification (IA, IB, IIA, IIB, III, IV—see text) and corresponding "T" groupings from the TNM system. (Copyright privileges do not apply to these drawings. Permission for reproduction is given by the American Joint Committee for Cancer Staging and End Results Reporting, which specifically wishes these drawings to remain in the public domain.)

Stage O—carcinoma in situ—no invasion; Stage I (A and B)—limited to cervix proper; Stage II (A and B)—spread to upper vagina or parametria; Stage III—spread to lower vagina and/or laterally to the pelvic wall; and Stage IV—spread outside pelvis proper, bladder or rectal invasion, or metastatic nodes.

**Cytology.** Most value accrues from smears in the *normal-appearing cervix.* Although a positive or suspicious cervical smear does not constitute a definitive diagnosis in the cervix, it is an absolute indication for further studies, such as four-quadrant biopsy, conization, and careful follow-up. The preferred method of obtaining a smear consists in swabbing the external os with a cotton-tipped applicator, or scraping it with a wooden spatula and then smearing the material on two slides that are immediately dropped into 95% alcohol as a fixative. As mentioned before, this smear precedes the bimanual examination.

**Endocervical scraping smear.** This is probably a good routine and is especially indicated for all symptomatic patients. One obtains cytologic material from the endocervix with a tiny curet.

**Biopsy.** Punch biopsies with a sharp, biting forceps (Fig. 16) give us a definitive diagnosis of any abnormality, lesion, or iodine-negative area of mucosa. Whereas

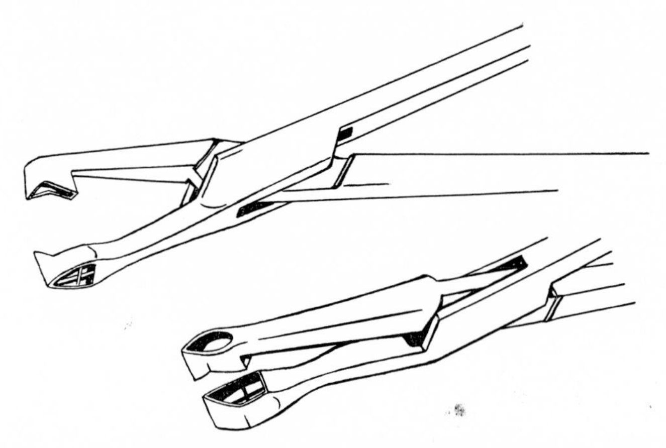

**Fig. 16.** Preferred type of biopsy instrument. Open, sharp-pointed, sharp-edged jaws interdigitate and accurately secure an undistorted sliver of tissue exactly where desired. It also facilitates biopsy of lesions of the skin and mouth.

smears are appropriate for surveying all cervices, biopsies are reserved for abnormal cervices and have value in assessing the slightest irregularity. Four, or as many as six to eight, biopsies around the circumference of the cervix, if processed carefully, can survey a cervix nearly as well as a conization. The colposcope helps considerably in selecting biopsy sites. The colpomicroscope aids investigative studies of cervical lesions in large clinics. If a biopsy shows invasive cancer, conization is unnecessary.

**Conization.** When carcinoma in situ appears in a cytologic smear or biopsy, cold knife conization generally follows to determine if invasive cancer also accompanies the precursor lesion. Multiple "quadrant" biopsies, if carefully spaced, may suffice. Some gynecologists advocate conization after two consecutive smears that show dysplasia, the term given to cellular atypia theoretically approaching full-blown carcinoma in situ. In taking a cone, one cores out the full circumference of squamocolumnar junction and most of the endocervical canal. This can be a formidable procedure because of the bleeding, and can later result in cervical stenosis.

**Fractional curettage of the endocervix.** Sometimes smears and biopsies prove negative, but abnormal bleeding or discharge persists. In such instances a dilatation and curettage must be performed, but one must keep a fractional, sequential separation of the specimens for accurate diagnosis. One first scrapes the endocervix, then scrapes the lower and then the upper endometrial cavity, and finally does cervical biopsies if these are indicated, keeping all these tissues in separate bottles.

**Endoscopy.** When cancer is present or especially when one contemplates surgery, the complete diagnostic study includes cystoscopy and sigmoidoscopy. Usually only slight puckering or bullous edema of the mucosa marks the site of cancerous invasion of the outer walls of bladder or rectum, but these signs are not diagnostic of cancerous invasion.

**X-ray studies.** An *intravenous pyelogram* forms a part of a complete cervical cancer work-up. Hydronephrosis, abnormal curves in the normal course of the ureters (from metastatic nodes), may appear in these films. Retrograde pyelograms may be needed to confirm suggested irregularities. Pelvic lymphography and venography still fall in the class of experimental tools.

**Laboratory studies.** We require at least two studies—blood counts to find anemia, if present, and a blood urea nitrogen to further assess kidney function (which may be impaired from chronic ureteral blockage).

### Differential diagnosis

Many small, insignificant cervical changes can resemble early invasive cancer: (1) eversion of the endocervical mucosa, especially in the lacerated cervix, (2) traumatic ulcerations, (3) inflammations such as with *Trichomonas*, (4) "cervical erosions," and (5) decidual reaction of pregnancy in the cervical mucosa. All may need biopsy to differentiate them from cancer.

*Chronic cervicitis* also mimics early cancer, but possesses a fibrotic character with a hypertrophied, chronically inflamed cervix.

*Cervical polyps* are usually present at the external os on a stalk and are well circumscribed and nonulcerated—a picture seldom produced by cancer. They have no more cancer potential than a normal endocervix.

Tuberculosis and syphilis of the cervix are rare.

*Cancer of the corpus* extending down into the cervix needs biopsy and fractional curettage for differentiation.

*Cervical endometriosis* from implantation of fragments shed from above can cause a hemorrhagic submucosal lesion with persistent metrorrhagia.

## PREVENTIVE MEASURES

1. *Yearly cervical smears* on all females over 20 years, or beginning at the age of marriage, will prevent cancer by discovering and treating precancer and by accomplishing earlier case finding of invasive cancer. When initiated in a whole population such a plan selects out the cancers and in situ lesions in a few years. The majority of women who will have had several consecutive negative smears may then wait longer intervals for their smears, such as every 2 or 3 years. Ideally, pelvic examinations by doctors should accompany smears, but this is impractical in screening a large population and would limit the cancer-preventive result of such screening.

2. Female promiscuity and very early intercourse seem firmly linked to cervical cancer; its avoidance might help prevent neoplasia.

3. Special attention to clean habits by the uncircumcised male may reduce cancer by lowering smegma exposure of the cervix; clean practices in all phases of sexual intercourse also seem worthwhile.

## TREATMENT PRINCIPLES

1. *X-ray therapy* constitutes the most accepted treatment for cancer of the cervix.

2. Irradiation needs ideal circumstances to be successful; if excessive pelvic deformity, vaginal abnormality, uncontrolled pelvic infection, or previous surgery

prevent an ideal treatment plan, one needs to consider primary surgery instead. Surgeon-radiotherapist consultations are of help just as in the mouth and throat because the types of cancer and problems of treatment by irradiation and surgery are generally similar in both areas.

3. A combination of intracavitary (cervical canal and uterine cavity) radium and external x-ray therapy serves as the basic plan. Del Regato states that radium plays a major role in early cases; external therapy does the major job in advanced cases.

4. Surgery can cure nearly as many Stage I and early Stage II lesions as x-ray therapy, but surgeons trained to do this tedious, extensive dissection are few, and the urinary complications run high in the best of hands.

5. Radical pelvic (exenterative) surgery provides the only hopeful treatment for recurrent cancer or cancers with bladder or rectal invasion and for the few patients with extensive radionecrosis.

6. Retreatment with x-ray after a first full course achieves little benefit as a rule.

7. Treated cancer patients need to make follow-up visits for the rest of their lives, every 2 to 3 months for 3 years, and every 6 months from then on.

8. Total hysterectomy plus a vaginal cuff adequately treats carcinoma in situ in older women. Younger women may have a conization and, if no invasive cancer shows up, can bear children, provided they submit to close follow-up with periodic smears.

9. Modern chemotherapy does not offer much worthwhile palliation in cervical cancer.

## COMMON ERRORS

1. Poorly planned and poorly executed radiotherapy jeopardizes the chance for cure.

2. If the patient undergoes total hysterectomy and the specimen contains unsuspected invasive cancer, as sometimes happens due to inadequate diagnostic studies and procedures, ideal treatment is impossible.

3. Many recurrent cancers receive retreatment with x-ray, often constituting overdosage. This compromises possible surgical success later and has little chance of curing the patient.

4. Many practitioners omit conization when smears or biopsies show carcinoma in situ. This risks error *2* above.

5. Many physicians prevent their patients from having an exenteration for recurrent cancer because they have not seen successes with this surgery. They fail to appreciate that most such patients (who are mothers in their 40's, with young children) would gladly accept the risk and deformity of pelvic exenteration for a 25% chance of survival.

6. Failure to follow patients closely prevents the detection of recurrence at the earliest possible time.

## PROMISING DEVELOPMENTS FOR THE FUTURE

1. The popularization of cervical cytology for all women over 20 will effectively reduce cervical cancer to a negligible public health problem, even though by

itself cytology will never entirely eliminate cervical cancer. A few cancers will always grow and spread too quickly for early detection and some may show no precancerous phase. Several pilot studies of mass cervical smear screening have already demonstrated the reduction of cervical cancer incidence by nearly half and a doubling of the percentage of early Stage I cases. This is modern medicine's most outstanding contribution to cancer control; when all large communities undergo mass screening it will surely save many more lives than the vaccine for poliomyelitis. Hammond and Seidman estimate that various cervical cancer control measures, principally cytologic testing, have spared nearly 200,000 women in the past 33 years.

2. Cryosurgery holds interest as a measure of ablating cervical and endocervical precancerous lesions.

## PROGNOSIS

Of all the major cancers, cervical cancer perhaps carries the best overall prognosis. More than half of all patients achieve permanent control of their neoplasms. We list the prospects for various stages of disease according to the widely used international classification of staging, which is also easily convertible to the TNM staging system (Chapter 34):

| | |
|---|---|
| Stage O ($T_0$) | 100% 5-year survival |
| Stage I ($T_1$) | 75% 5-year survival |
| Stage II ($T_2$) | 55% 5-year survival |
| Stage III ($T_3$) | 35% 5-year survival |
| Stage IV ($T_4$) | 7% 5-year survival |
| All stages | 55% 5-year survival |

Nearly one patient of every four with recurrent cancer may survive through pelvic exenteration (Brunschwig and Daniel and Bricker). Positive pelvic lymph nodes constitute a poor prognostic sign, but not a hopeless one. Several studies report salvaging 20% of patients with node metastases.

### REFERENCES

Ackerman, L. V., and del Regato, J. A.: Cancer, ed. 3, St. Louis, 1962, The C. V. Mosby Co., pp. 982-1032.

Bricker, E. M.: Management of recurrent cancer of the cervix, Postgrad. Med. **35:**145-149, 1964.

Brunschwig, A., and Daniel, W. W.: The surgical attack upon gynecologic cancer, Proceedings of Fourth National Cancer Conference, Philadelphia, 1961, J. B. Lippincott Co., pp. 343-347.

Clinical staging system for carcinoma of the cervix, American Joint Committee for Staging and End Results Reporting, Feb., 1964.

Erickson, C. L., and Sprunt, D. H.: The duration of intraepithelial and preclinical squamous cell carcinoma of the uterine cervix, Proceedings of Ninth International Cancer Conference, Tokyo, Oct., 1966, Berlin, 1967, Springer-Verlag, p. 1044.

Fletcher, G. H., Rutledge, F. M., and Chau, P. M.: Policies of treatment in cancer of the cervix uteri, Amer. J. Roentgen. **87:**6-14, 1962.

Frick, H. C., II, Atchoo, N., Adamsons, K. J., and Taylor, H. C., Jr.: Efficacy of chemotherapeutic agents in management of disseminated gynecologic cancer, Amer. J. Obstet. Gynec. **93:**1112-1121, 1966.

Gray, L. A., editor: Dysplasia, carcinoma in situ and microinvasive carcinoma of the cervix uteri, Springfield, Ill., 1964, Charles C Thomas, Publisher.

Hammond, E. C., and Seidman, H.: Progress in the control of cancer of the uterus, Arch. Environ. Health **13:**105-116, 1966.

Jeffcoate, T. N. A.: Cervical cytology, Brit. Med. J. **2:**1091-1094, 1966.

Kottmeier, H. L.: Current treatment of carcinoma of the cervix, Amer. J. Obstet. Gynec. **76:**243-251, 1958.

Lundin, F. E., Christopherson, W. M., Mendez, W. M., and Parker, J. E.: Morbidity from cervical cancer: effects of cervical cytology and socio-economic status, J. Nat. Cancer Inst. **35:**1015-1025, 1965.

Papanicolaou, G. N.: A general survey of the vaginal smear and its use in research and diagnosis, Amer. J. Obstet. Gynec. **51:**316-324, 1946.

Pederson, B. L., and Jeffries, F. W.: Cervical carcinoma in situ, Obstet. Gynec. **26:**725-730, 1965.

Stallworthy, J.: The malignant uterus yesterday, today, and tomorrow, J.A.M.A. **195:**465-470, 1966.

Wall, J. A., Collins, V. P., Hudgins, P. T., Kaplan, A. L., and Adams, R. M.: Carcinoma of the cervix, Amer. J. Obstet. Gynec. **96:**57-63, 1966.

Chapter 20

# Cancer of the body of the uterus

Throughout a woman's fertile life the epithelial lining of the uterus undergoes profound cyclical changes in response to hormones. As we might expect from studying tumors of other endocrine target organs (thyroid, breast), most tumors of the uterine endometrium react markedly to hormones.

## INCIDENCE AND DISTRIBUTION

Cancer of the endometrial lining of the uterine cavity occurs less often than cancer of the cervix and comprises 2% of female cancers. Unaccountably, the incidence appears to be rising. This neoplasm accounts for 95% of uterine body cancers, and sarcomas account for the remaining 5%. No noteworthy geographic variations exist as far as we know. Endometrial cancer typically attacks infertile, postmenopausal women of high socioeconomic status, just the opposite from cancer of the cervix. Peak age of incidence comes at around 60 years.

## ETIOLOGY

### External initiating agents

Again in complete contrast to the picture of cervical cancer, endometrial cancer develops more often in unmarried, nulliparous women who would contact fewer external substances introduced through the vaginal tract than most other women. Environmental agents would have difficulty reaching the endometrial canal anyway. We cannot now implicate any environmental or external triggering agents in the genesis of this cancer. The uncommon endometrial sarcomas seem to show a high association with prior pelvic irradiation for other conditions.

### Predisposing factors

Although environmental carcinogens play no known role, several constitutional abnormalities, all related to excess estrogenic hormone, clearly do characterize the women likely to acquire endometrial cancer. The disease tends to develop in anovulatory women, those whose menstrual cycles have been irregular, women with endometrial hyperplasias, women with a late menopause, and women with estrogen-secreting ovarian tumors (20% of granulosa-theca cell tumors have associate endometrial cancers), and the disease has been correlated in some cases with prolonged exogenous estrogen administration. Endometrial cancer patients also show a strong tendency to be obese, to be hirsute, to have diabetes or a diabetic glucose tolerance curve, and to have hypertension—all conditions possibly connected with hormonal imbalance. This tumor might be considered one manifestation of a polyglandular endocrinopathy. Women subjected to oophorectomy in early life seldom acquire endometrial cancer; the same is true in women with breast cancer.

Three fourths of these cancers occur ten or more years *postmenopause,* reflecting the long period of "stage setting" needed for this complex endocrinopathy to work. This pattern also resembles the one often described in breast cancer patients. McKay stresses prolonged anovulation as the common denominator of the precursor events, which makes us wonder about the long-term effect of the contraceptive "pill."

## PATHOLOGY

Two gross types of endometrial carcinoma develop: (1) the *discrete* tumor mass that may be sessile or polypoid and is usually exophytic and growing into the cavity (sometimes it also infiltrates the musculature by the time of diagnosis) and (2) the *diffuse* variety that involves the entire cavity with a thin, pale, friable layer of tumor exuding mucus and blood.

Rarely *leiomyosarcomas* will arise from the common uterine myoma (fibromyoma, leiomyoma), causing these rubbery tumors to become reddish and softer. Even more unusual are the *malignant mesodermal mixed tumors* and other *endometrial stromal sarcomas* (fibromyxosarcoma, carcinosarcoma) that grow from a broad pedicle, usually on the posterior wall of the fundus. The mesodermal mixed tumors derive from the epithelium of the müllerian duct. (A summary of data on *hydatid mole, chorioadenoma destruens,* and *choriocarcinoma*—all neoplastic conditions of the trophoblast—will be found at the end of this chapter.)

Spread of cancer of the endometrium occurs slowly and relatively late and allows the primary tumor to become locally bulky without metastasis. It often grows directly through the myometrium to the serosa, involves intestines or bladder, and can seed implants on the peritoneal surfaces. Or it may invade the broad ligaments. Twenty percent metastasize to pelvic lymph nodes, 10% mestastasize to ovaries, and occasionally inguinal nodes harbor metastases that arrive by way of lymphatics in the round ligaments. Blood-borne emboli grow to metastases in lungs and liver late in the clinical course. The sarcomas also tend to grow as expanding local tumors, generally do not metastasize to regional nodes, and travel by the bloodstream as a late phenomenon.

Under the microscope most of the adenocarcinomas of the endometrium show moderate differentiation, although a full range of morphology from almost normal-appearing endometrium to complete anaplasia occurs. It is believed that any invasion or displacement of the endometrial stroma indicates definite carcinoma, a criterion which plays a key role in the numerous cases in which hyperplasia must be distinguished from cancer.

### Precancerous lesions

Gore and Hertig have demonstrated that *carcinoma in situ* of the endometrium commonly precedes invasive cancer, just as in the cervix. They believe that cancer never arises from normal epithelium. Some authorities trace the histogenesis of endometrial cancer from endometrial cystic hyperplasia through adenomatous hyperplasia to carcinoma in situ to invasive cancer, both in serial human biopsies over a period of years and in experimentally induced animal tumors. The first of these lesions, cystic hyperplasia, certainly can be reversed by curettage or medication and does not qualify as precancerous, since approximately one in 100 patients with it develops cancer.

*Adenomatous hyperplasia* causes us more concern because a sizable proportion proceed, after several years, to the in situ stage. Carcinoma in situ itself, sometimes termed "atypical hyperplasia" or "severe adenomatous hyperplasia," qualifies as a definite precursor lesion. Many of these progress to invasive cancer in an average period of 6 to 8 years. Often found in the same uterus with, and adjacent to, invasive carcinoma, the in situ stage deserves the same careful attention and eradication as does cervical cancer in situ. No typical gross appearance characterizes carcinoma in situ; it is a microscopic diagnosis. As yet we cannot clearly define the role estrogens play in its development.

Cancer may arise now and then from the endometrial polyps that occur so commonly in association with endometrial cancer (35% of endometrial cancer patients also have polyps). But polyps probably stem from the same antecedent conditions as do cancers. Polyps appear to be precursors about as infrequently as they do in the rectum.

## NATURAL HISTORY

Malignant tumors of the uterine cavity usually manifest themselves after the menopause at an age when vaginal bleeding or a thin, watery discharge are definitely abnormal and usually cause alarm. If nothing is done, however, the tumor grows at a slow rate, doubling its size in 6 months or so, and perhaps taking several years to penetrate through the serosa to the outside of the uterus. As the cancer enlarges, bleeding may increase to hemorrhage, pieces of necrotic tumors may extrude and be passed vaginally, or menstrual "cramps" can occur from retained blood in the cavity. Pain in the back, hips, or thighs develops with further intrapelvic expansion, and when the mass becomes large enough, compression of the bladder and rectum may occasion frequent, painful urination or constipation. Patients often live 4 or more years in comfort; death usually comes from uncontrolled local complications such as infection or massive hemorrhage.

## DIAGNOSIS

**History.** Because the main complaint engendered by this tumor is recognized as a danger signal by most women, postmenopausal vaginal bleeding leads them to an early visit to the physician. Premenopausal irregular bleeding largely stems from benign conditions, but in the postmenopausal period 50% of bleeding patients harbor malignant or premalignant tumors. Bleeding can be an early or a late sign. Only 10% of patients will complain first of abnormal vaginal discharge.

**Physical examination.** As an office routine, speculum examination of the cervix and a cytologic smear come first. Then on bimanual pelvic examination one feels for uterine enlargement, asymmetry, fixation, and adnexal masses that could represent associated ovarian neoplasms.

**Cytology.** Cervical smears will pick up desquamated endometrial tumor cells in only 50% to 70% of the endometrial tumor cases. We need a more dependable screening test for endometrial cancer. In approaching the most accurate diagnosis possible in the office, we can employ endometrial aspiration smears in all cases of unexplained bleeding; these smears yield an accuracy of 85%. Used together with office diagnostic procedures directed at the cervix (smear, Schiller test, biopsy), these procedures can achieve over 90% accuracy in uterine cancer diagnosis. Endometrial aspiration can be done frequently and easily, if practiced, and in some instances a good preparation by aspiration can save the patient a formal dilatation and curettage in hospital, be less traumatic, and cause less risk of cancer spread.

**Dilatation of the cervix and curettage of the uterine cavity.** General anesthesia in the hospital is needed for this procedure, which produces a definitive diagnosis if office endometrial biopsy has not done so. In cases in which a cervical smear is positive and the cervix normal, it constitutes the equivalent of a full biopsy survey of the cavity. It can by bypassed only when aspiration gives a good specimen and the clinical picture is clear. Fractional curettage, described before, yields accurate information about the extent of the tumor. At the time of curettage, with the patient asleep and completely relaxed, the physician has a good chance to perform a more informative bimanual pelvic examination in the obese patient.

**X-ray studies.** X-ray studies contribute little to this diagnosis.

**Laboratory studies.** Laboratory tests also are of little importance in diagnosis, although eight of nine patients with endometrial cancer exhibit high vaginal cornification indexes.

### Differential diagnosis

*Submucous myoma* will cause abnormal bleeding, but it can be readily diagnosed by combining manual examination and curettage. These tumors tend to shrink after the menopause. However, some reports show that one third of endometrial cancers have an incidental myoma too. Therefore a full office work-up, including endometrial aspiration smear, constitutes the only way to detect the true source of abnormal bleeding.

*Endometritis* and *endometrial polyps* can easily be differentiated, grossly and microscopically, from cancer.

*Adenocarcinoma of the endocervix* and endometrial cancer with cervical extension can be distinguished from each other by careful clinical and histologic study.

## PREVENTIVE MEASURES

Ablation of the severe hyperplasias and carcinoma in situ by curettement or medication in the young and hysterectomy in older women can prevent some endometrial cancers. This implies wide use of endometrial aspiration smears to diagnose the precancerous states.

## TREATMENT PRINCIPLES

1. A combination of preoperative irradiation and surgery generally prevails as the ideal method.

2. The first step usually consists of intracavitary radium, followed in 4 to 6 weeks by the second step—total abdominal hysterectomy, bilateral salpingo-oophorectomy, plus a generous vaginal cuff.

3. Patients unsuitable for operation because of medical complications or wide tumor extension receive full irradiation as complete treatment. Some experts prefer x-ray therapy alone as definitive treatment.

4. Patients unsuitable for ideal irradiation because of a suspicion of ovarian tumor, multiple large myoma, persistent pyometra, etc. can often be treated quite successfully with surgery alone.

5. Massive progesterone dosage for uncontrolled cancer or distant metastasis seems worthwhile, especially in well-differentiated tumors that are likely to be responsive. (The rationale for such treatment is that progesterone causes maturation of normal endometrium and actually causes similar changes in many endometrial neoplasms.) Both Delalutin and Provera prove effective.

6. Irradiation receives first trial in isolated or vaginal recurrences.

7. Surgery is needed, as a rule, for leiomyosarcomas, which do not respond well to x-ray therapy.

8. Dilatation and curettage plus progesterone and nonsteroidal estrogens can be tried, with close follow-up, in younger patients with carcinoma in situ of the endometrium. Hysterectomy provides the best measure for older women with this lesion.

## COMMON ERRORS

We often fail to appreciate the importance of adenomatous hyperplasia and the value of close follow-up care with endometrial smears and biopsies for women with this condition.

## PROMISING DEVELOPMENTS FOR THE FUTURE

1. Refinements of the endometrial smear technique, plus added data about hyperplasias, may occur to make this as accurate a screening technique as cervical cytology.

2. A study of hormonal adjuvants to x-ray therapy and surgery is now under way and shows some promise of improving the total results of treatment.

## PROGNOSIS

The outlook in general is quite good for endometrial cancer. A tumor that spreads slowly and a patient population that responds readily to first symptoms combine to give physicians a satisfactory therapeutic advantage. Two thirds of patients present with localized cancers. Luckily, the kind of surgery and x-ray therapy needed here do *not* involve difficult, expensive, or unavailable techniques.

As a round figure, 60% of patients survive 5 years. The Mayo Clinic reports 80%. Factors auguring for a poorer prognosis include anaplastic tumors, deep invasion of the myometrium, cervical extension, large uterine cavity, metastases, and tumors that have grown quite large in older women whose medical complications prevent ideal treatment.

In incurable cases, massive progesterone therapy has induced "objective remissions" in 30% of patients.

A TNM system of clinical staging, not unlike that for cervix, probably serves best for future reports (see Chapter 34).

## CHORIOCARCINOMA OF THE CHORIONIC VILLI (TROPHOBLASTIC DISEASE)

An extremely interesting but rare group of tumors develop now and then from the products of conception; these neoplasms respond remarkably well to chemotherapy. Since they represent medicine's first and, perhaps, only cure of cancer with drugs and since they do occur *in* the uterus, we have elected to treat them in this chapter, but separately.

Choriocarcinoma of the trophoblastic tissues seldom occurs in the United States, but it does occur with some frequency in China, the Philippine Islands, and Indonesia. Authorities suggest that its occurrence is related to a large number of pregnancies in rapid succession. A full range of benign to malignant tumor varieties develop, from the harmless hydatidiform mole through the locally invasive chorioadenoma destruens to the metastasizing, fully malignant choriocarcinoma; the whole group bears the name trophoblastic disease (Hertz and associates). The metastasizing cancerous form seems to evolve from benign moles in half of the instances and follows either abortions or term pregnancies in the rest. Despite the fact that villi are not recognized in fully developed choriocarcinoma, the chorionic villi are considered to be the tissue of origin in all forms of trophoblastic disease.

Diagnosis of these tumors ensues from recognition of typical cystic structures that pass from the uterus in cases of mole and from uterine curettage specimens in chorioadenoma and carcinoma. High *urinary chorionic gonadotrophin* titers from the tumor's production of this hormone frequently help establish the diagnosis and indicate response to treatment.

This cancer exhibits great sensitivity to x-ray therapy and to drugs (methotrexate). Strangely, choriocarcinoma of the testicle does not respond to methotrexate, although it demonstrates more sensitivity to other drugs (actinomycin D) than many cancers. Choriocarcinoma of the chorion also frequently undergoes spontaneous regression, both of the primary site in the uterus and in the lung metastases. Hertz and associates at the National Cancer Institute have established long-term clinical control in over half of these cancers with metastases by drug therapy, supplemented at times with surgery. Their work serves as the authoritative, possible life-saving source of management details for any woman with choriocarcinoma or chorioadenoma.

### REFERENCES

Aaro, L. A., Symmonds, R. E., and Dockerty, M. B.: Sarcoma of the uterus, Amer. J. Obstet. Gynec. **94:**101-109, 1966.

Ackerman, L. V., and del Regato, J. A.: Cancer, ed. 3, St. Louis, 1962, The C. V. Mosby Co., pp. 959-981, 1035-1037.

Gore, H., and Hertig, A. T.: Carcinoma in situ of the endometrium, Amer. J. Obstet. Gynec. **94:**134-155, 1966.

Hahn, G. A.: The endometrium. In Nealon, T. F., Jr., editor: Management of the patient with cancer, Philadelphia, 1966, W. B. Saunders Co., pp. 739-757.

Hecht, E. L., and Oppenheim, A.: The cytology of endometrial cancer, Surg. Gynec. Obstet. **122:**1025-1029, 1966.

Hertz, R., Ross, G. T., and Lipsett, M. B.: Chemotherapy in women with trophoblasic disease: choriocarcinoma, chorioadenoma destruens and complicated hydatidiform mole, Ann. N. Y. Acad. Sci. **114:**881-885, 1964.

Javert, C. T.: Cancer of the endometrium. In Postgraduate course on malignant disease in the female pelvis, Chicago, October, 1967, American College of Surgeons 53rd Clinical Congress.

McKay, D. G.: A review of the status of endometrial cancer, Cancer Res. **25:**1182-1187, 1965.

Wall, J. A., Collins, V. P., Kaplan, A. L., and Hudgins, P. T.: Adenocarcinoma of the endometrium, Amer. J. Obstet. Gynec. **97:**787-799, 1967.

Chapter 21

# Cancer of the ovary

Many different tissues compose the ovary—germ cells, endocrine-producing cells, inert supporting cells, and epithelial cells. Therefore we find in the ovary a variety of benign and malignant neoplasms—in fact, such a variety that they defy easy classification. As we would expect in any endocrine gland, many of the ovarian tumors produce hormones and involve hormonal relationships in their etiology.

## INCIDENCE AND DISTRIBUTION

Ovarian cancer has been on the increase during this century in the United States and now approaches 5% of all female cancers. Its mortality rate equals that of cancer of the cervix, although its incidence rate remains lower. For no clear reason Scandinavia shows an occurrence rate twice as high as North America, whereas a relatively low incidence prevails in Chile and other parts of South America and in Japan.

Only one in every six ovarian tumors is malignant. Most carcinomas develop so as to be diagnosed between the ages of 40 to 60 years. A small group of interesting benign and malignant neoplasms present in infancy and childhood (see below).

## ETIOLOGY

### External initiating agents

No definite clues exist here for human tumors. X-rays, some hormones, and other exogenously applied agents produce ovarian tumors in mice by direct action on the ovaries (reduction of the number of follicles), but no evidence indicts these agents in the causation of cancer in man. Theoretically, external agents could also act indirectly by causing an imbalance in the reciprocal ovarian-pituitary hormonal relationship, but we know of no particular agent that merits suspicion in this respect.

### Predisposing factors

In animals a variety of internal functional manipulations will induce ovarian tumors; all of these have in common one basic alteration—lowered steroid production and the secondary increase of pituitary gonadotrophins. By analogy such a hormonal imbalance may possibly act as a disposing influence in humans. Such a concept receives support from the fact that most ovarian cancers occur around the time of the menopause when ovarian function declines, gonadotrophin levels rise, and the menstrual rhythm ceases. In the dysgerminomas of childhood an accompanying maldevelopment of the sex organs indicates that a profound *embryologic disturbance* formed a background for these tumors. No doubt the other rare ovarian neoplasms of childhood occur with antecedent irregularities of fetal development as well.

## PATHOLOGY

Remembering that most ovarian tumors are benign and that the distinction between benign and malignant growths may give great difficulty at times, we must accord considerable attention to the benign neoplasms of the ovary. Most of the numerous classifications for ovarian neoplasms serve mainly as aids to prognosis, such as groupings by type of hormone secreted, by anatomic extent of spread, or by the histologic grade of the tumor. But only a *histogenetic* classification helps us to understand tumors, and we intend to present a reasonable formulation of this "cell of origin" grouping, despite controversy over some points.

According to Abell, *four histogenetic categories* deserve our attention: tumors derived from (1) *germinal epithelium,* (2) *germ cells,* (3) *specialized stroma,* and (4) *nonspecialized stroma.*

**Germinal epithelium.** Tumors of the germinal (surface) epithelium of the ovary are usually cystic, comprise most of the common neoplasms, and occur during a woman's reproductive years and up to the age of 65; the older the woman, the greater the chance of cancer. Five subclasses exist:

1. *Serous tumors* account for 40% of all ovarian neoplasms; half of them are malignant and half occur bilaterally. Cancers in this subgroup show greater invasiveness and aggressiveness than most other kinds. Examples are the *serous cystadenoma* and serous papilloma and their malignant counterparts, *serous cystadenocarcinoma* and *papillary serous carcinoma.*

2. *Mucinous tumors* are less common than the serous tumors, with a predominant cell type that resembles the mucin-secreting endocervical cell. (Some physicians believe these tumors have a teratomatous origin and that the mucinous cells represent intestinal epithelium.) Characteristically multicystic, they can attain a huge size. Mucinous cancer behaves less dangerously than the serous kind; examples are the *mucinous cystadenoma* (90%) and *mucinous cystadenocarcinoma* (10%).

3. *Endometrioid tumors* grow as fairly well-differentiated neoplasms resembling endometrial tissue; benign *cystomas* and malignant *cystadenocarcinomas* both occur. These cancers behave even better than the mucinous cancers.

4. *Brenner tumors* may come from (a) Walthard's cell rests, (b) metaplasia of germinal epithelium, and (c) metaplasia in a preexisting mucinous tumor. They are uncommon and nearly always benign; they grow from the hilum of the ovary as solid, nonfunctioning, silent neoplasms.

5. *Mixed tumors* and *unclassifiable* carcinomas are usually solid tumors.

**Germ cells.** Tumors of germ cells of the ovary include teratomatous growths, many of which are the common *"dermoid" cysts.* These neoplasms resemble tumors of similar origin in the testicle and arise from somatic differentiation of the multipotential germ cells. If the primitive, undifferentiated cell has matured very little when forming a neoplasm, an aggressive, *malignant embryonal teratoma* results that comes to our attention during childhood because of rapid growth pattern. When the cell matures fully, benign, usually cystic growths evolve with mature structures from ectoderm, mesoderm, and entoderm frequently present (dermoid cyst). Since mature teratomas are benign, they frequently escape detection until later life.

Three classes of *germ cell neoplasms* occur:

1. *Dysgerminoma,* a malignant tumor of childhood, is often associated with sexual maldevelopment, but is without specific endocrine secretion itself.

2. *Teratomas* develop quite frequently, with varying degrees of differentiation from embryonal to mature, cystic to solid; they are most often benign. *Dermoid cysts* comprise one of the commonest of benign ovarian tumors; malignant embryonal teratomas are rare.

3. *Mixed varieties* occur, including malignant types.

**Specialized stroma.** Tumors of specialized ovarian stroma consist of those that often produce steroid hormones. Three subgroups warrant attention:

1. *Granulosa-theca cell* neoplasms generally secrete estrogen and cause precocious puberty in childhood and excess feminization in adults. Sometimes they manufacture other hormones as well, which result in masculinizing signs; however, precocious virilization never stems from ovarian neoplasms, but from adrenal tumors. After the menopause, granulosa cell tumors may cause recurrence of uterine bleeding and endometrial hyperplasia, and they have often been associated with endometrial carcinoma (Chapter 20). These growths deserve treatment as low-grade malignant tumors, although only one in five shows histologic cancer.

2. The rare *Sertoli-Leydig* cell group of tumors arise from sex-cord elements and mesenchyme in the hilar region of the ovary and resemble "opposite number" tumors of the testes. The Leydig cell produces testosterone, causes masculinization, is always benign, favors menopausal ages, and occurs in dysgenetic ovaries. The *Sertoli cell tumor,* by its estrogen production, causes feminization in adults and precocious puberty in children, and likewise appears in abnormally formed ovaries.

3. *Arrhenoblastomas* are rare tumors, arise from rete ovarii, often contain a mixture of the first two types, are unilateral, and are usually benign although occasionally malignant. As a result of several homones they elaborate, either kind of sex character exaggeration may appear clinically.

**Nonspecialized stroma.** Tumors of nonspecialized ovarian stroma arise from the supportive, vascular, and mesodermal tissues of the ovary. They include the common fibromas as well as occasional leiomyomas, angiomas, and a few malignant solid tumors. One interesting syndrome—the Meigs' syndrome—appears in postmenopausal women and consists of a fibroma of the ovary, massive ascites, and hydrothorax. Surprisingly, the effusions disappear after removal of the benign fibroma. This picture may also occur with other ovarian neoplasms. Recently

Burkitt's tumor (African lymphoma) has been found in the ovaries of African female children, usually with other systemic manifestations of lymphoma.

In addition to these four general groups of tumors, many mixtures of all of these types can develop, particularly unclassified solid carcinomas that often behave most aggressively.

Eighty percent of ovarian tumors are cystic; most of these are benign. The remaining 20% grow as solid tumors; most of these are malignant (Fig. 17). Ovarian cancers tend to develop bilaterally in 20% of patients, although it may prove hard to distinguish a primary with metastasis to the opposite ovary from synchronous bilateral cancers. The benign cystic tumors grow to moderate or huge size rather silently. Cells desquamate into the peritoneal space from the normal ovary, from benign tumors, and from cancers. Scant evidence exists for evolution from benign to malignant tumors. However, malignant cells first appear to pile up in the *inside* of a cystic tumor, not on the outside, and then as the cancer progresses it ruptures or grows through to the peritoneal surface from the inside. Cancers spread by attachment to, and invasion of, adjacent structures, such as tubes, uterus, sigmoid and rectum, and small bowel and bladder; they also spread by transperitoneal seeding. Lymphatic metastases can occur to pelvic and aortic nodes, as well as blood-borne metastases to lungs and liver. These latter extensions occur more commonly with the serous cancers.

*Pelvic peritoneal seeding* with small, cauliflower-like nodules close to the primary or in the cul-de-sac, with some ascites, typically characterizes ovarian cancer by the time most of the cases come to diagnosis. One rare type of spread encountered in some appendiceal tumors occurs from rupture of mucinous, cystic carcinomas. Massive peritoneal proliferation of mucin may result from this—*pseudomyxoma peritonei.*

Another distinctive syndrome appears in the ovary—the *Krukenberg tumor.* This is the name given to an ovarian mass when a cancer of the stomach or colon selectively metastasizes to the ovary and gives a clinical picture exactly like that of the primary ovarian cancer, usually with ascites and occasionally even with abnormal ovarian hormone production. The ovary can act to "attract" metastases, and any ovarian neoplasm, primary or secondary, can sometimes develop a functioning stroma.

### Precancerous lesions

None have yet been identified.

## NATURAL HISTORY

Generally an ovarian tumor grows silently and slowly for some years. Benign tumors can go undetected for many years unless their pedicle twists acutely to produce an abdominal emergency, or unless they develop intracystic hemorrhage or rupture. Hormone secretion may also give the diagnostic signal, as when excess estrogen causes precocious puberty in children or brings on abnormal vaginal bleeding, breast pain, and breast enlargement in adults (granulosa cell tumors). Benign cystic lesions may attain huge size resembling advanced pregnancy.

Symptoms eventually develop from pressure of the bulk of a continually enlarging tumor mass. Lower abdominal pain, swelling, dysuria, and constipation may gradually arise with pressure on, and invasion of, organs adjacent to the ovaries. Malignant tumors then progress further to produce weight loss, anorexia, the appearance of multiple abdominal masses from omental metastases, partial small bowel obstruction, ascites, and metastases in lungs, mediastinum, or lower neck. Vaginal bleeding may occur from uterine invasion. Death usually occurs as a result of terminal pneumonia after a long, wasting, downhill course.

## DIAGNOSIS

Today 75% of ovarian cancers reach an incurable stage by the time of diagnosis.

**History and physical examination.** Symptoms from ovarian cancer usually mean incurability, although exceptions occur among the histologic borderline cancers. A story of gradually worsening lower abdominal aching, pain, and swelling or a change in bowel or urinary habit suggest a spreading pelvic tumor—possibly ovarian. Abnormal vaginal bleeding, backache, the finding of an abdominal or pelvic mass, or ascites alert us also to consider ovarian cancer. An asymptomatic adnexal mass forms the only clue to a contained, curable cancer.

Feminizing tumors (granulosa cell) cause precocious puberty in childhood, disordered menses in the premenopausal woman, abnormal vaginal bleeding, endometrial hyperplasia, and swollen breasts in the postmenopausal female. Dysgerminomas may have associated genital maldevelopment or menstrual irregularity. Cystic teratomas (dermoid cysts) seldom engender symptoms. Brenner tumors and fibromas generally come to diagnosis by pelvic examination after the menopause.

No more important method exists for diagnosing ovarian tumors than the careful *bimanual pelvic examination,* often best carried out under general anesthesia in obese women or those otherwise difficult to examine. But even here it cannot detect the early stages of cancer; the clinician must rely on knowledge and suspicion.

**X-ray studies.** *Plain abdominal films* may help diagnose some tumors that contain characteristic calcifications; teeth may occasionally determine that a cyst is a teratoma; dermoids also show distinctive soft tissue densities; psammoma bodies can aid in identifying cystadenomas or cystadenocarcinomas. Sigmoidoscopy, *barium enema, upper gastrointestinal x-ray studies,* and *chest films* constitute proper preoperative work-up procedures for any pelvic mass. Rectosigmoid cancers can mimic ovarian tumors; stomach and colorectal cancers can metastasize to the ovary and so simulate a primary ovarian tumor.

**Cytology.** Cervical smears may help somewhat since ovarian cells can migrate down the tubes and through the uterine tract. Graham states that 40% of ovarian cancers may be so diagnosed. A more logical maneuver is to perform *cul-de-sac aspiration* (culdocentesis) to obtain smears for cytologic study. Such cytologic material may show cells of ovarian cancer before metastases and seeding occur. Malignant cells in ascitic fluid generally, but not always, mean incurable spread.

**Culdoscopy.** The visualization of the ovaries through a small "scope" inserted into the cul-de-sac via the posterior fornix of the vagina may aid in diagnosis; a biopsy can often be secured in cases of cul-de-sac seeding.

**Laboratory studies.** Laboratory studies may prove useful; for example, urinary chorionic gonadotrophin determination can eliminate pregnancy as a differential diagnosis or the finding of excess urinary estrogenic hormones may pinpoint granulosa cell tumors.

*Laparotomy.* Notwithstanding the above-mentioned aids, laparotomy usually is needed for the final diagnosis. Here a knowledge of the gross pathology of ovarian tumors proves invaluable because decisions concerning the various diagnostic and therapeutic maneuvers often depend on such knowledge. In cases in which the tumor has not broken through the cystic wall, the whole ovary may be cleanly removed for frozen section or permanent diagnosis, according to the wishes of the pathologist. In instances of solid tumors, metastases, seeding, or gross papillary excrescences on the surface of the mass or where some obvious normal ovarian tissue remains adjacent to tumor, wedge biopsy can serve as well. Aspiration of fluid from cystic tumors will occasionally make the important distinction between serous and mucinous tumors; a thin transudate characterizes serous growths and a thicker, slimy aspirate comes from the mucinous tumors.

## Differential diagnosis

*Physiologic cysts* of the ovary—*follicle* and *corpus luteum* cysts—can usually be identified at operation. Clinically, however, any cystic adnexal mass less than 5 cm. in diameter in a premenopausal woman can be observed for 3 weeks on the presumption that it represents one of these types of functional cysts and that it may regress.

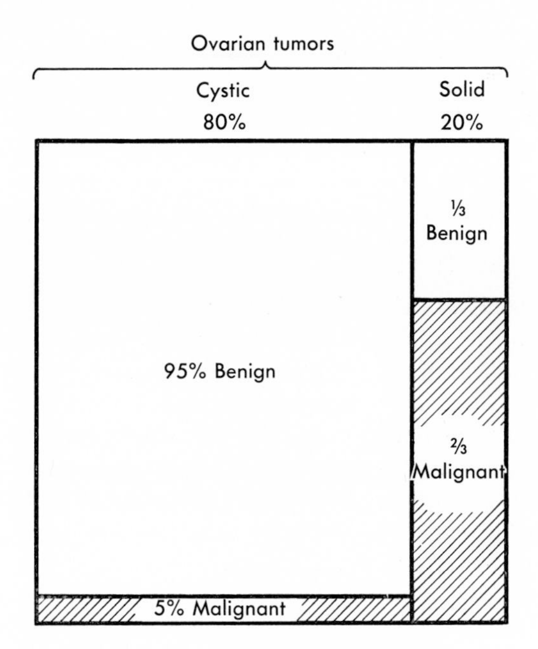


**Fig. 17.** Relative risk of cancer in cystic and solid ovarian masses.

*Leiomyomas* (fibroids) can duplicate the feel of an ovarian neoplasm on pelvic examination. In fact, they occur concomitantly with one third of ovarian tumors. Many laparotomies are performed with a working diagnosis of uterine fibroids when the true pathology concerns an ovarian growth. An x-ray film can sometimes show the partial calcifications typical of fibroids. The main distinguishing feature, of course, concerns attachment to the uterus. The fibroid feels attached; the ovarian tumor generally is separate from the body of the uterus.

*Hydrosalpinx, pyosalpinx,* and *tubo-ovarian abscess* differ from tumor by history of gonococcal infection, the actual presence of uterine tract infection, or by the tenderness of the masses.

*Endometrial cysts* (chocolate cyst) frequently occur from endometrial implants on the ovary and can be distinguished from other neoplasms by gross examination after local removal.

*Metastatic carcinoma* of the breast, of the colorectum, and of the uterus may also simulate primary ovarian neoplasms (20% of malignant ovaries).

*Cancer of the sigmoid colon* may be palpated in an adnexal position and be mistaken on pelvic examination for a tumor of the ovary. Only sigmoidoscopy and barium enema can make the preoperative distinction.

*Ectopic pregnancy* needs only the completion of a laboratory study for chorionic gonadotrophins to differentiate it from tumor.

*Cancer of the fallopian tube* develops rarely (usually at the fimbriated ends of the tube) so that distinction from ovarian tumor ultimately depends on histology.

*Presacral meningoceles, chordomas,* or other neurogenic neoplasms may also rarely complicate the diagnosis.

A *pelvic kidney* also feels like an adnexal tumor.

## PREVENTIVE MEASURES

No measures presently merit attention. Prophylactic oophorectomy to prevent cancer constitutes questionable medical practice, since statistically it would not reduce the incidence of ovarian cancer by any significant amount.

## TREATMENT PRINCIPLES

1. Management of the *adnexal mass:*
   a. *Premenopausal*—if cystic and under 5 cm., observe; if solid, operate regardless of size; over 5 cm., operate.
   b. *Postmenopausal*—any abnormal mass, operate.
   c. *Mass with endometrial hyperplasia*—operate.
2. *Surgery* generally constitutes the initial treatment for all ovarian tumors.
3. Whenever possible one tries to establish a *firm diagnosis first* by resection of an ovary or a wedge biopsy because the extent of surgery will, of course, differ with benign and with malignant tumors.
4. The extent of surgery may be curtailed in some benign and borderline malignant tumors of childhood or during female reproductive years; postmenopausal surgery seldom needs to be conservative.

5. The surgeon removes one or both ovaries for benign tumors, depending on the likelihood of bilaterality. (Half of serous cystadenomas become bilateral.) Dermoid cysts can often be excised with preservation of some ovarian tissue. In contrast, papillary serous cystadenomas may look benign histologically, but behave in a malignant fashion clinically; therefore they may warrant more radical removal.

6. *Total hysterectomy* and *bilateral salpingo-oophorectomy* generally comprise treatment for malignant tumors and steroid-producing neoplasms. Removal of the omentum can often prevent later ascites. With incurable spread of tumor in the abdomen, partial removal gives palliation only if 90% or more of the cancer can be excised; removal of lesser amounts yields little benefit.

7. *X-ray therapy* generally follows surgery for malignant tumors and probably contributes to some cures when used postoperatively, since most ovarian cancers are "radiosensitive." Irradiation helps to contain or destroy irremovable peritoneal seedings or adjacent organ metastases. The frequent scattered location of tumor masses among the abdominal viscera, however, does not allow optimum x-ray dosage to individual deposits.

8. Some cancers are biologically indolent, which permits occasional beneficial surgical excisions of a single recurrent mass.

9. *Systemic chemotherapy,* usually with one of the alkylating groups of drugs, is proving quite helpful for temporary, or sometimes long-term, control of inoperable cancer. Many cancers regress under these drugs. They probably deserve to be chosen as the first mode of treatment after noncurative surgery. Half of the patients so treated respond.

10. Intraperitoneal radioactive isotopes can achieve tumor regression and relief of ascites when metastases are tiny, but therapists are using them less today because of radiation complications.

## COMMON ERRORS

1. The physician may tend to "give up" if he cannot cure the patient surgically. Near total excisions, persistent chemotherapy, and judicious x-ray therapy can produce months or years of useful life.

2. Ovaries may be unnecessarily sacrificed by surgeons poorly schooled in the gross pathology of physiologic cysts and the various benign neoplasms of the ovary.

## PROMISING DEVELOPMENTS FOR THE FUTURE

We learn more about chemotherapy every year, and this modality will undoubtedly play an increasingly large role in the therapeusis of this usually advanced cancer that seems quite "drug sensitive."

## PROGNOSIS

Because many cancers of the ovary fall in the "unclassified" group, the criteria of histologic grade of the cancer and the anatomic extent or degree of spread of the tumor constitute the two most reliable prognostic indicators. The outlook varies all the way from 85% 5-year survivals in Stage I, Grade I to 0% for Stage IV,

Grade IV types. The most common histogenetic type, serous cancers, average around 25% 5-year survivals because most cannot be diagnosed in early stages. Solid and undifferentiated cancers have poorer prognosis, but cancers confined to one or both ovaries have a 60% survival rate.

In "borderline" malignant tumors, such as papillary cystadenomas or granulosa cell tumors, in mucinous cancers confined within the capsule of the cyst, and in dysgerminomas, the outlook is excellent.

**REFERENCES**


Abell, M. R.: The nature and classification of ovarian neoplasms, Canad. Med. Ass. J. **64:** 1102-1124, 1966.

Ackerman, L. V., and del Regato, J. A.: Cancer, ed. 3, St. Louis, 1962, The C. V. Mosby Co., pp. 922-959.

Frick, H. C., II, Atchoo, N., Adamsons, K., Jr., and Taylor, H. C., Jr.: Efficacy of chemotherapeutic agents in management of disseminated gynecologic cancer, Amer. J. Obstet. Gynec. **93:**1112-1121, 1966.

Graham, J. B.: Cancer of the ovary. In Postgraduate course on malignant disease in the female pelvis, Chicago, 1967, American College of Surgeons 53rd Clinical Congress, pp. 81-85.

Grillo, D., Steinmier, R. H., and Lowell, D. M.: Early diagnosis of ovarian carcinoma by culdocentesis, Obstet. Gynec. **28:**346-350, 1966.

Kottmeier, H. L.: Ovarian cancer—diagnosis and treatment, Med. Col. Virginia Quarterly **3:** 47-53, 1967.

Marchant, J.: Ovary—some basic considerations. In Raven, R. W., and Roe, F. J. C., editors: The prevention of cancer, New York, 1967, Appleton-Century-Crofts, pp. 269-272.

Masterson, J. G.: Cancer of the ovary. In Postgraduate course on malignant disease in the female pelvis, Chicago, 1967, American College of Surgeons 53rd Clinical Congress, pp. 92-93.

Nealon, T. F., Jr.: The ovary. In Nealon, T. F., Jr., editor: Management of the patient with cancer, Philadelphia, 1966, W. B. Saunders Co., pp. 719-738.

Nolan, J. F.: Cancer of the ovary. In Postgraduate course on malignant disease in the female pelvis, Chicago, 1967, American College of Surgeons 53rd Clinical Congress, pp. 90-91.

Richardson, G. S.: Cancer of the ovary. In Postgraduate course on malignant disease in the female pelvis, Chicago, 1967, American College of Surgeons 53rd Clinical Congress, pp. 86-89.

Rutledge, F., and Burnes, B. C.: Chemotherapy for advanced ovarian cancer, Amer. J. Obstet. Gynec. **96:**761-772, 1966.

Tweedale, D. N., and Peduson, B. L.: Serous neoplasms of the ovary, Amer. J. Med. Sci. **249:**701-717, 1965.

Van Orden, D. W., McAllister, W. B., Zerne, S. R., and Morris, J. McL.: Ovarian carcinoma, Amer. J. Obstet. Gynec. **94:**195-202, 1966.

Chapter 22

# Cancer of the vulva and vagina

We return now to a consideration of the relatively uncomplicated stratified squamous epithelium of the vulva and vagina that produces a uniform type of cancer. This squamous or epidermoid type resembles those described in the skin, lip, and mouth.

## INCIDENCE AND DISTRIBUTION

Even by combining these two adjacent regional tumors for the sake of brevity, we have a group of uncommon cancers. Most reviews of all publications on these sites succeed in collecting only a few hundred cases. Together they comprise approximately 5% of gynecologic cancers; the vulval carcinomas far outnumber the primary vaginal cancers. No reliable data on racial distribution are available, although many reports seem to show a predominance in American Negroes.

## ETIOLOGY

### External initiating agents

By analogy to what we know of cancers of the skin, lip, and mouth, external chemical carcinogens certainly could produce vaginal and vulval cancers. Multiple cancers develop relatively often in the lower female genital tract, particularly cancer of the cervix followed by vulval or vaginal cancers.

### Predisposing factors

Data on predisposition arise from clinical impressions rather than definitive studies. Vulval cancers occur in old women with long-standing pruritus vulvae, whose vulvas show atrophy, thickening, dryness, and irregular and abnormal pigmentations. Over one half of vulval cancers come to diagnosis associated with some one of the venereal diseases or clinical leukoplakia. No internal predispositions are known.

## PATHOLOGY

Cancer of the vulva usually grows slowly as a differentiated squamous cancer of the labium majus; it may appear ulcerating or papillary and exophytic, may bleed, and metastasizes to inguinal lymph nodes. A few adenocarcinomas reportedly arise from Bartholin's glands.

Vaginal carcinoma develops as an undifferentiated *epidermoid cancer* in the upper third of the vaginal tube (often on the posterior wall). It presents as an indurated ulcer and expands to involve the whole lining, the cervix, bladder, or rectum. Metastases first appear in the deep pelvic (hypogastric) lymph nodes. Sarcoma botryoides arises from the vagina in young female children on rare occasions.

### Precancerous lesions

*Four* specific types of *intraepithelial carcinoma* of the vulva have been described—*Bowen's disease,* erythroplasia of Queyrat, *squamous cell carcinoma in situ,* and extramammary Paget's disease. Individually rare, together they constitute a large enough group to emphasize the frequency and importance of in situ cancer, its multicentricity, and its common association with, as well as potential for, invasive cancer in the vulva and adjacent perineal skin. Red, raised plaquelike changes in the epithelium and also the whitish heaping up of hyperkeratosis and leukoplakia comprise the gross signs denoting the precancerous vulva, which, like in situ cervical lesions, has an average age of diagnosis about 10 years younger than the average age of invasive cancer.

Descriptions of carcinoma in situ of the vagina also appear quite often and determine the need for removal of a cuff of vaginal mucosa in surgery for carcinoma in situ of the cervix.

## NATURAL HISTORY

A postmenopausal woman with longstanding pruritus and weeping eczema of the vulva (perhaps one who also has diabetes and is obese) may one day feel a hard, painless plaque or a slightly tender ulcer in the labial skin. This may slowly spread over the surface, deepen, enlarge, or flower outward as a large warty external growth. Over a period of 6 months the growth increases in size, but because of the looseness and flexibility of the labia, there is no deep fixation. However, the ipsilateral inguinal and femoral lymph nodes may swell and become harder than those on the opposite side after a few more months. The local mass finally ulcerates, weeps, and oozes blood so badly that the patient becomes a nursing problem, eventually dying of cachexia brought on by pain, anorexia, inanition, bleeding, and local infection. Distant metastases to liver, lungs, brain, and bones may occur if the patient survives long enough.

There is no external evidence of vaginal cancer; *bleeding* or vaginal discharge first occur, but deep pelvic pain from infection of the cancerous ulcer usually develops relatively late after the tumor has invaded the paravaginal tissues. Uncontrolled local disease follows much the same course as other discharging, infected, bleeding pelvic cancers.

## DIAGNOSIS

**History and physical examination.** Vulval cancer needs only to be observed by the physician for suspicion of cancer to occasion the pursuit of a diagnostic workup. Any thickened, dry, pruritic vulval skin, any warty excrescence, or certainly any weeping excoriation or ulcer alerts us to the need for biopsy. Any ulcer or mass in the vaginal wall also demands suspicion and diagnostic attention.

**Biopsy.** Several bites with a sharp punch biopsy forceps can easily secure a definite histologic diagnosis in these accessible regions. The need for multiple biopsies in these locations is occasioned by the frequent simultaneous occurrence of multiple and multicentric precancers and cancers.

**Other diagnostic procedures.** Cytology, laboratory studies, and x-ray films play no special part other than the routine study of any potential cancer patient.

### Differential diagnosis

The following conditions need differentiation from carcinoma of the vulva: (1) the so-called *venereal lesions,* which can appear cancerous—condyloma acuminatum, granuloma inguinale, and lymphopathia venereum; (2) the *chronic vulvar dystrophies,* which elicit itching, a mottled pigmentation, and thickening of the vulva (kraurosis vulvae); (3) lichen sclerosus, herpes simplex, fungal infections, eczematoid changes from chronic vaginal discharge, and self-inflicted trauma of scratching; (4) chronic nonspecific *ulcers* and pyogenic granuloma; and (5) leukoplakia, which is precancerous as in the mouth and on the lower lip.

Vaginal tumors result more commonly from metastases from primaries in the cervix and endometrium, ovaries, or, occasionally, the rectum than from a primary vaginal mucosal neoplasm. Therefore a careful study to exclude other pelvic tumors must precede the firm establishment of a diagnosis of vaginal cancer. If the tumor is an adenocarcinoma, it is probably metastatic from elsewhere rather than being a rare Bartholin gland cancer.

## PREVENTIVE MEASURES

1. Local medications to eradicate dermatoses and prevent vulval itching might prevent the progression of precancerous lesions to invasive cancer.
2. Wide *excision* of all *precancerous dermatoses*—Bowen's disease or simple intraepithelial carcinoma—would prevent the invasive stage. When extensive changes are present in the vulval mucosa and skin, excision may entail conservative vulvectomy to eradicate multiple foci.
3. Biopsy (or narrow excision for diagnosis) of all papillomas, warts, growing moles, granulomas, ulcers, hard or white spots, or subcutaneous nodules achieves prevention in the sense that precancer and invasive cancer may thereby be diagnosed at an early stage and easily cured.

## TREATMENT PRINCIPLES

1. For vulval cancer a *radical vulvectomy* plus bilateral inguinal and femoral node dissection comprises the only fully curative treatment. Many authorities insist on bilateral intrapelvic node dissections as well, but age and medical complications in these elderly women often argue for compromise with this extensive surgical plan. However, it would seem that in the past, surgical compromises have been far too conservative with resultant prompt local recurrences, which yield greater morbidity than from radical surgery and generally lead to death. Fifty percent of patients have positive ipsilateral inguinal nodes involved on diagnosis and 20% show bilateral involvement.
2. X-ray treatment for cancer of the vulva constitutes "second best" treatment, since this tissue tolerates irradiation poorly.

3. Irradiation provides fairly reliable treatment for primary vaginal cancer as a rule; since most of these arise in upper parts of the tube near the vault, they can be treated somewhat like cancer of the cervix. Combinations of preoperative irradiation and surgery may prove helpful. However, in selected patients with cancers in the lower third of the vagina, wide surgical removal may be preferable as it is in the vulva.

4. X-ray treatment can palliate uncontrolled local cancer.

5. The occasional patient with advanced vulval or vaginal cancer will benefit from one of the pelvic exenterative operations, since both of these epidermoid tumors remain localized to the perineum and pelvis for relatively long periods.

## COMMON ERRORS

1. The diagnosis is often missed by a single biopsy.

2. Failure also occurs sometimes from overconservative excisional surgery that permits local recurrences or does not remove a sufficient amount of the "condemned" vulvar epithelium.

## PROMISING DEVELOPMENTS FOR THE FUTURE

1. *Cryosurgery* promises to give a more definitive eradication of precancerous lesions than cautery.

2. Trained radiotherapists with better equipment can plan more effective irradiation than has been possible in the past.

3. The long delay period before diagnosis in these cancers may be shortened in the future by a trend away from false modesty in women.

## PROGNOSIS

Approximately one patient in three survives 5 years with present therapy. When lymph nodes are negative, survivals in vulval cancer approach 80%. More than half the patients who are able to undergo radical vulvectomy and lymphadenectomy survive.

### REFERENCES

Abell, M. R.: Intraepithelial carcinoma of the epidermis and squamous mucosa of the vulva and perineum, Surg. Clin. N. Amer. **45:**1179-1198, 1965.

Ackerman, L. V., and del Regato, J. A.: Cancer, ed. 3, St. Louis, 1962, The C. V. Mosby Co., pp. 1041-1059.

Collins, C. G., and Barclay, D. L. The vulva and vagina. In Nealon, T. F., Jr., editor: Management of the patient with cancer, Philadelphia, 1966, W. B. Saunders Co., pp. 790-810.

Edsmyr, F.: Carcinoma of the vulva, Acta Radiol. **217**(supp.):1-135, 1962.

Green, T. H., Gardner, H. L., Twombly, G. H., Riva, H. L., Collins, J. H., and Barbar, H. R. K.: Cancer of the vulva and vagina. In Postgraduate course on malignant disease in the female pelvis, Chicago, 1967, American College of Surgeons 53rd Clinical Congress.

Kaufman, R. H., and Gardner, H. L.: Intraepithelial carcinoma of the vulva, Clin. Obstet. Gynec. **8:**1035-1049, 1965.

Mickal, A., Andonie, J. A., and Dougherty, C. M.: Squamous cell carcinoma of the vulva, Obstet. Gynec. **28:**370-374, 1966.

Rutledge, F. N.: Cancer of the vulva and vagina, Clin. Obstet. Gynec. **8:**1051-1079, 1965.

Smith, F. R.: Clinical management of cancer of the vagina, Ann. N. Y. Acad. Sci. **114:**1012-1019, 1964.

Chapter 23

# Cancer of the bladder

The transitional epithelium lining the urinary bladder serves to contain and store urine, a relatively simple function. Tumors from it are of a broadly uniform kind, not unlike tumors of the squamous-lined organs in other areas of the body.

## INCIDENCE AND DISTRIBUTION

Bladder cancer constitutes 3% of all human cancers and occurs three times more often in men than in women. It generally develops around the age of 60. Rates in Europe and in the United States run fairly even and equal; a low rate prevails in Japan, Sweden, and New Zealand, whereas a very high incidence of bladder cancer occurs in Egypt, presumably because of a high attack rate of bilharziasis.

## ETIOLOGY

### External initiating agents

The urinary bladder comprises an ideal organ in which to study the effect of stasis on the localization of cancer. Bladder tumors greatly exceed the number of tumors higher in the urinary excretory tract, a situation related to stasis, just as rectal cancers outnumber those of equal segments higher in the intestinal tract.

A great deal of experimental, chemical, and clinical study has been devoted to demonstrating the precise chemical structure of carcinogens responsible for many occupational bladder cancers, and this work has, by comparison with similar efforts in other regional cancers, been brilliantly successful. There seems little doubt that the aniline dye compounds, beta-naphthylamine, para-aminodiphenyl, and benzidine, play a major role in the cancerous sequence in many human bladders. With regard to this sequence, some believe that the ultimate carcinogen is 2-amino-1-naphthol. Investigators generally contend that the breakdown products of the ingested dye compounds are excreted in the urine in an inactive state, but that they are converted to a carcinogenic compound by the action of the enzyme glucuronidase in the bladder, and that the active end product is the 2-amino-1-naphthol. No doubt other compounds may also be found in the bladder that act as carcinogens (coming from ingested compounds of occupational or other origin). These studies constitute medicine's most complete description of chemical carcinogenesis from external agents.

Study of the breakdown products of indigenous tryptophan metabolism (orthohydroxyamines) show that they may be major initiating carcinogens, the counterparts of the exogenous aniline compounds, and might thus account for "spontaneous" bladder cancers where no occupational exposure exists. Some evidence also links tobacco use with bladder cancer (Clemmesen and associates), presumably from the concentrated prolonged contact of bladder mucosa with metabolized products of the carcinogenic chemicals in absorbed cigarette smoke condensate. It seems well established that the infecting organism of bilharziasis is the external factor responsible for the high incidence of bladder cancer in Egypt and in other countries where this also occurs.

### Predisposing factors

Obviously from the observations made above on the products of tryptophan metabolism, the metabolic pathway that overproduces the orthohydroxyamines to the extent of inciting bladder cancer must be considered an abnormal one. Although we cannot at present regard the mechanism as proved, there exists the strong possibility that abnormal or excess tryptophan metabolites initiate or promote cancer. Tobacco smoking may indirectly promote this type of cancer by its effect on enhancing tryptophan abnormality (Kerr and associates).

## PATHOLOGY

Many bladder tumors seem to begin as *papillomas,* or *Grade 1 transitional cell carcinomas,* which are the same for clinical purposes. They often develop at *multiple* sites, mostly in or near the bladder base. Usually these tumors can be traced to origin in the normal transitional epithelium or from adjacent carcinoma in situ. As they grow and invade the bladder musculature, they appear to undergo progression to higher grades, become ulcerated and flatter, and take on anaplastic forms at the periphery and at the base of the polypoid or papillary masses. Treat-

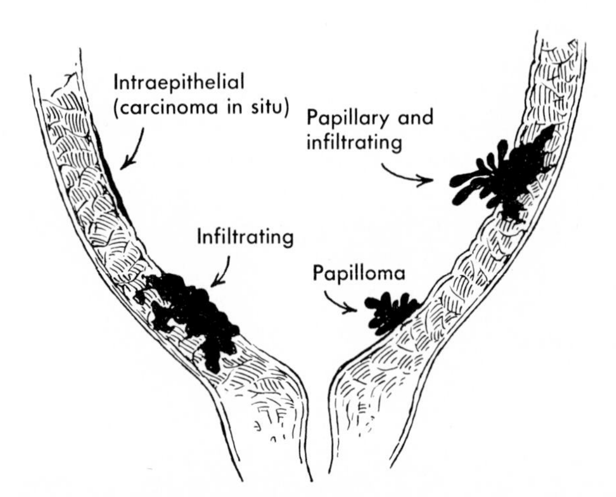


**Fig. 18.** Several different growth patterns in the bladder showing tendency of tumors to occur near the bladder base. (Modified from Pugh, R. C. B.: In Wallace, D. M., editor: Tumors of the bladder, Edinburgh, 1959, E. & S. Livingstone Ltd.)

ment and prognosis depend on the extent of invasion of muscle layers of the bladder wall (Figs. 18 and 19). Bladder tumors display a strong tendency to seed themselves to other locations of the urothelium, despite local destruction or removal.

Whether cancers begin as differentiated tumors and progress, or whether they begin as highly anaplastic and invasive from the start, two gross forms appear to the clinician viewing them through the cystoscope: (1) *papillary* and (2) *solid* cancers. Histologically, there are generally three recognized groups of transitional cell carcinoma: (1) the *papilloma,* (2) the *differentiated carcinoma,* and (3) the *undifferentiated* or anaplastic tumor. *Squamous* or epidermoid varieties occur less frequently; the latter cancers grow as flat, invasive neoplasms. The rather uncommon *adenocarcinomas* often have a cystic or glandular cystitis as a concomitant.

Metastases develop commonly when the cancer has invaded the muscle layers, occurring in the hypogastric lymph nodes and later in the para-aortic lymph nodes, but it is not uncommon for lymphatic metastases to skip the regional lymph nodes in their progress. Distant deposits in liver, lungs, and bone are frequent.

### Precancerous lesions

We have already commented on the very high malignant potential of the *bladder papilloma;* it is regarded by most urologists as a low-grade cancer. Perhaps this lesion bears some resemblance to the villous adenoma of the rectum, except that the bladder papilloma develops more commonly than any other bladder neoplasm. It has a tendency to occur at multiple sites over many years and to recur persistently despite local destruction; the patient with papillomas needs lifelong scrutiny because papillomas often undergo progression to invasive cancer.

*Carcinoma in situ* of the bladder is a real entity but very hard to find by itself. It causes no symptoms and consists of a microscopic surface change limited to the epithelium so that no characteristic gross appearance gives it away to the cystoscopist. Even fluorescence studies fail to reveal it in some cases (Melamed and associates). It is a microscopic diagnosis made by cytologic study of urine specimens or by histologic examination of biopsy material done for other gross lesions when carcinoma in situ happens to be adjacent. Not enough cases have been studied by themselves to give us guides as to the frequency of progression to invasive cancer, but Koss and associates have followed workers exposed to para-aminodiphenyl, a potent carcinogen, and find over half of carcinoma in situ lesions progressed to invasive cancer in a period of 7 years. They estimate that the total period of existence of the in situ stage may be twice that long.

## NATURAL HISTORY

*Hematuria* ushers in the sequence of events in bladder cancer, either gross, massive or microscopic, but the amount of this persistent bleeding bears no relation to the type or size of the tumor. Papillomas progress very slowly and produce few symptoms or signs except hematuria; but the more anaplastic, ulcerating tumors soon invade the bladder musculature. The latter progress relatively fast and cause frequency of urination, dysuria, and sometimes steady pain unrelated to urination. The more malignant varieties bleed less profusely than the papillomas or papillary types of cancer. Obstruction of one or both ureteral orifices occurs after variable periods of time in most cancers, leading to upper urinary infection, flank pain, fever, chills, and acute and chronic pyelonephritis, with resultant kidney failure and uremia following in due time. Sometimes massive hematuria yields clots that obstruct the urethra and cause acute urinary retention; occasionally cancer involves the bladder base and urethra to produce urinary incontinence. Untreated patients live an average of 13 months after first symptoms.

## DIAGNOSIS

**History.** Often *gross hematuria* that is painless first causes the patient to seek medical advice; this one symptom may signify a papilloma or an invasive cancer, but it always demands a urinary diagnostic study for tumor. Other urinary symptoms, such as frequency, hesitancy, painful urination, burning, etc., are less specific and suggestive because they result from infection or prostatic hypertrophy more often than from neoplasm, but they occur if the growth has progressed into the bladder musculature to such an extent as to interfere with function, or if the growth is so located as to block a ureteral orifice or the urethral opening.

**Physical examination.** Tumors must grow fairly large to be palpated on physical examination; rectal or vaginal *bimanual palpation* can sometimes detect a firm mass at the base. With a large, palpable mass one must assess the degree of fixation to the bony pelvis or surrounding organs, and this is best done under anesthesia for complete muscular relaxation.

**Urinalysis.** For microscopic detection of red *blood cells,* urinalysis will help screen persons and select out those suspected of bladder tumors. Microscopic hematuria, as well as gross hematuria, always demands a full tumor study of the patient. This, in conjunction with urine cytology, constitutes a very effective tumor screening method.

**Cytology.** Cytology performed on the urine yields the best lead to asymptomatic tumors. False positives seldom are reported; if the pathologist finds malignant cells, some neoplastic process is sure to be present somewhere in the urinary tract, most often in the bladder. If the growth consists only of an in situ, intraepithelial lesion, it may very likely escape detection by gross observation. Most invasive cancers can be found easily, as outlined below, once the positive urine cytology has alerted one to the certain presence of neoplasia. Bladder washings may also help secure exfoliated cells for cytologic study. Urinary cytology could well become as successful a screening test for genitourinary cancer as the cervical smear has for cancer of the cervix.

**Cystoscopy.** The basic maneuver in bladder diagnosis is cystoscopy, enabling the examiner to see and inspect all areas of the lining in great detail and with some magnification. Biopsies can be performed through the cystoscope, and a firm diagnosis of cancer can be established. One needs multiple biopsies and deep bites at the base of the tumor where it meets the wall to assess fully the type and extent, since tumors exhibit a variety of patterns.

**X-ray studies.** X-ray cystography proves of value in estimating the relative extent of a tumor. *Excretory urography, retrograde pyelography,* and chest films need to accompany any bladder cancer study to look for other urinary tract tumors, upper tract obstruction, and metastases.

**Laboratory studies.** *Renal function studies* in the laboratory must supplement a complete study, especially when obstruction of urinary flow is suspected.

### Differential diagnosis

Many conditions initiate the common presenting symptom of bladder cancer, which is hematuria. In many instances the blood arises from disease in the kidney or, occasionally, the ureter, but in most it comes from primary bladder disease. Nonneoplastic bladder conditions that produce hematuria are *bladder stones,* chronic interstitial *cystitis, tuberculosis,* prostatic inflammations, and infections. We generally depend upon cystoscopy and biopsy and sometimes on culture for diagnosis and differentiation of these conditions from tumors.

Other tumors that need distinguishing from cancer are *carcinoma* of the *prostate, carcinoma* of the *cervix, carcinoma* of the *rectum,* especially those that have invaded the bladder, *cancer* of the *female urethra,* rare benign soft part tumors such as hemangioma, neurofibroma, and leiomyoma, and their malignant counterparts. Careful pelvic and rectal bimanual examinations, plus cystoscopy and biopsy will usually clarify the true diagnosis.

## PREVENTIVE MEASURES

1. Strict industrial safeguards in dye and many other chemical industries, both by law and by private managerial supervision, must be carried out. Much has been accomplished in these lines in England and, to a slightly lesser extent, in the United States. Cystoscopic and urinary cytologic follow-up studies for life on all workers that have contact with known carcinogens, or suspected carcinogens, constitutes common-sense preventive medicine. Strict control of worker exposure has proved impossible in some industrial processes, and the only solution sometimes may be the substitution of a new industrial chemical process for an old, possibly carcinogenic one.
2. Development of suitable bioassay methods to screen new and unknown chemical compounds for carcinogenic potential seems essential, since "spontaneous" bladder cancer remains fairly frequent and lethal, and present data suggest that exogenous chemicals, whose nature is at present unknown, constitute the most likely initiators.
3. Urine *cytology,* as a screening, universally applied test, should be able to detect precancer and cases of asymptomatic cancer.
4. Perhaps patients with bladder papillomas should quit smoking.

## TREATMENT PRINCIPLES

1. *Papillomas* (Stage 0) may be destroyed by thorough fulguration through the cystoscope, but the patient needs lifelong follow-up by cystoscopy and cytology.
2. A urologist-radiotherapist conference on all lesions except papillomas makes sense.
3. Stage A cancers of low grade may sometimes be fulgurated. Segmental cystectomy may be used if the lesion is single, removed from the ureteral orifices,

and histologically a transitional cell type with sharp borders that change abruptly to normal mucosa. Histologically low-grade papillary tumors are not suitable for this. Because of the high expectancy of new tumors, lifelong follow-up will be required, probably with periodic biopsy.

4. Stage B-1 tumors of low grade probably represent the group that would profit most from total cystectomy, perhaps with consideration of *preoperative x-ray therapy.* Urinary diversion by construction of an ileal conduit provides a manageable bladder substitute. Cystectomy suits the bladder with many scattered superficial cancers.

5. Stages B-2 and higher, and highly undifferentiated tumors, are probably not curable by surgery. *Supervoltage irradiation* offers control in some instances. Orthovoltage, interstitial radium, and intracavitary radioactive sources have limited usefulness and success.

6. Chemotherapy has not yielded much help in cancer of the bladder.

## COMMON ERRORS

1. Poor patient follow-up on papillomas, which allow multiple recurrences to progress to invasive cancer before the progression is recognized, accounts for many failures.

2. We sometimes make the mistake of underassessing the degree of penetration of the bladder wall by the tumor, which results in inadequate treatment.

## PROMISING DEVELOPMENTS FOR THE FUTURE

1. X-ray angiography to better assess the extent of bladder wall invasion by tumor would be an immense aid in planning treatment.

2. Topically applied thio-TEPA or another chemotherapeutic agent to eradi-

| | $T_1$ | | $T_2$ | | $T_3$ | | | $T_4$ |
|---|---|---|---|---|---|---|---|---|
| STAGE | O | A | $B_1$ | $B_2$ | C | $D_1$ | $D_2$ | $D_3$ |
| Mucosa | | | | | | | | |
| Submucosa | | | | | | | | |
| Muscularis | | | | | | | | |
| Fat | | | | | | | | |
| Nodes | − | − | − | − | − | + | + | |
| Pelvic | − | − | − | − | − | + | + | |
| Aortic | − | − | − | − | − | − | + | |

**Fig. 19.** Staging of bladder cancer with corresponding T groups from the TNM system. Invasion of the prostate gland by a bladder cancer constitutes a poor prognosis but this is not indicated here. Such prostatic invasion would call for a stage of $D_2$ ($T_3$) or $D_3$ ($T_4$). (Modified from Marshall, V. F.: Cancer **9**:543, 1956.)

cate abnormal bladder epithelium could perhaps prevent multiple tumors in the future life of the predisposed or industrially exposed individual.

3. Patients will profit from better cooperation between the urologist and the radiotherapist in every case of cancer; combined preoperative x-ray therapy and surgery promises to increase survival rates in the future.

4. Some substance similar to saccharolactone (which has been tried but found unsuccessful) may be discovered to inhibit the carcinogenic activator enzymes in the bladder, such as glucuronidase.

## PROGNOSIS

*Papillary* tumors, of course, have a good outlook, whereas *infiltrating* cancers carry a poor prognosis. Papillomas (Grade 1 transitional cell carcinomas) carry an 85% 5-year survival rate despite their multiplicity of foci. Stage A and Stage B-1 tumors can achieve a 60% 5-year survival. Grade 2 and Grade 3 infiltrating carcinomas (Stages B-2, C, D-1, and D-2) achieve only 20% 5-year survival.

Survivals vary greatly from series to series depending on the number of papillomas included. In general, bladder cancer has been discouragingly hard to cure.

### REFERENCES

Ackerman, L. V., and del Regato, J. A.: Cancer, ed. 3, St. Louis, 1962, The C. V. Mosby Co., pp. 819-841.

Allen, T. D., moderator: Panel discussion on tumors of the bladder, Urol. Survey **16:**2-16, 1966.

Arduino, L. J.: Chemotherapy in urologic cancer, Surg. Clin. N. Amer. **45:**1352-1364, 1965.

Berman, H. I.: Urinary diversion in the treatment of carcinoma of the bladder, Surg. Clin. N. Amer. **45:**1495-1508, 1965.

Bryan, P. T., Brown, R. R., and Price, J. M.: Studies in the etiology of bovine bladder cancers, Ann. N. Y. Acad. Sci. **108:**924-937, 1963.

Clemmesen, J., Lockwood, K., and Nielsen, A.: Smoking habits of patients with carcinoma of the urinary bladder, Danish Med. Bull. **5:**123-128, 1958.

DeWeerd, J. H., and Colby, M. Y., Jr.: Bladder carcinoma—combined radiotherapy and surgical treatment, J.A.M.A. **199:**109-111, 1967.

Kerr, W. K., Barkin, M., Livers, P. E., Woo, S. A. C., and Menczyk, Z.: The effect of cigarette smoking on bladder carcinogens in man, Canad. Med. Ass. J. **93:**1-7, 1965.

Koss, L. G., Melamed, M. R., Ricca, A., Melick, W. F., and Kelly, R. E.: Carcinogenesis in the human urinary bladder, New Eng. J. Med. **272:**767-778, 1965.

Masina, F.: Segmental resection for tumors of the urinary bladder, Brit. J. Surg. **52:**279-283, 1965.

Melamed, M. R., Grabstald, H., and Whitmore, W. F., Jr.: Carcinoma in situ of bladder, J. Urol. **96:**466-471, 1966.

Pugh, R. C. B.: The pathology of bladder tumors. In Wallace, D. M., editor: Tumors of the bladder, vol. II, London, 1952, E. & S. Livingstone Ltd., pp. 116-156.

Schilling, R. S. F.: Symposium on Occupational Bladder Cancers, Section of Occupational Medicine, Proc. Roy. Soc. Med. **59:**1247-1254, 1966.

Veenema, R. J., Girgis, A. S., Dean, A. L., Jr., and Uson, A. C.: Chemotherapy in bladder carcinoma, Proc. Nat. Cancer Conf. **5:**295-301, 1964.

Wise, H. M., and Fainsinger, M. H.: Angiography in the evaluation of carcinoma of the bladder, J.A.M.A. **192:**1027-1031, 1965.

Chapter 24

# Cancer of the kidney

Several diverse cells and tissues with widely varying functions compose the kidney. Its tumors therefore present a considerable variety; the three main groups are the parenchymal tumors, the kidney pelvis tumors, and Wilms' tumors of childhood.

## INCIDENCE AND DISTRIBUTION

Kidney tumors constitute 1% or 2% of cancers; they occur in males three times as often as in females and generally between the ages of 50 and 70. An embryoma, Wilms' tumor, accounts for many of the various childhood cancers. For reasons unknown, rates for renal carcinomas are lowest in Japan and highest in Denmark. England reports a higher incidence among the higher socioeconomic groups. Occurrence of renal cancer among males shows a slight recent increase—a statistic without a ready explanation at the present time.

## ETIOLOGY

### External initiating agents

Although many agents, including viruses, produce renal cancer in laboratory animals, virtually no correlations exist between externally applied substances and the increase of human renal cancer. A large number of substances that we have mentioned in relation to other sites remain under suspicion, especially those incriminated in bladder cancer. These might as easily initiate tumors of the renal pelvis because stasis of concentrated urine occurs to some extent in the kidney pelvis as well as the bladder. Some agents that are being studied in relation to human renal neoplasms are liver carcinogenic compounds, such as dimethylnitrosamine, the aflatoxins, lead compounds, cycasin from the tropical cycad plant, fungicides (hexachlorobenzene), inhaled tobacco smoke, exogenous estrogens, ionizing radiations, and adenoviruses 12 and 18. At present, however, no agent constitutes a proved threat. Since bilateral renal parenchymal cancers are rare, external agents may not be as important in renal cancer as in other sites. One would normally expect a fair incidence of bilaterality in cancers where ingested agents play the main role.

### Predisposing factors

Certain metabolites of *tryptophan metabolism,* such as 3-hydroxyanthranilic acid reportedly occur in increased amounts in the urine of kidney cancer patients and also in patients with bladder cancer (Chapter 23). Some authors invoke hormonal imbalance, particularly that of *excess estrogens,* as a background for the origin of parenchymal cancers; hormonal alterations then might explain the spontaneous or otherwise unexplained regression of some renal cancer metastases. Grabstald has reviewed the indirect evidence for the role of endogenous steroids in the origin of human renal cancer: cholesterol esters are found in tubular epithelial cells of adenomas, probably precancerous lesions; adenomas develop more often in diabetics with hypercholesterolemia; renal cancer has a definite sex preponderance for males and for persons with hormonal adenomas elsewhere; and some recent records show favorable clinical responses of human kidney cancer to doses of progestational hormones.

In the case of Wilms' tumors of childhood a high incidence of other congenital anomalies occurs, but these can hardly be considered causative. They merely accompany these nephroblastomas and emphasize their probable genesis during the life of the fetus in utero. *Renal calculi* frequently accompany tumors of the kidney and ureter in contrast to the lack of a stone-cancer association in the human bladder. No one has satisfactorily explained this.

## PATHOLOGY

Four fifths of kidney cancers are *adenocarcinomas* of the renal parenchyma, arising presumably from cells of the convoluted tubules. They grow at extremely varying rates by replacing and compressing the normal parenchyma and finally by distorting the kidney pelvis as well; they remain well circumscribed, as opposed to basically infiltrating tumors of other organs, and often become bulky masses in a generally enlarged kidney. These cancers have been called "hypernephromas." Microscopically three varieties develop—the *papillary diffuse,* the *granular cell,* and the *clear cell* type.

Adenomas of the parenchyma occur with some frequency as small, circumscribed yellowish cortical masses, well-encapsulated, that can only be distinguished from cancer by the microscope. Adenocarcinomas metastasize by invading veins, but usually not until they have reached the critical size of 5 cm. in greatest diameter. Notoriously they form tumor thrombi in the main renal veins. Consequently lung metastases develop frequently, which have an almost characteristic snowball-like appearance on an x-ray film. These adenocarcinomas also show a predilection for metastasizing to bones, and solitary brain metastases are not uncommon. But they can travel as well by the paracaval and para-aortic lymphatics to regional lymph nodes.

A second but smaller group of renal cancers, the *epidermoid growths of the renal pelvis,* comprise 10% of kidney tumors. They would be more appropriately discussed with bladder cancer because they arise from a common type of urothelium that lines the urinary drainage tract from pelvis to bladder and they seem to show a more or less common etiology, behavior pattern, and gross appearance. Many kidney-pelvis cancers are papillary at first, are quite often multiple, and sometimes exhibit secondary and tertiary papillomatous neoplasms in the ipsilateral ureter. Benign papillomas frequently accompany the papillary invasive pelvic tumors; whether they reflect an underlying widespread change in the epithelium or represent seeding from a single site, we do not know. Papillary cancers metastasize seldom and late and spread via lymphatics when they do. The less frequent ulcerating, flat, invasive epidermoid cancer spreads early via lymphatics to the regional lymph nodes.

Less frequent than the two groups mentioned above, *Wilms' tumors* comprise a large segment of childhood growths, arising as they do from embryonic nephrogenic tissue. They usually come to diagnosis before the child reaches 7 years of age. They may grow rapidly; in many cases they become quite large, distend the kidney capsule, and finally rupture through to invade and involve the perirenal tissues, the large bowel, liver, vena cava, or vertebrae. A microscopic mixture of cells, Wilms' tumors appear composed of most of the various cell types representing the normal fetal kidney such as striated muscle, glomeruli, smooth muscle, connective tissue, etc.

The following unusual and interesting abnormalities develop on occasion from renal parenchymal cancers: secondary polycythemia, due perhaps to tumorous elaboration of an erythropoietic substance; secondary hyperparathyroidism, stemming apparently from a parathormone-like substance in some cancers; and rarely a salt-losing syndrome.

### Precancerous lesions

Renal *adenomas* in the parenchyma seem closely linked to adenocarcinomas in animals and man; they constitute the only lesion that might develop into invasive cancer, but proof of this progression is lacking. *Papillomas* of the epithelium of the kidney, pelvis, and ureter definitely qualify as premalignant, just as they do in the bladder. *Leukoplakia* of the renal pelvis sometimes accompanies stones and chronic infection and may develop into cancer.

## NATURAL HISTORY

*Hematuria* clinically ushers in about half of the adult renal cancers; *pain in the flank* from the primary tumor begins the illness in some of the others. Often the primary cancer may remain asymptomatic and seed *metastases* to distant sites that then cause the initial symptoms for the patient, such as cough, bone pain, or any of a variety of central nervous system irregularities. The general pattern of growth is slow, but marked variations and fluctuations occur. Some renal parenchymal cancers have been followed by x-ray films for 10 years or more and are then found to be still operable and resectable for cure without evidence of metastases. As the tumor grows a mass may be felt in the flank, or blood clots may block the ureter with resulting severe colicky pain. Low-grade fever of tumor origin and anemia sometimes develop. The progression pattern of the primary and various widespread metastases is most irregular, with the average patient dying of cancerous catabolism (cachexia) in 4 to 5 years.

Prolonged *painless hematuria,* often with anemia, presages the tumors of the renal pelvis. With these tumors, infection occurs frequently with bouts of fever and chills, and death usually supervenes from severe unrelieved kidney sepsis.

On the other hand, Wilms' tumors generally come to diagnosis by virtue of the palpation of the bulky tumor masses in the abdomen; seldom do these tumors cause hematuria, although sometimes they cause pain. Lung metastases develop commonly and then anorexia, weight loss, and cachexia follow.

## DIAGNOSIS

**History.** A history of hematuria always raises the question of urinary tumor, with marked variation in intensity of the bleeding constituting a common characteristic of kidney cancer. Occasionally costovertebral angle *tenderness* and *pain* result from blood clots in the renal pelvis and ureter or from invasion by the tumor of the perirenal tissues. The "classic triad" of hematuria, pain, and flank mass seldom presents all at once in renal cancer (10% of the cases). In one third no symptoms at all are present. Fever, weight loss, hypertension, and edema of the ankles are less common symptoms. The systemic symptoms of fever, weight loss, and fatigability are much more common in clear cell tumors as opposed to the granular cell variety, and they are not related to metastases nor to tumor necrosis and hemorrhage.

**Physical examination.** *Palpation* of the kidney tumor becomes possible when the tumor is large or when the whole kidney enlarges from infection or hydronephrosis and pushes the tumor mass down and forward for bimanual appreciation. However, hydronephrosis and infection are not the main causes of the tumor mass with renal parenchymal tumors; it occurs from unexplained generalized parenchymal hypertrophy. Hypertension frequently develops with Wilms' tumors. One third of renal cancers show distant metastases on diagnosis, mainly in lungs, in bones, and sometimes in the skin.

**Urinalysis.** In contrast to bladder tumors, one third of renal cancers do not show even microscopic red blood cells. However, *proteinuria* occurs in over 90% of the instances.

**Cytology.** Cytologic study performed on urinary sediment has given disappointing results in cases of kidney parenchymal cancer. Cortical tumors do not exfoliate cells or else hyperplasia of the tubular epithelium can mimic cancerous cells so that both false negatives and false positives frequently result. Tumors of the renal pelvis and ureter, however, unless they are very well differentiated (papillomas), usually desquamate and can be regularly detected by cytology.

**X-ray studies.** X-ray films of various types usually give the most diagnostic information about kidney tumors. A preliminary "flat film" serves as a baseline comparison picture, to be followed by an excretory urogram (intravenous pyelogram). This constitutes the most revealing overall study. Then a retrograde pyelogram done at cytoscopy gives a clearer picture of the pelvis and calyces. By these three x-ray studies, the source of bleeding, kidney function, and distortions of the pelvis may be determined and the conclusions on each combined to form a reasonable picture of the pathology. *Arteriography* (selective renal angiography) has recently proved even more helpful in delineating kidney masses and in distinguishing cysts (no vessels) from cancers (many bizarre vessels). Good renal arteriograms may be almost diagnostic, showing typical vascular puddling. *Nephrotomography* also helps. Because of the tendency of renal cancers to metastasize to bones, any bone tumor found by x-ray film carries a suspicion of being metastatic from the kidney.

**Renal scanning.** Renal scanning with radioisotopes (mercury) may assist in locating tumorous areas in a kidney.

**Biopsy.** Some clinicians recommend needle aspiration of large kidney tumors; by this method spread of cancer cells is kept to a minimum. Seldom does one do open biopsies at operation for fear of jeopardizing cure in favorable cases. The diagnosis must be established with 90% certainty on clinical or radiographic grounds, and then the pathologist makes this 100% on the resected specimen. When the mass is irremovable, one does biopsy the tumor, of course.

**Laboratory studies.** Adjunctive information about the cancer is given by laboratory studies. Anemia occurs in one third of patients and an elevated erythrocyte sedimentation rate is helpful on occasion. Most tumors are moderately advanced on diagnosis and show an elevated sedimentation rate. Elevated urinary lactic dehydrogenase and alkaline phosphatase levels sometimes occur, and polycythemia or hypercalcemia can occasionally be found. Some authors report abnormal plasma C-reactive protein with renal carcinoma.

**Operation.** The definitive diagnosis comes at operative exploration that is made because of the strong suspicion of cancer. If curative resection can be done, one avoids exposure of the actual tumor capsule to preclude tumor seeding.

## Differential diagnosis

A *single renal cyst* can simulate cancer; arteriography best helps differentiate them. Alkaline phosphatase levels in the urine are said to be elevated with cancer, but not with simple cysts. Some cancers (the papillary cystadenocarcinomas) develop large cystic, necrotic areas. But exploration is often needed because about 5% of solitary cysts have associated cancers. If bloody fluid is found on needle aspiration of a cyst, solid tumor most likely coexists and exploration becomes necessary. (The nature of multicystic or polycystic kidneys is generally well revealed on x-ray films.)

*Necrotizing renal papillitis,* often found in diabetics, can imitate the pyelographic distortions of tumor.

*Pyelitis* with clots in the pelvis may give diagnostic difficulty and necessitate repeated pyelograms.

*Cancers of the right colon* present right flank masses, but barium enema studies clarify the diagnosis.

*Tumors of the adrenal gland,* lying on top of the kidney, are unusual. They present an impossible task of differentiation short of operation, unless they are functional and chemical studies suggest their diagnosis.

*Splenic enlargements or tumors,* although rare, simulate a left renal tumor on physical examination; they move on respiration, however, and the differentiation can usually be made on the basis of an x-ray film.

*Kidney stones* may coexist with an enlarged kidney and cause hematuria, but the pain of stone, unlike cancer, changes with activity, urination, or rest.

*Retroperitoneal tumors* of various kinds will, of course, mimic cancer of the kidney, such as childhood neuroblastomas (frequent metastases to bone), lymphosarcoma (usually with peripheral lymphadenopathy), or the undifferentiated soft part sarcomas that will need an operation and biopsy to make the distinction.

A *pancreatic cyst* may simulate a kidney cancer.

## PREVENTIVE MEASURES

No preventive measures can qualify for a definite recommendation at this time; evidence of causative agents and mechanisms is still only tentative and suggestive.

## TREATMENT PRINCIPLES

1. *Surgery (radical thoracoabdominal nephrectomy)* provides the best treatment for curable patients with parenchymal adenocarcinoma. Approaches to secure the vessels first before manipulation of the tumor and wide removal outside Gerota's fascia, staying away from the growing surface of the cancer, constitute techniques of importance.

2. *Irradiation* enters into the treatment of kidney cancers in the form of postoperative therapy, either routinely or for instances of inadequate margin, and for inoperable patients. But its value in instances of inadequate or borderline-adequate removal has not by any means been proved. Irradiation gives definite palliation for recurrence or distant metastases. Preoperative x-ray therapy may increase successes to some extent, but this has not been fully evaluated as yet.

3. *Nephrectomy* and *ureterectomy* comprise the surgical attack preferred for renal pelvic cancers because of the frequency of multiple pelvic and ureteral tumors. Extremely careful follow-up study of these patients is necessary to detect possible bladder tumors later in the life of the patient.

4. Increasing success in controlling *Wilms' tumors* arises from recently applied combinations of x-ray treatment, immediate surgery, and chemotherapy with actinomycin D.

5. *Chemotherapy* in general has shown disappointing results in renal cancers. A few regressions of metastases have occurred. Cytoxan achieves a few more responses than the other common drugs.

6. Pulmonary resection of solitary renal cancer metastases occasionally succeeds in gaining a long-term survival.

7. Palliative nephrectomy or resection of the primary in the face of distant metastases contributes questionable benefit to the patient. It probably gives real palliation only when it relieves local symptoms. The hope is faint for spontaneous regression of metastases by removal of the primary.

## COMMON ERRORS

Inadequate work-up of patients constitutes the main error. Exploration and wide exposure and manipulation of the tumor to make a diagnosis that could almost unequivocally be established by careful preoperative angiographic studies may jeopardize cure.

## PROMISING DEVELOPMENTS FOR THE FUTURE

1. A beginning has been made in identifying possible external etiologic agents in kidney cancer. The certain pinpointing of a major causative agent and its elimination from the environment seems our best hope for the future.

2. Increasingly wide use of selective renal arteriography in urologic work-ups will improve diagnosis.

## PROGNOSIS

1. Renal parenchymal adenocarcinomas have a relatively good prognosis, since nearly half of the patients survive 5 years or more. However, many such tumors possess a slow growth pattern and recurrences between 5 and 10 years frequently develop. The best outlook accompanies those cancers with a high degree of differentiation, a low number of mitoses, a gross size of less than 7 cm. in diameter, and no vein invasion, either grossly into the renal vein or microscopically into capillaries, and those cancers that show clearly defined borders. Also, clear-cell tumors carry a much better outlook than granular-cell types.

2. Epidermoid and papillary cancers of the kidney pelvis carry a poorer prognosis—less than 20% survive 5 years.

3. Most patients with Wilms' tumors survive more than 5 years today, a great improvement due largely to the addition of actinomycin D to our armamentarium. Collins has convincingly shown that a child who survives well a length of time equal to his age at diagnosis plus 9 months has no further risk of recurrence.

### REFERENCES

Ackerman, L. V., and del Regato, J. A.: Cancer, ed. 3, St. Louis, 1962, The C. V. Mosby Co., pp. 793-819.

Arduino, L. J.: Chemotherapy in urologic cancer, Surg. Clin. N. Amer. **45:**1352-1364, 1965.

Arner, O., Blanck, C., and von Schreeb, T.: Renal adenocarcinoma, Acta Chir. Scand. **346**(supp.)**:**1-51, 1965.

Bloom, H. J. G.: Cancer of the kidney. In Raven, R. W., and Roe, F. J. C., editors: The prevention of cancer, New York, 1967, Appleton-Century-Crofts, pp. 226-236.

Bottiger, L. E., Blanck, C., and von Schreeb, T.: Renal carcinoma, Acta Med. Scand. **180:** 329-338, 1966.

Collins, V. P.: The treatment of Wilms' tumor, Cancer **11:**89-94, 1958.

Grabstald, H.: Renal-cell cancer, New York J. Med. **64:**2539-2545, 2659-2671, 2771-2782, 1964.

Kark, W.: A synopsis of cancer, Baltimore, 1966, The Williams & Wilkins Co., pp. 84, 140.

Malament, M.: The diagnosis of renal cyst versus renal carcinoma, Surg. Clin. N. Amer. **45:** 1377-1392, 1965.

Stewart, B. H., and Meaney, T. F.: Diagnosis and treatment of renal neoplasm—a fresh approach, Cleveland Clin. Quart. **33:**45-57, 1966.

Chapter 25

# Cancer of the prostate

Primarily a gland of external secretion related to sexual function, the prostate responds in various ways to hormones. As in the breast, the neoplasm arising from the prostatic glandular tissues and cells shows varying degrees of hormone dependence.

## INCIDENCE AND DISTRIBUTION

Prostatic cancer is a disease of old men; 95% of patients are over 60 years of age and the incidence rises steeply with each decade after 60. It constitutes 5% of all cancers and 10% of cancers in males over 50. Cancer of the prostate is exceeded in incidence only by two sites—lung and colorectum. Asymptomatic, latent cancers of the prostate can be detected at autopsy in 15% of older men, a far greater frequency than that of clinically detected prostatic cancer. The disease occurs 15 times as frequently in the Union of South Africa as in Japan, with the United States and European rates falling in the middle ranges when compared to the rest of the world. Rates are low in Israel, China, and Italy. Apparently this cancer increases each year due to man's increasing longevity.

## ETIOLOGY

### External initiating agents

No such agents have come to light for animals or man. Like breast cancer, pancreatic cancer, and tumors of other solid secretory glands, prostatic cancer seems to arise without outside initiating agents.

### Predisposing factors

Benign prostatic hypertrophy does not appear to play any etiologic role in cancer. Hypertrophy occurs in the lateral lobes exclusively, whereas cancer usually starts in the atrophic glandular epithelium of the posterior lobe. Benign hypertrophy is a common condition and often coexists with cancer, but it does not cause it.

No evidence exists for any familial predisposition to prostatic cancer, and the testimony for certain racial proclivities remains inconclusive. Undoubtedly the presence of testosterone as a stimulating agent for prostatic glandular epithelium comprises a necessary background for cancer, since early castration of both animals and humans seems to eliminate the disease and induced mouse cancer transplants will only grow in the presence of testosterone. But no one knows whether or not androgens need to be present in excess to predispose the individual, or if perhaps a more complicated, indirect pituitary-testis-adrenal imbalance prevails. Basically androgens and estrogens are antagonistic in action on the prostate; testosterones stimulate the glands to produce secretion, and estrogens counteract this but stimulate the fibromuscular tissue to hypertrophy (benign prostatic hypertrophy). Estrogen has a similar effect on uterine musculature (fibroids).

## PATHOLOGY

The hidden location and small size of the prostate gland militates against easy detection of cancer. However, one gross pathologic characteristic does help the clinician—most cancers arise in the *posterior lobe,* which lies flat against the rectum. Also, nearly all cancers are *subcapsular.* Therefore the majority of cancers present just under the surface for the rectal examining finger to feel. The physician can feel most cancers when they are quite tiny, far less than 1 cm. in diameter.

Practically all cancers are *adenocarcinomas.* Two subtypes occur—(1) the common small-cell variety, which grows fast, invades early, and metastasizes quicker than (2) the well-differentiated type, which generally follows a more indolent course. A rare leiomyosarcoma, rhabdomyosarcoma, or lymphoma develops in the prostate. Epidermoid cancers, found occasionally, probably arise from urethral epithelium.

The capsule of the gland consists of a condensed layer of connective-elastic tissue and muscle. Cancer usually develops just under this capsular layer and so invades it early. Just outside the capsule, between it and the heavy prostatic fascia (Denonvilliers' fascia), lie many nerves and a profuse prostatic plexus of veins. These structures, too, succumb to early invasion by cancer after it penetrates the capsule, and the copious communication of venous networks with the vesical plexus, the other pelvic plexuses, and finally with Batson's vertebral vein system accounts for the frequent systemic metastases from prostatic cancer. The adjacent seminal vesicles often suffer involvement and local invasion of the urethra and bladder neck, with urinary obstruction, occasionally occurs, but this develops late in the tumor's growth when it has attained some bulk. With an advanced tumor, partial or complete blockage of one or both ureters can also take place. Invasion of the rectum, although it lies quite close, seldom develops because of the heavy prostatic fascial barrier. Lymphatic involvement of pelvic groups of nodes ensues equally quickly with venous spread. Often *bony metastases to the pelvis, lumbar spine, and femora* occur early, and the next most frequent sites are the lungs, liver, the aortic nodes, and then the mediastinal nodes. Multiple cancers often arise in the prostate (15% to 20%).

Because of the great frequency of benign prostatic hypertrophy (lateral lobes), half of the prostatic cancers coincide with benign hypertrophy in the same gland, but the two lesions appear distinct and separate. If cancer accidentally shows up in an enucleation for benign hypertrophy, one can assume that most of the cancer still remains with the patient in the subcapsular rim that does not come

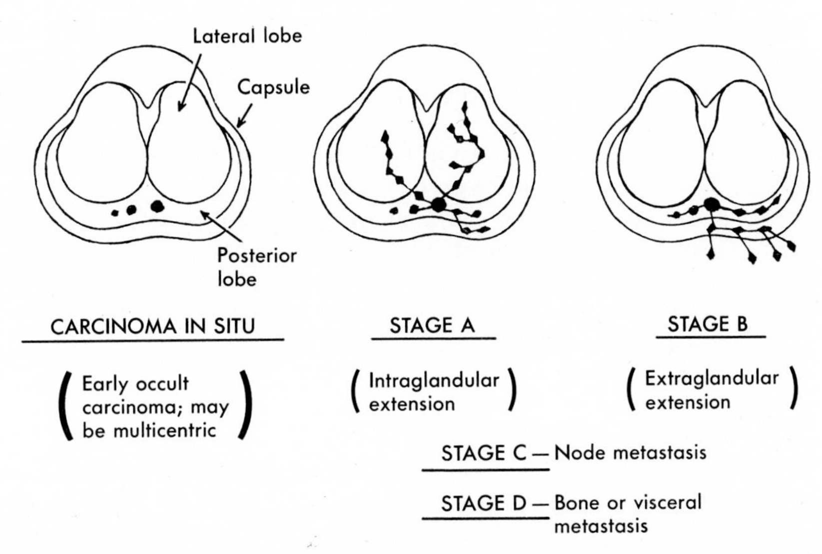


**Fig. 20.** Stages of prostatic cancer. (Modified from Melicow, M. M.: J. Urol. **95:**791, 1966; copyright 1966, The Williams & Wilkins Co., Baltimore.)

out with simple enucleation of hypertrophic nodules. These nodules are composed of hyperplasia, rather than neoplasia, of both stromal and glandular elements of the lateral lobes and middle lobe. Usually multiple, they tend to increase in number and size as men become older until the majority of males over 75 harbor them. They possess clinical importance only because they obstruct the flow of urine from the bladder.

## Precancerous lesions

The distinction between normal, active epithelium and "early" well-differentiated cancer of the prostate can be extremely difficult, just as in the thyroid. Various histochemical studies have been undertaken to try to simplify the matter. Carcinoma in situ appears to constitute a real entity in the prostate gland; according to McNeal, it may only precede a certain segment of carcinomas. Defined differently by others (Melicow), hyperactive microacini, without normal basement membranes separating them, may or may not represent a precancerous change. Nevertheless, the identification of these lesions is somewhat academic in so inaccessible a location as the prostatic capsule where any precancer would escape easy identification by any screening method.

# NATURAL HISTORY

As in the case of cancers of the breast, cancers of the prostate vary tremendously in their natural untreated course. In some patients anaplastic growths progress rapidly to widespread bone, lung, and liver deposits and cause death within half a year from first symptoms, whereas other patients harbor slow-growing tumor foci with few symptoms for 10 or 15 years before death.

Symptoms from prostatic cancer only occur when the growth is widespread locally—local pain from perineural extension and urethral or bladder neck obstruction with consequent frequency, urgency, cystitis, pyelitis, etc.—or has metastasized to bone with consequent bone pain. "Early" small cancers produce no symtoms.

In some series, 80% of patients show distant metastases on diagnosis and 90% to 95% are incurable because of distant or local spread. Two years approximates an average length of life from diagnosis for most of these men, if untreated; some men die in 6 months, others live for 10 years or more. Many die of local tumor effects, such as urinary obstruction and unrelieved upper urinary tract infection and renal failure; even more men die from the effects of distant metastases—constant debilitating bone pain, secondary anemia, overmedication, cachexia, etc.

## DIAGNOSIS

**History.** As stated above, small *curable cancers* in the prostate are silent and cause no symptoms. Frequency of urination, dysuria, nocturia (all signs of prostatism), pelvic pain, and urinary retention all stem from advanced local tumor growth. Hematuria occurs seldom and very late in the tumor's course and it may arise from a high fibrinolysin titer of tumor origin. Bone pain from metastases frequently is the first complaint.

**Physical examination.** Physical examination contributes to the diagnosis of prostatic cancer mainly through digital *rectal examination.* A silent, discrete, usually hard, but sometimes soft, nodule felt in the rectal aspect of the prostate gland, felt best with the patient in the knee-chest position, immediately raises the suspicion of cancer. Half of such nodules prove to be cancers. They can be felt by careful palpation as small as 0.5 cm. in greatest diameter. A large tumor may be less discrete, hard, more diffuse, obliterating the normal outline of the gland, and may be felt to invade the seminal vesicles. Large, stony-hard, bosselated cancers are obvious.

A routine yearly digital rectal examination constitutes the only screening test now possible for prostatic cancer. Reliance on symptoms or other tests leads to no early clues whatsoever.

**Biopsy.** Because the physician generally has only one chance to detect a curable neoplasm, biopsy always follows the palpation of a nodule; watching and waiting contribute nothing but hopelessness. One can use several biopsy techniques, the best and easiest being the *transperineal,* Silverman *needle biopsy,* which can be done in the office but is often done in the hospital for convenience. Mellinger advocates taking five cylinders of tissue at each biopsy session to eliminate false negatives. Often one needs to conduct several biopsy sessions because the smaller and more curable the cancers, the harder it is to make a correct diagnosis. With practice the physician becomes quite accurate with needle biopsy. Two dangers are perforations of the rectum and of the bladder.

Transrectal needle biopsy gives some complications without any added accuracy and requires a 24-hour rectal preparation. Open perineal biopsy scars and contaminates the field with tumor cells if radical prostatectomy has to follow later, but it does yield some added accuracy by exposing to vision the nodule in question. Histologic confirmation sometimes results from transurethral resection specimens, but this route applies only to tumors large enough to obstruct the urethra or bladder neck.

**Cytology.** Since small cancers will not exfoliate and even with vigorous prostatic massage (potentially a cancer-seeding maneuver), and since many large cancers do not shed cells into the prostatic secretion, cytology plays no part in early diagnosis. In addition to the many false negatives, false positives occur with infection of the gland.

**X-ray studies.** X-ray films contribute little to diagnosis of the primary mass in the prostatic gland, but they alone can detect and characterize the predominantly osteoblastic bone metastases from prostatic cancer. Only Paget's disease of bone mimics these typically dense metastatic lesions on an x-ray film. An excretory urogram (intravenous pyelogram) can both evaluate kidney function and survey the pelvic bones for metastases with the same films.

**Cystoscopy.** Cystoscopy can supply evidence in advanced cancers invading the bladder base; the examiner can also use the "scope" as resistance against which to palpate the prostate.

**Laboratory studies.** Various kinds of laboratory determinations help us to estimate the extent of the cancer. One particular test, the *serum acid phosphatase* (the first chemical test for any cancer, described by Gutman and associates), shows an abnormal elevation in the presence of most cases of metastases from prostatic cancer. Thirty percent of patients with metastases do not exhibit this elevation. Therefore a normal level does not rule out the possibility of metastases, but a positive elevation *definitely rules them in*—metastases must be present. A chance finding of an elevated acid phosphatase in any asymptomatic patient also unequivocally establishes the diagnosis of prostatic cancer. Elevations from other causes are rare (liver and renal disease), and generally only recent prostatic massage or prostatic manipulation can give a false rise. The procedure is too complicated for small laboratories to perform. Serum specimens can best be preserved and shipped to central, large laboratories. This enzyme also falls and rises with remissions and exacerbations of the cancer under treatment.

Alkaline phosphatase levels rise with the osteoblastic activity going on at the periphery of bone metastases as well as when bone heals a cavity from a dying cancer deposit. Therefore the course of prostatic cancer under treatment can be followed by periodic determinations of both acid and alkaline phosphatases.

Occasional laboratory findings include myelophthisic anemia from bone marrow metastases, a high serum fibrinolysin titer, pyuria, hematuria, or azotemia from kidney infection and kidney failure.

Prout and associates have demonstrated significant changes in two isozymes of serum lactic dehydrogenase with remission and relapse of prostatic cancer. These enzymic fluctuations may help follow results of treatment and predict the efficacy of new chemical treatments.

### Differential diagnosis

*Benign prostatic hypertrophy* may prove difficult to distinguish from cancer at times, but it generally forms a rubbery mass, is not absolutely fixed, is symmetrical, occurs in the lateral lobes of the gland, and causes urethral obstruction initially.

*Infarction* can exactly mimic cancer, even with elevated acid phosphatase. Biopsy must decide.

Prostatic *calculi* can be found on x-ray films; they may on occasion coexist with cancer.

Carcinomatous invasion from primary bladder cancer (squamous or transitional cell) and primary rectal cancer (mucin producing), the rare primary squamous cancer in the urethra, or occasionally a metastatic rectal shelf deposit from cancer of the gastrointestinal tract may present in or near the prostate gland and cause confusion.

Chronic *prostatitis* localized, or a granuloma, may also simulate cancer, but they are generally tender and soft.

## PREVENTIVE MEASURES

Unfortunately, the only known method of preventing this cancer consists of prepubertal castration of all males, a wholly unacceptable measure. This would bring the human race to an end. Slight inroads into the problem could possibly come from prophylactic removal of the thin compressed posterior lobe of the prostate when the patient has an operation for benign hypertrophy of the lateral lobe.

## TREATMENT PRINCIPLES

1. *Surgery (radical prostatectomy)* performed by either the perineal or retropubic approach, constitutes the only curative method today. One applies it to two groups of patients: (1) those who have had a suprapubic operation for benign hypertrophy wherein occult carcinoma or carcinoma in situ showed up unexpectedly and (2) patients harboring a localized nodule of prostatic cancer without spread outside the movable tissue and no x-ray, chemical, or other evidence of distant metastases. Such cases occur rarely because these small, asymptomatic cancers are difficult to diagnose. The operation includes resection of the prostatic capsule, Denonvilliers' fascia, the vesical neck, and the seminal vesicles. Impotence nearly always results from the operation, but otherwise few functional defects result.

2. All other treatment aims only at palliation. *Supervoltage x-ray therapy* directed at the prostate may achieve improvement superior to other methods of irradiation for locally invasive (Stage III) lesions, but this modality has not yet been well evaluated. Irradiation provides excellent palliation for isolated bone metastases as well as for other soft tissue lesions causing symptoms.

3. Prostatic cancers generally seem stimulated in their growth by the administration of testosterone. Therefore *castration* (orchiectomy) to eliminate androgens of testicular origin secures the quickest relief of local and distant metastatic symptoms. Reportedly, 70% of patients show improvement in a few days, since most prostatic cancers are hormone dependent when diagnosed. Frequently local cancer "melts away," metastases disappear, pain abates, anemia improves, and appetitie returns as a result of this measure. Variable as the length of remission may be—months to years, with an average of 20 months—relapses always occur in time as cancers lose their endocrine responsiveness.

4. *Estrogen administration* may counteract the tumor-stimulating effect of androgens (if testicles are still intact or if the adrenals are producing testosterone). Thus palliation and perhaps greater longevity may accrue to some patients treated with estrogen. The exact mechanism of action and benefit from this agent remains obscure. Various sequences of castration, estrogen administration, or both together form different treatment plans favored by different clinics. Most authorities, however, believe that estrogen alone is inferior to orchiectomy or to a combination of the two; they seem to agree that estrogen alone contributes little to the disease in relapse.

5. Recently a trend has developed to treat the Stage III (locally incurable) and Stage IV (distant metastasis) patients only if they have definite symptoms; this trend is based on the belief that no present evidence indicates any increased longevity from any palliative measure, and that therefore one must save the hormonal manipulation for symptomatic relief only. Our impression remains that a vigorous employment of both castration and estrogen achieves some added useful life in most cases.

6. Interstitial radioactive gold ($Au^{198}$) has been employed extensively by Flocks as an adjunct to local surgery and as treatment for locally inoperable cancers. It has definite advantages in selected cases.

7. Adrenalectomy, hypophysectomy, chemotherapy with cytolytic drugs, and the systemic use of $P^{32}$ (for bone metastases) have proved disappointing in the main.

8. Cortisone administration provides useful relief in cases of relapse from androgen control therapy.

9. Transurethral resection relieves bladder outlet obstruction in instances of large local cancers.

## COMMON ERRORS

1. Omission of the rectal examination on routine physical examination.
2. Observation only of prostatic nodules, without biopsy.
3. Failure to carry out radical prostatectomy in cases where unexpected cancers appear in the specimen of a suprapubic enucleation.

## PROMISING DEVELOPMENTS FOR THE FUTURE

1. *Yearly rectal examination* for all men over 40 could duplicate the 50% cure rate achieved by this measure in the armed forces. This would be a considerable improvement over the present 5% cure rate obtained in the civilian population by our traditional habit of examining people only when they are ill.

2. Refinements in histochemical and electron microscopic distinctions between normal cells, precancerous cells, and frankly cancerous cells will undoubtedly make "early" diagnosis more of a reality in the future.

## PROGNOSIS

We must temper decisions about ideal treatment of "early" cancers because of reports such as that of Barnes, who treated nearly 60 patients with curable cancer by conservative palliative measures and secured a 15-year survival rate of

31%. "Early" cancer may somehow equate with biologically indolent cancer; treatment may not influence the course as much as we like to think.

In general, somewhat more than half of the patients suitable for radical prostatectomy survive 5 years and about 30% survive for 10 years.

Patients with low grade tumors, older patients, and those who respond to androgen control measures live longer than the average. Seven to 10% of untreated patients survive 5 years. Among treated patients (and these usually consist mostly of people treated with hormonal alteration therapy), the overall survival rates for all patients in all stages approach 40% at 5 years and 20% at 10 years.

**REFERENCES**

Ackerman, L. V., and del Regato, J. A.: Cancer, ed. 3, St. Louis, 1962, The C. V. Mosby Co., pp. 841-866.

Barnes, R. W.: Nonoperative treatment of operative carcinoma of the prostate, Proc. Nat. Cancer Conf. **5:**323-326, 1964.

Belt, E.: Carcinoma of the prostate, Proc. Nat. Cancer Conf. **5:**327-329, 1964.

Bertelsen, S.: Transrectal needle biopsy of the prostate, Acta Chir. Scand. **357:**226-231, 1966.

Dixon, F. J., and Moore, R. A.: Tumors of the male sex organs. In Atlas of tumor pathology, Sect. 8, Fasc. 31B and 32, Washington, D. C., 1952, Armed Forces Institute of Pathology.

Eisenberg, H., and Heise, H.: End-results in cancer of the prostate and the urinary bladder, 1940-1959, Proc. Nat. Cancer Conf. **5:**331-340, 1964.

Fergusson, J. D.: Cancer of the prostrate. Raven, R. W., and Rose, F. J. C., editors: The prevention of cancer, New York, 1967, Appleton-Century-Crofts, pp. 257-261.

Flocks, R. H.: Interstitial irradiation therapy with solution of Au198 as part of combination therapy for prostatic cancer, J. Nucl. Med. **5:**691-705, 1964.

Frankus, L. M.: Some comments on long-term results of endocrine treatment of prostatic cancer, Brit. J. Urol. **30:**383-388, 1958.

Gutman, A. B., Gutman, E. B., and Robinson, J. N.: Determination of serum "acid" phosphatase activity in differentiating skeletal metastases secondary to prostatic carcinoma from Paget's disease of bone, Amer. J. Cancer **38:**103-108, 1940.

Huggins, C.: Endocrine-induced regression of cancer, Nobel foundation lecture, Science **156:** 1050-1053, 1967.

Jonsson, G.: Geriatric urology, Acta Chir. Scand. **357** (supp.):59-70, 1966.

Kark, W.: Synopsis of cancer, Baltimore, 1966, The Williams & Wilkins Co., pp. 178-182.

Kirchheim, D., Niles, N. R., Frankus, E., and Hodges, C. V.: Correlative histochemical and histological studies on thirty radical prostatectomy specimens, Cancer **19:**1683-1696, 1966.

McNeal, J. E.: Morphogenesis of prostatic carcinoma, Cancer **18:**1659-1666, 1965.

Melicow, M. M.: Cancer of the prostate, J. Urol. **95:**791-800, 1966.

Mellinger, G. T.: Carcinoma of the prostate, Surg. Clin. N. Amer. **45:**1413-1426, 1965.

Prout, G. R., Jr., Macalalay, E. V., Jr., and Dennis, L. J.: A comparison of serum LDH and its fourth and fifth isozymes in patients with prostatic carcinoma before and after treatment and during relapse, Proc. Nat. Cancer Conf. **5:**311-321, 1964.

Scott, R. J.: Needle biopsy of the prostate, J.A.M.A. **201:**958-960, 1967.

Tjaden, H. B., Culp, D. A., and Flocks, R. H.: Clinical adenocarcinoma of prostate in patients under 50 years, J. Urol. **93:**618-621, 1965.

Chapter 26

# Cancer of the testis

The testis comprises the male counterpart of the ovary, but differs from the female gland in many ways. One difference lies in the relatively greater abundance of germ cell tissue—seminiferous convoluted tubules—and relatively less stroma than the ovary. Tumors of the testicular tissues are thus predominantly germ cell tumors; they exhibit less variety than ovarian tumors and nearly all of them are malignant.

## INCIDENCE AND DISTRIBUTION

Testicular cancers are not common and comprise less than 1% of all cancers. They become evident in the young male adult, however, and assume clinical importance because they account for more cancers in the male between the ages of 29 and 34 than any other type of cancer. No geographic or racial predilections are apparent, although this cancer seems rare in Negroes.

## ETIOLOGY

### External etiologic agents

No reports suggest any outside activator substances as causative agents. These primarily germ cell tumors, coming to a clinical level of appreciation at relatively early ages, must originate from developmental and internal abnormalities.

### Predisposing factors

Despite the testis serving as the male reproductive manufactory, which is normally responsive to hormones (principally gonadotrophins), amazingly little demonstrable relation between testicular tumors and hormones exists. No very obvious hormonal imbalance precedes their development in man, although speculation abounds that deficient testicular interstitial cell production of testosterone causes oversecretion of gonadotrophin by the pituitary and sustained hyperplasia of testicular cells. Seldom do these tumors produce hormones, except for the choriocarcinomatous elements that secrete gonadotrophins.

*Cryptorchidism* and testicular cancers are associated, but not necessarily causally connected. Neoplasms reportedly develop ten to fifty times more often in the undescended testis than in the normal one. Burrows and Horning believe that the environmental temperature difference between the normal descended testis and the abnormal undescended gland causes crucial deficiency of testosterone that leads to excess interstitial cell–stimulating hormone (ICSH) and thus tumor production. However, orchiopexy after puberty, like circumcision after puberty, does not reduce the tumor incidence. The evidence for a direct causative effect of maldescent itself does not completely convince us. Probably lack of descent of the testis constitutes one sign of an abnormal testis to begin with; a gland is therefore more prone to neoplasia from other, earlier, and more basic influences than location alone provides. Perhaps excess interstitial cell–stimulating hormone is a contributory background cause. Also, if such an excess of pituitary hormone were a major predisposing condition, Leydig cell tumors should be common; actually they are rare.

Another predisposing cause often cited is trauma to the testis. The fallacy of injury as an etiologic factor becomes apparent when we learn that abdominal testes show cancer four times more often than inguinal testes, the latter being the more traumatized. Injury occurs more easily to a tumor-containing testis, and hence the clinical connection arises. In short, we know little about the etiology of the testicular tumors, and therefore we call them "developmental."

## PATHOLOGY

Four principal classes of testicular tumor deserve our attention:

| | |
|---|---|
| *Seminoma* | 40% |
| *Embryonal carcinoma* | 28% |
| *Teratocarcinoma* | 27% |
| *Choriocarcinoma* | 2% |
| (Nongerminal tumors) | 2% |

Nearly half of testicular cancers show mixtures of these four basic types. The main clinical significance of classification lies in deciding which of the four types predominates because treatment and prognosis depend upon this classification. Dixon and Moore believe that seminomas constitute a distinctly separate variety of tumor that arises from the epithelium of the seminiferous tubules, whereas the other three (embryonal, teratocarcinoma, and choriocarcinomas) arise from a common totipotential germ cell and possess a close interrelationship with each other. The frequencies, mixtures, and growth behavior of seminoma compared to the other three support this general idea. Seminoma, the most common type of all, exhibits a startling concentration of frequency of occurrence between the ages of 40 and 45 years, whereas teratocarcinoma occurs evenly between the ages of 20 and 40. Most tumors in ectopic testes are seminomas. Second primary cancers in the opposite testicle occur more often than in the normal male population.

Nearly all tumors of the testis have counterparts in the ovary; seminomas correspond to dysgerminomas and embryonal carcinomas; teratocarcinomas, choriocarcinomas, and the rare Leydig cell tumors occur in both ovaries and testes under the same names. Differences appear in degree of malignancy and in frequency of recurrence. Teratomas are frequent and benign in the ovary, whereas they are infrequent and nearly always malignant in the testis. No testicular tumors corresponding to ovarian cystadenomas or granulosa-theca cell tumors have been described.

Childhood tumors of the testis are quite uncommon and generally are classified as embryonal or teratocarcinoma types.

Benign neoplasms rarely arise in the testis, but when present they consist of nongerminal kinds of tumor, principally capsular fibromas or interstitial cell tumors (Leydig cell tumors).

Spread of testicular cancer by local invasion is sharply limited because of the heavy tunica albuginea of the testis; it requires long-standing growth or a tumor with great aggressive potential to penetrate this tunica. Metastases occur first via the rich lymphatic network of the testes. Interestingly, the first echelon of lymph nodes draining the testicle lie along the aorta just below the renal pedicles, a route generally parallel to the venous drainage pathways of the testicle. (Node dissections, therefore, begin at the lower aortic–vena cava area and concentrate about the renal pedicles.) When cancers involve the epididymis, the external iliac nodes may be the first involved. Blood-borne metastases develop somewhat later in the tumor's course and have become established in lungs and liver in most cases that come to autopsy.

### Precancerous lesions

No such lesions have been described for human testicular cancer, although noninvasive seminomas have been identified in the dog and in sheep.

## NATURAL HISTORY

The growth rate characterizing most testicular neoplasms may be called slow to moderate, but we lack accurate documentation. A few cancers progress rapidly from first symptoms to death within a year because of widespread metastasis on diagnosis. A painless slight enlargement with hardness and heaviness of one testicle first calls attention to the gland. This gradually progresses in 6 months or so to a larger mass that may cause a dull aching because of the added testicular weight and increased sensitivity of the abnormal testis. Metastasis generally develops within 6 months of the first symptom, although it may require several years for metastatic lesions to manifest themselves. Metastatic symptoms stem from large retroperitoneal lymph nodes obstructing ureter or vena cava; or cough, hemoptysis, and dyspnea may indicate lung metastases. Death approaches by way of ureteral blockage, infection, and uremia from kidney failure, or through the familiar mechanism of cachexia from the catabolic effect of large amounts of widespread, growing tumor.

## DIAGNOSIS

**History.** Symptoms that may bring the patient to the physician seldom come from small tumors. Sensitivity of the testicle and aching pain or palpation by the patient of a nodule ensue when the tumor reaches moderate size. Nevertheless, the physician soon learns to pay close attention to any testicular complaint in young adult males because almost all testicular masses are cancerous. Occasionally, metastases cause the first complaints, such as lumbar pain or tenderness, fever, anorexia, vomiting, or recent development of a cough. Rarely, choriocarcinomas produce sufficient gonadotrophins to cause gynecomastia and nipple pigmentation; or the rare interstitial cell tumor may cause virilization.

**Physical examination.** The typical tumor-containing testicle feels *enlarged, heavy, and painless.* Careful palpation of the testes naturally forms an essential part of any complete physical examination, mainly to search out asymptomatic tumors. Hydroceles accompany neoplasms often enough to justify removing the fluid from these cystic masses to facilitate palpation for tumor. Tumors do not transilluminate, but hydroceles do. Occasionally very large retroperitoneal lymph node metastases around the lower aorta may be felt by abdominal examination.

**X-ray studies.** X-ray films must be done to study the patient for possible metastases; *excretory urography,* and sometimes retrograde pyelography will often reveal para-aortic lymph node enlargement by showing ureteral deviations, and *chest films* may detect pulmonary metastases. Venograms and lymphangiograms may also help find nodal spread, but they are more complicated to perform.

**Laboratory studies.** Specific laboratory studies consist mainly of the *urinary gonadotrophin* determinations; elevated levels occur with nearly half of the cases of all four types of cancer because of the frequent histologic mixtures of the various types. Choriocarcinoma usually causes the greatest elevation. Persistent high levels after an orchiectomy has been performed can be fairly certain evidence of metastases; this finding helps the physician considerably if such metastases are not otherwise detectable. Elevated sedimentation rates after treatment may likewise indicate occult metastases.

**Operation.** Removal of the testis constitutes the main definitive diagnostic measure. Wedge and needle biopsies seldom give the pathologist enough tissue for a reliable diagnosis or a reliable classification of the tumor, and they also risk tumor spread in the local tissues. However, biopsies can serve to rule out tumor in cases of inflammatory or benign lesions.

### Differential diagnosis

*Orchitis* is acute in onset and tender.

*Hematomas* and *hematoceles* occur associated with trauma; no easy differential test exists except watching or biopsy.

*Tuberculosis* involves the epididymis rather than the testicle proper and often shows calcification on x-ray film and beading of the vas deferens, along with pulmonary tuberculosis or tuberculous prostatitis.

*Hydroceles* transilluminate, but may overlie tumors.

## PREVENTIVE MEASURES

In view of our ignorance of mechanisms causing testicular cancer, we have no cancer preventive measures. Many authorities believe that orchiopexy for an undescended testis should be accomplished before the age of 6, mainly to secure normal spermatogenic development that would be damaged if the operation were delayed longer. This measure also hopefully prevents a somewhat increased risk of cancer in that testis. A second maneuver that could conceivably prevent some cancers consists in the operative removal of any permanently atrophic testis. Some evidence suggests the idea that atrophic glands become cancerous more often than normal ones; abdominal testes, those remaining atrophic or becoming so after orchiopexy, or those atrophic following trauma probably warrant removal.

## TREATMENT PRINCIPLES

1. Surgery always constitutes the first step of the treatment plan. *Orchiectomy,* complete, with removal of all tunic and fascial investments of the testis, early clamping of the cord before manipulating the tumor, and high ligation and excision of the spermatic cord and vessels within the inguinal canal, constitutes the proper approach. All specialists recommend this operation for all testicular tumors. Further treatment depends upon the histology.

2. Pure *seminomas,* or predominantly seminomatous neoplasms, then require thorough radiotherapy to the potential metastatic node-bearing areas in the abdomen and pelvis, without further surgery. Radiotherapy also proves beneficial for distant blood-borne deposits, since this tumor typically responds well to x-ray therapy.

3. *Embryonal carcinomas* and *teratocarcinomas* as a group generally benefit from *retroperitoneal node dissections* if no distant metastases are present. If positive nodes appear in the operative specimen, the contralateral nodes also undergo

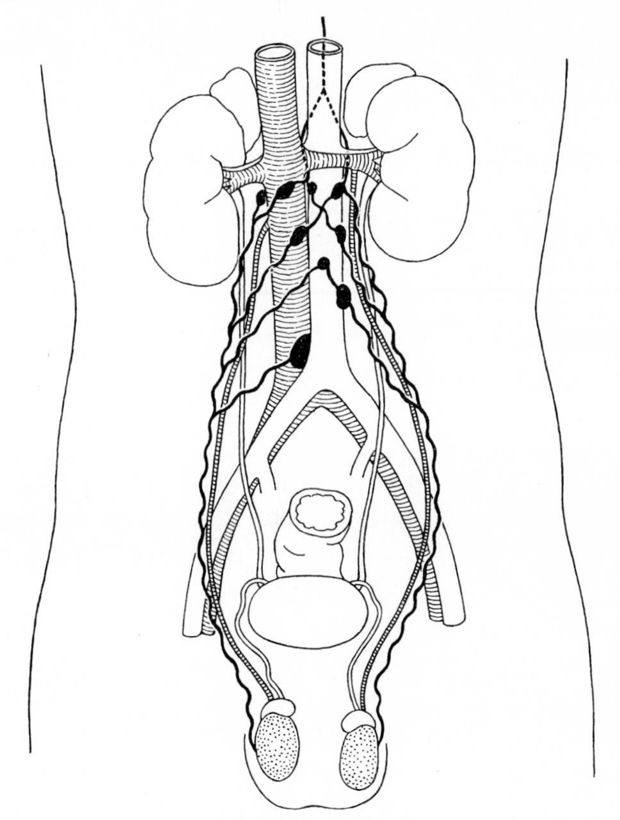

**Fig. 21.** First nodal group in lymphatic drainage pathways from the testes lie along the vena cava and aorta near the renal pedicles. (From Ackerman, L. V., and del Regato, J. A.: Cancer, ed. 3, St. Louis, 1962, The C. V. Mosby Co.)

removal, and postoperative radiotherapy to the retroperitoneal bed is generally advisable. Irradiation constitutes effective therapy for isolated, especially symptomatic, distant metastases.

4. Those few tumors composed mainly of choriocarcinoma are so aggressive that, after orchiectomy, further surgery on regional nodes seems a wasted effort. Combination chemotherapy may be best; the most effective drug (also the most toxic) is actinomycin D. The outstanding success of drug control for choriocarcinoma in the female supports this decision. X-ray therapy to localized metastatic areas may also help. Small choriomatous components in tumors possessing a predominance of other types of cells should not, however, preclude curative attempts along the lines outlined for embryonal carcinoma and teratocarcinoma.

5. Combined triple-drug chemotherapy for distant metastases has achieved significant control in a number of cases of all tumor types; *actinomycin D* seems mainly responsible for this effect. *Chlorambucil* appears the drug of choice for distant metastases from seminoma.

## COMMON ERRORS

1. As with some other cancers, we fail often in applying our best diagnostic acumen. First of all, we often do not examine all testes carefully, if at all. Second, we allow hydroceles and perhaps a history of trauma to divert us from a full-scale study of a testis that may contain tumor. Last, we fail to teach the lay public any technique of self-examination.

2. Errors of treatment seldom occur today. Most urologists receive thorough grounding in the management of testicular tumors. However, a 10% to 15% added advantage is given to patients by retroperitoneal node dissection in suitable cases; the added advantage of this operation seems more often withheld than offered.

## PROMISING DEVELOPMENTS FOR THE FUTURE

A vigorous administration of preoperative and postoperative prophylactic chemotherapy as a regular, routine measure may result in increased salvage in the future.

## PROGNOSIS

1. *Seminomas* have the best outlook—75% 5-year survivals and 65% 10-year survivals. Dixon and Moore report 90% 5-year survivals. Salvage remains quite possible with metastases to nodes and even to distant sites.

2. *Embryonal carcinomas, teratocarcinomas,* and *choriocarcinomas* carry a reduced salvage rate; grouping them together, as is often done, 35% 5-year salvage may represent a fairly average figure. One report shows half of these tumors with node metastases to have been salvaged. Teratocarcinoma survival may be somewhat better.

3. Factors that worsen the prognosis consist of elevated gonadotrophin levels in the urine, pretreatment pain, positive retroperitoneal nodes, vascular invasion, penetration of the tunica albuginea, and Leydig cell hyperplasia in the normal testicular tissue of the specimen.

**REFERENCES**

Ackerman, L. V., and del Regato, J. A.: Cancer, ed. 3, St. Louis, 1962, The C. V. Mosby Co., pp. 867-887.

Burrows, H., and Horning, E. S.: Oestrogens and neoplasia, Springfield, Ill., 1952, Charles C Thomas, Publisher, pp. 59-66.

Dixon, F. J., and Moore, R. A.: Tumors of the male sex organs, In Atlas of tumor pathology, Sect. VIII, Fasc. 31B and 32, Washington, D. C., 1952, Armed Forces Institute of Pathology, pp. 48-120.

Guthrie, J.: Testicular cancer. In Raven, R. W., and Roe, F. J. C., editors: The prevention of cancer, New York, 1967, Appleton-Century-Crofts, pp. 265-268.

MacKenzie, A. R.: Chemotherapy of metastatic testis cancer, Cancer **19:**1369-1376, 1966.

Murphy, J. J., and Schoenberg, H. W.: In Nealon, T. F., Jr., editor: Management of the patient with cancer, Philadelphia, 1966, W. B. Saunders Co., pp. 715-717.

Notter, G., and Ranudd, M. E.: Treatment of malignant testicular tumors, Acta Radiol. (Ther.) **2:**273-301, 1964.

Staubitz, W. J., Jewett, T. C., Jr., Magoss, I. V., Schenk, W. G., Jr., and Phalakornkule, S.: Management of testicular tumors in children, J. Urol. **94:**683-686, 1965.

Willis, R. A.: Teratomas. In Atlas of tumor pathology, Sect. VIII, Fasc. 9, Washington, D. C., 1951, Armed Forces Institute of Pathology, pp. 7-58.

Chapter 27

# Sarcomas of soft (mesodermal) tissues

Grouping together all tumors of mesodermal tissue origin creates quite a heterogeneous group. Neoplasms derived from muscle, fat, connective tissue, and blood vessels that lie between skin and bones tend to behave, however, in surprisingly similar ways despite the diversity of their parent tissues. However, tumors of the same tissue of origin, for example, fibrous tissue, can vary greatly in behavior. Because they are comparatively rare tumors, however, they must be considered in a single chapter for the sake of convenience.

## INCIDENCE AND DISTRIBUTION

Of all malignant tumors the soft part sarcomas comprise only about 1%. Approximately 20 benign neoplasms arise from these soft tissues for every malignant tumor. With a few exceptions these sarcomas exhibit no sex, racial, or geographic preference in their occurrence, nor in general do they limit themselves to any particular age group, except that sarcomas as a rule tend to afflict persons at slightly younger ages than the common carcinomas.

## ETIOLOGY

### External initiating agents

Although one half of the body weight lies in the soft part tissues, tumors develop rather seldom in these tissues, possibly because their cells divide less frequently than do epithelial cells (thus reducing the chance for progression of the tumor process) or possibly because deposition and storage of carcinogenic external agents does not take place in them. Many carcinogenic chemical compounds have produced fibrosarcomas and other sarcomatous varieties in animals. It is of particular interest to note the development of sarcomas after the implantation of inert plastic films or sheets in the subcutaneous tissues of animals. However, no external agents have been linked to human sarcomas except the association of pleural mesotheliomas with asbestos exposure. There are also scattered reports of fibrosarcomas occurring in irradiated tissues.

Trauma, often invoked by medical and legal proceedings as possibly causative, has never been satisfactorily demonstrated to be a primary initiating factor. That it may occasionally aggravate an already existing but clinically hidden tumor can never be categorically denied. And trauma may localize a metastasis by causing an intravascular clot that traps circulating cancer cells. Arising under the skin and often on extremities, soft part tumors exactly fit the layman's idea of a cancer that must have some relation to injury. And since injuries occur so often on extremities, it is perhaps natural that many lawsuits are instituted, claiming injury caused a sarcoma, despite the lack of scientific support for such a concept.

### Predisposing factors

No internal predisposition has ever been suggested as a causative factor.

## PATHOLOGY

Stout lists *eighteen different malignant soft part tumors,* many of which occur so rarely as to be seen only once or twice in a physician's lifetime. Our purpose in this résumé will be served by trying to describe a few of the common types with only mention of the others. *Fibrosarcoma, liposarcoma, rhabdomyosarcoma,* and *synovial sarcoma* are the more common varieties. Occasional examples of *leiomyosarcoma* outside the uterus and gastrointestinal tract, hemangioendothelioma, myxosarcoma, alveolar soft part sarcoma, malignant mesenchymoma (mixed sarcomas), malignant mesothelioma, plasmacytoma, and lymphangiosarcoma may be seen. The list of individual benign tumors that require differentiation from the malignant ones are of even greater variety (thirty-eight types). Only by grouping them by tissue of origin, according to Stout, can we manage to discuss them at all. The lipomatoses, fibromatoses, myxomatoses, xanthomatoses, and angiomatoses constitute the five main benign categories.

*Fibrosarcoma* is the commonest sarcoma, comprising at least one third to one half of the whole group, depending upon individual choice of nomenclature by pathologists. Occurring usually on the extremities or the trunk in persons between the ages of 30 and 60, these neoplasms arise from subcutaneous fibrous connective tissue, fascial sheaths over muscle, nerve sheaths, periosteum, or scars. They seem encapsulated, but have only compressed surrounding tissue to form a pseudocapsule. Most tumors are well differentiated, and nearly all show reticulin fibers under the microscope. Fibrosarcomas characteristically invade local tissues, defying ordinary excisional eradication, and metastasize late via the bloodstream, usually to the lungs, but sometimes to local nodes (20%). A continuous spectrum of fibrous neoplasms exists from the benign keloids, fibromas, and palmar fibromatoses (Dupuytren's contraction), through desmoids and another intermediate, locally invasive proliferation called pseudosarcomatous fasciitis, to the next more malignant group of dermatofibrosarcoma protuberans, the well-differentiated fibrosarcoma that invades locally but seldom metastasizes, then on to the poorly differentiated, highly lethal types. Sometimes a nodule of multiple neurofibromatosis will progress to a sarcoma.

*Liposarcoma* generally develops next in frequency, coming in any area of the body where fatty tissues lie, although usually developing from deeper fat deposits in the thigh, groin, and retroperitoneum. Generally the patients are males and older than victims of fibrosarcoma. This tumor arises de novo, but hardly ever from the common, benign lipoma. Sometimes attaining huge size, especially in the retroperitoneal and perirenal areas, these tumors also have pseudocapsules and come in well-differentiated and poorly differentiated types; most contain varying amounts of myxoid elements that led to the term *myxoliposarcoma* in times past. They can be of multicentric origin; they feel firm, nodular, but not stony hard, and invade locally, insidiously, and widely. About half of the more anaplastic tumors spread to lungs, pleura, and liver. Nodal metastases may occur (10%).

*Rhabdomyosarcoma* constitutes the third most frequent group and usually affects males on their extremities; however, they appear deeper in the limb than fibrosarcoma, since they presumably arise from skeletal muscle underneath fascia. Presenting as deep, semifixed, softish masses, which may contain areas of hemorrhage and necrosis, these tumors behave like the preceding fibrosarcomas and liposarcomas by invading much wider than can be grossly detected. They metastasize via the blood vascular system, but seldom by the lymphatics. The fully malignant type as described above is usually called a pleomorphic rhabdomyosarcoma. Two other subtypes bear mention. (1) The *embryonal* rhabdomyosarcoma, a highly malignant tumor of childhood, appears in the head and neck area quite often, in the genitourinary tract, or in the pelvis, but seldom on the extremities. Probably in this group we should include the sarcoma botryoides of the gynecologic tracts in infants. (2) The *alveolar* type of rhabdomyosarcoma affects older children and young adults and occurs at random at any site in the body.

*Granular cell myoblastoma* deserves mention in discussing muscle origin neoplasms. This tumor generally develops in the tongue, and most cases are only locally invasive and nonmetastasizing. They are important because they may be confused with squamous cancer.

*Synovial sarcoma* is a seldom encountered tumor of the knee and ankle regions. It arises next to the joint capsule, bursa, or tendon sheath, but, strangely, seldom involves the synovial lining of the joint itself. To palpation it is a solid, hard, well demarcated, deeply fixed tumor; it attacks young adults (average age 32 years), grows slowly, and metastasizes most often to the lungs, and in at least 10% of instances to regional nodes as well. Children with these tumors fare better than adults.

(Reticulum cell sarcoma behaves and responds to treatment more like lymphoma than like a soft part tumor and will be considered among the lymphomas, as will plasmacytoma and mycosis fungoides. Leiomyosarcomas occur so rarely outside the uterus, the stomach, and the small bowel that they will not be further described here. The various angiosarcomas are too rare for detailed description, as is the alveolar soft part sarcoma.)

## Precancerous lesions

No true soft part precancers exist, so far as we know. The progression of benign fibrous, fatty, or muscular tumors to malignant tumors has rarely been described; the occasional transformation of fibroma to fibrosarcoma after repeated recurrences impresses most authorities as an unsupported assumption based on an erroneous initial diagnosis.

## NATURAL HISTORY

Several generalizations bear emphasis in regard to the course of these various sarcomas. They often start on extremities, grow slowly, with periods of rapid growth, and appear as painless lumps under the skin without ulcerations. A few synovial sarcomas begin with pain, however, before the mass appears. Local excision, no matter how carefully done, constitutes inadequate treatment and the sarcomas recur locally in a year or so, spreading in tissue planes at considerable distance from their grossly detectable margins. Lung metastases eventually develop and local pain begins from the expanding bulk of the primary tumor. Weight loss and inanition supervene, followed by a terminal pneumonia. Mean duration of detectable tumor before treatment is 1 to 2 years; mean survival in the patients dying of tumor metastases usually is about 5 years.

Despite the discouraging course of the above "average" case, the commonest sarcomas prove quite favorable in outlook; three fourths of fibrosarcomas are in the well-differentiated group that persist locally but seldom metastasize and need not cause death. Therefore individualization of each tumor is mandatory. The detailed study and assignment of histogenesis of each of these sarcomas constitutes the most important single measure in determining the patient's management and survival.

## DIAGNOSIS

**History.** Whenever a patient gives a story of a slowly enlarging, painless firm-to-hard subcutaneous mass, the conscientious physician does well to have sarcoma in mind from the start as he examines and advises. As in many other types of cancer, there are no early "tip-off" symptoms or signs—the *lump* is the symptom and the sign. One exception to this occurs in one fourth of synovial sarcomas that begin with pain before a lump appears. Patients as a rule allow the lump to increase for 6 months to 1 year or more before seeking attention, so that it has generally attained at least a 3 or 4 cm. diameter by the time the physician sees it. If the mass lies in the retroperitoneal space, it will perhaps have attained great bulk before attracting notice. One important point in the physical examination merits our attention—by having the patient alternately contract and relax the underlying muscles, one can decide about fixation of the mass to fascia and about location *within* a muscle group.

**Biopsy.** Open wedge biopsy for any mass greater than 2.5 cm. constitutes the first and cardinal measure in diagnosis of these subcutaneous neoplasms. The reader may be surprised that we recommend the risk of cutting into what may be a highly malignant tumor deep in body tissues and so spreading cancer cells in the wound. The answer is that we accept this risk because the risk of total excision for diagnosis is greater. We accept the risk and minimize it by careful technique, by meticulous hemostasis, and by avoiding local anesthesia that may distend and open up tissue planes for spread. No matter how he may try not to do so, the surgeon invariably cuts into and through *microscopic* tumor when doing any total excision before a diagnosis is made. Therefore, he really spreads cancer over a wider surface of tissue than he would with a wedge biopsy. Without a diagnosis of sarcoma, the surgeon can never do the somewhat mutilating wide dissection necessary for proper treatment—this surgery is morally and legally indefensible before he knows what kind of tumor he is dealing with. Therefore, just as with melanoma, two operations are always inevitable—the first a small biopsy for diagnosis and the second a planned resection for cure. No matter how widely the first diagnostic excision may be, it can *never* be adequate to treat a fully malignant sarcoma. In other words, the surgeon cannot spare the patient the two operations. So the gentle, careful open wedge biopsy serves best and spreads cancer the least.

*Needle biopsy* can seldom be relied on. These neoplasms give the average pathologist enough trouble in classification when large sheets of tumor configurations are available. Since determining exact histogenesis as far as possible means more than any other single measure for deciding on treatment, the physician only harms the patient in trying to spare him a formal biopsy procedure.

**X-ray studies.** In larger tumors x-ray study may be helpful. Synovial sarcomas sometimes possess typical calcifications. Arteriography often demonstrates the increased and tortuous vascularity of malignant tumors that sometimes contain arteriovenous shunts and can help establish relationships to nearby bone. X-ray films can also eliminate the possibility of primary bone tumor, a frequent alternative in differential diagnosis.

## Differential diagnosis

*Sebaceous cyst* (epidermoid cyst, wen) develops most often on the scalp, face and neck, or the back; it has a dimpled attachment to the skin at one hair follicle, usually feels soft, smooth, and doughy. Sarcomas seldom possess these features.

*Lipomatoses,* the common lipoma, should be easy to diagnose as a rule; they feel quite typically soft, discrete, freely movable, usually lie in the superficial subcutaneous fatty layer, and are extremely smooth. Lipomas tend to be multiple and to develop when patients are gaining weight.

*Fibromatoses* include a number of fibrous tissue proliferative conditions that must undergo the most rigorous histologic scrutiny, as a rule, to be distinguished from fibrosarcoma. Some lesions are clinically apparent, however, as *keloids* of dark-skinned persons or the spontaneous fibrous thickenings of the skin *(fibroma durum).* The abdominal desmoid that occasionally develops in the abdominal wall of pregnant women has an essentially benign character, never metastasizes, and seldom recurs after excision. Other lesions lie in between benignancy and malignancy, such as the infiltrative juvenile *fibromatosis of children* and the less common *pseudosarcomatous fasciitis* of childhood. Wedge biopsy makes the distinction. Some fibromas are called sarcoma but never metastasize, such as the multinodular *dermatofibrosarcoma protuberans.* A *nodular fasciitis* also occurs on upper extremities and on the trunk which has local infiltrative power and grows rapidly like a sarcoma. Neurofibromas generally occur in multiple fashion over the trunk (von Recklinghausen's neurofibromatosis); any neurofibroma that grows quickly deserves biopsy for detailed diagnostic study.

*Myxomatoses—ganglion cysts* of the wrist area and *Baker's cysts* of the popliteal space—are, of course, completely benign formations with no malignant potential. Rarely a myxomatous cyst with thin walls, containing a gelatinous, or viscid, clear substance will develop in the fascial planes elsewhere in the body; these lesions behave more like locally malignant tumors than the ordinary ganglion cyst and should be classed with the more favorable forms of malignant sarcomas.

*Xanthomatoses* include the common *xanthomatous giant cell* tumors attached to tendons on extremities, often associated with hyperlipidemia. *Giant cell tumors of tendon sheath origin* of fingers and hand constitute another common variety of benign neoplasm belonging here. *Giant cell tumors* of the gums are closely related. The dark, hard, raised skin growths developing on the thighs and legs, often called a *sclerosing hemangioma,* probably represents a fibrous xanthoma, quite benign, deserving excision if enlarging.

*Angiomatoses,* benign vascular neoplasms, appear most often in or under the skin shortly after birth as *capillary* or *cavernous hemangiomas.* As a rule the congenital capillary type will spontaneously disappear as the child grows older. *Glomus tumors,* painful vascular proliferations under the fingernails of females, have been identified as hemangiopericytomas by Stout. Tumors of the lymphatics generally occur as single, large cystic masses in the lower neck of young children—cystic hygroma—but growth is usually self-limited. Many benign angiomatoses constitute mixtures of lymphangiomas and hemangiomas. Total removal of congenital angiomatoses in youngsters presents a danger because essential structures can inadvertently suffer permanent damage, since there is so much bleeding in them, the margins are uncertain, and essential anatomic structures such as nerves are quite tiny. Such damage is not acceptable in treating benign tumors.

*Solitary myositis ossificans* sometimes evolves in traumatized skeletal muscle with the resultant growth of actual cartilage or bone in the soft tissue; it ceases enlargement on its own after a time and probably is not a true neoplasm.

## PREVENTIVE MEASURES

When we know more of the causes of sarcomas, we can then plan prevention. Protective means are already being devised for shielding workers and others from asbestos dust contact.

## TREATMENT PRINCIPLES

1. The *first principle* of treatment has already described above—open *wedge biopsy* under general anesthesia with meticulous hemostasis and care not to open tissue planes unnecessarily. We always close the biopsy wound tightly without drainage.

2. The *second principle* of treatment involves a *definitive resection* of soft tissue, planned anatomically after some thought (usually with an anatomy textbook for reference), widely to encompass the biopsy wound from skin to its depths without entering it, to remove the *insertion* and *origin* of all *muscles* that

may be touching the tumor or whose fascial covering may be touching the tumor. This necessarily destroys some motor function in many cases, but amputation need only be done in circumstances of sarcomas at joints or adherent to bone where no adequate soft tissue margin would obtain with less radical surgery. Therefore, some amputations must be done, but they are not always necessary as initial treatment.

3. The histologic appearance of the tumor and the pathologist's opinion as to tumor behavior play a considerable part in shaping the excisional plan, in addition to the exact anatomic location of the growth.

4. Regional node dissections probably should be performed if a monobloc, in continuity operation can be done, or if nodes are clinically suspicious.

5. Radiotherapy constitutes a poor substitute for wide excisional surgery, because most soft-part sarcomas do not respond very well to irradiation. But when surgery is refused, or when the initial tumor or postsurgical recurrence cannot be operated upon, x-ray therapy may control the local neoplasm. A few sarcomas prove surprisingly sensitive.

6. Combined regional isolation perfusion and radical surgery on an extremity with sarcoma succeeds in controlling some advanced and recurrent sarcomas.

## COMMON ERRORS

Physicians fall into errors in the management of these tumors so often that any review of a number of cases will reveal in most instances something that was less than ideal.

1. A poor histologic classification by the pathologist has in the past frequently misled the clinician in planning his treatment. Usually the error was in underdiagnosis of the malignant potential of the tumor. Because of Stout's work, these sarcomas are better understood today.

2. An enucleation or narrow excision of a large sarcoma, rather than a neat wedge biopsy, has often resulted in the *"disturbed tumor bed" syndrome.* Here the surgeon unwittingly and unavoidably cuts through microscopic tumor that consists of highly viable cells at the growing edge of the sarcoma in the belief that he is "getting around it." Sarcoma cells thus freed from their "bed" are then carried by uncontrolled hemorrhage along wide tissue planes so that even subsequent very radical excision cannot encompass them. This may convert a tumor curable by wide resection into one curable only by amputation. Of course, the physician commits this mistake in the belief that he is doing the right thing, that he is avoiding the very pitfall he wishes to prevent. Cutting into a sarcoma for biopsy certainly can be dangerous, but it is the preferable measure when every other measure to secure a diagnosis is more dangerous.

3. Even with a correct diagnosis of a fully malignant soft-part sarcoma that may metastasize, individual surgeons have so little experience with these relatively unusual neoplasms that they often fail to carry resection to the necessary limits—removal of all possibly involved muscles from origin to insertion.

## PROMISING DEVELOPMENTS FOR THE FUTURE

No immediate breakthrough seems destined to occur in this type of neoplasia.

## PROGNOSIS

In no other group of tumors has planned radical surgery paid dividends higher than in the soft-part sarcomas. Scattered reports from clinics without special interest in such tumors show poor survival figures. On the other hand, the group at Memorial Hospital in New York, led by Pack and Ariel, with a unified concept of management, achieves an overall 40% 5-year survival—nearly twice the survival generally seen elsewhere. James reports 27% survival in a collected series from various institutions.

Well-differentiated tumors of every histogenetic variety fare better than undifferentiated growths. Those on the upper limbs have a better outlook than those on the lower. Fibrosarcomas constitute the most favorable histologic group; liposarcomas have nearly as good a prospect, according to a recent report from the Mayo Clinic. Rhabdomyosarcoma and synovial sarcoma have the worst outlook. Those neoplasms treated by initial wedge biopsy and then planned resection in a second procedure carry the best outlook. Node metastases reduce the prognosis to the range of 10%.

### REFERENCES

Ackerman, L. V., and del Regato, J. A.: Cancer, ed. 3, St. Louis, 1962, The C. V. Mosby Co., pp. 1181-1202.

Bowden, L.: Clinical management of soft part sarcoma, Ann. N. Y. Acad. Sci. **114:**1047-1060, 1964.

Cadman, N. L., Soule, E. H., and Kelly, P. J.: Synovial sarcoma: analysis of 134 tumors, Cancer **18:**613-627, 1965.

Delaney, W. F., Nealon, R. F., Jr., and Pierucci, L.: The soft tissues. In Nealon, T. F., Jr., editor: Management of the patient with cancer, Philadelphia, 1966, W. B. Saunders Co., Chap. 28.

Horn, R. C., Jr.: Sarcomas of the soft tissues, J.A.M.A. **183:**511-515, 1963.

James, A. G.: Cancer diagnosis manual, New York, 1961, American Cancer Society, Inc.

Krementz, E. T., and Shaver, O. T.: Behavior and treatment of soft tissue sarcomas, Ann. Surg. **157:**770-784, 1963.

Lawrence, W., Jr.: Current status of regional chemotherapy. Part II. Results, New York State J. Med. **63:**2518-2534, 1963.

Pack, G. T., and Ariel, I. M.: Tumors of the soft tissues, New York, 1958, Paul B. Hoeber, Inc.

Reszel, P. A., Soule, E. H., and Coventry, M. B.: Liposarcoma of the extremities and limb girdles, J. Bone Joint Surg. **48A:**229-244, 1966.

Stout, A. P.: Pathological aspects of soft part sarcomas, Ann. N. Y. Acad. Sci. **114:**1041-1046, 1964.

Stout, A. P.: Tumors of the soft tissues. In Atlas of tumor pathology, Sect. II, Fasc. 5, Washington, D. C., 1953, Armed Forces Institute of Pathology.

Chapter 28

# Sarcomas of bone

Bone is a complex structure, composed of many kinds of bodily tissues but not epithelium. In consequence, its malignant tumors represent diverse varieties of sarcomas. However, the total number of such bone neoplasms remains quite small.

## INCIDENCE AND DISTRIBUTION

Bone cancer is generally considered rare; by including multiple (plasma cell) myeloma under bone tumors the whole group constitutes about 1% of all cancers. One third or more of this whole group generally occurs in adolescents and young adults—the primary osteosarcomas and Ewing's sarcomas. Most giant cell tumors appear in the young adult. Multiple myeloma generally emerges in middle-aged persons; this accounts for nearly half of all bone cancer. Malignant bone tumors in older persons may take the form of osteosarcomas arising in Paget's disease of bone.

Males predominate somewhat over females as victims of multiple myeloma, chondrosarcoma, reticulum cell sarcoma, and Ewing's sarcoma. We have no data on world-wide, geographic variations in distribution.

## ETIOLOGY

### External initiating agents

Little doubt remains that ionizing radiation can induce bone cancer, particularly radiations from the so-called bone-seeking radionuclides such as radium 226, radium 228, strontium 90, plutonium 239, and thorium 228; these radioactive metals and rare earths may occur in nature, but nuclear fission provides our main source today. They become more or less permanently deposited in bone after ingestion and their decay activity bombards bone with alpha and beta rays throughout life. Danger from external radiation seems mainly limited to damage to the hemopoietic marrow, with the main risk being that of leukemia (Chapter 30). Bone sarcomas from external irradiation have also been reported occasionally in various bone sites, particularly in the spine from x-ray therapy used in former days to treat ankylosing spondylitis. The main bone tissue danger, however, comes from radium poisoning and related isotopic overexposure, where the type of rays emitted, the location of the deposition of the substance in bone (endosteum, marrow cells, periosteum), and the dose and growth potential of the cells irradiated all play a part. Radium 226 appears to be 60 to 200 times more carcinogenic than strontium 90, but not as carcinogenic as plutonium or thorium, which are particularly concentrated in *endosteal* cells. The classic studies of Martland on radium watch-dial painters reminds us continually of the risk.

Radioisotopes, viruses, and carcinogenic chemicals have all produced a variety of bone sarcomas in laboratory animals as have intramedullary injections of metals such as beryllium. Therefore we cannot fail to be impressed by the importance of external agents in the carcinogenic complex of this group of cancers as well as in the many cancers discussed before.

### Predisposing factors

Three diseases predispose to a slight degree to malignant bone tumors—Paget's disease (osteitis deformans), hereditary multiple exostosis (deforming chondrodysplasia), and multiple enchondromatosis. The first develops in bones of older persons; 1% to 3% of these will evolve into osteosarcomas. The second begins to appear clinically in childhood and some believe 20% of such persons will eventually have chondrosarcoma in one or more of the many osteochondromas (exostoses). A rare childhood cartilaginous disturbance of bone growth, Ollier's disease, or multiple enchondromatosis, carries an increased risk of chondrosarcoma, even in the unusual locations of fingers and toes. Solitary exostoses rarely may become cancerous; central enchondromas of larger bones are suspected by some of occasional malignant degeneration.

Trauma probably rarely initiates neoplasia, but it may promote or aggravate an existing neoplastic process.

## PATHOLOGY

A list of the seven main malignant bone tumors appears below, along with tissues of origin:

| Neoplasm | Tissue of origin |
|---|---|
| 1. Osteosarcoma | Bone—osteoblasts, osteoclasts |
| 2. Chondrosarcoma | Cartilage—chondroblast |
| 3. Giant cell tumor<br>4. Fibrosarcoma | Connective tissue—fibroblast |
| 5. Plasma cell myeloma<br>6. Reticulum cell sarcoma of bone<br>7. Ewing's sarcoma | Reticuloendothelial marrow—primary reticular cells, plasma cells |

Many benign lesions and tumors, such as fibrous dysplasia, and osteochondromas probably really represent growth disturbances that are self-limited (regulated by the body's growth pattern) and without the character of true neoplasms. Benign tumors and abnormalities will be mentioned under differential diagnoses.

**Osteosarcoma.** These sarcomas are generally thought of as the typical ("osteogenic") bone tumors that develop in growing bone during the young, growth periods of life. They tend to occur in the ends of long, large bones (femur, tibia) where growing, proliferating cells are concentrated. Osteosarcomas contain *osteoid,* a substance produced by tumor osteoblasts; under normal conditions of bone production this osteoid then becomes mineralized for conversion into true bone. Highly aggressive, invasive metastasizing cancers, osteosarcomas generally destroy cortical bone as they invade and expand, raise the periosteum from the outer cortex, extend through this layer into the surrounding soft tissue, and after closure of the epiphyses invade the epiphyses but practically never invade the joint space. They often recur locally with conservative treatment and metastasize by the bloodstream, normally first to the lungs. Node metastases seldom occur. Predominantly osteoblastic and osteolytic types can be distinguished.

Three kinds of osteosarcoma compose the whole class: (1) the *central* one described above; (2) the less common *parosteal osteosarcoma* arising in the juxtacortical area, with a relatively indolent growth pattern and surprisingly good prognosis with adequate surgery; and (3) *osteosarcoma in Paget's disease* of bone, occurring in older persons who have osteitis deformans in the bone underlying the neoplasm, with a poor prognosis.

**Chondrosarcoma.** Chondrosarcomas arise from tumor chondroblasts and usually produce first a cartilaginous tumor tissue that may become calcified. When *primary* in previously normal bone they may follow an aggressive, destructive, quickly metastasizing course such as osteosarcoma; when *secondary,* from the cartilaginous cap of an exostosis at the end of long bones, particularly in the entity multiple cartilagenous exostosis, they can behave quite benignly, growing to huge dimensions in the soft tissues with minimal symptoms and only occasional, late lung metastases.

**Giant cell tumor.** In the ends of large, long bones (femur, radius, tibia) giant cell tumors also predominate. They begin in the epiphysis of the bone. They appear to arise from fibrous tissue of the bone marrow and have benign, borderline, and malignant varieties. Accurate histologic diagnosis is difficult. All of them must be regarded with suspicion in that they may progress from benign to malignant, or later on declare an original, hidden, malignant component. Half of the so-called benign giant cell tumors recur locally with conservative local treatment. From 10% to 20% of tumors on first diagnosis are frankly malignant.

**Fibrosarcoma.** The infrequent fibrosarcoma of bone does not differ in appearance or in the spectrum of clinical behavior from the soft tissue type, except in point of origin from within the medullary cavity from fibroblasts, most often distal femur and proximal tibia. Origin from periosteum is rare.

**Multiple myeloma.** The largest group of primary bone tumors—multiple *(plasma cell)* myeloma—presents a quite different picture from those mentioned above. It may have a single origin as a solitary plasma cell myeloma in soft tissue or in bone, a form of the disease which, although locally treated, nearly always generalizes later as a disease of multiple bones. Usually it is diagnosed at the stage of multiple bone marrow involvement, characterized by punched out, osteolytic lesions in different bones. Myeloma favors the flat bones (ribs, vertebrae, pelvis, and skull) with characteristic plasma cells composing the bulk of the malignant foci. Abnormal globulins occur in serum and urine (Bence Jones protein). It follows a gradually worsening course over months or several years, often featured by vertebral body collapse, consequent paralyses, other pathologic fractures, and anemia from marrow replacement. It rarely affects the lungs.

**Reticulum cell sarcoma.** This disease of bone is rare, may come on at any age, and resembles histologically the tumors described by this name under "lymphoma"; it metastasizes (or arises multifocally) in many, varied patterns, regionally and distantly, to other reticuloendothelial tissues and other bones as well as to the lungs.

**Ewing's sarcoma.** An undifferentiated malignant entity of probable reticular cell origin in the marrow, Ewing's sarcoma usually differs from other sarcomas by its origin in the *shaft* of long extremity bones in youngsters. It spreads along the shaft, widening the cortex, and then extends into and through the periosteum to reach the soft tissues. It carries a poor prognosis and metastasizes rapidly and variously to lungs, nodes, skull, and other bones.

### Precancerous lesions

As mentioned before, the following conditions carry a predisposition to the evolvement of sarcoma. They are listed in their order of degree of risk: (1) Paget's disease of bone; (2) hereditary multiple exostosis; (3) multiple enchondromatosis (Ollier's disease); (4) central enchondroma of large, long bones; and (5) single osteochondroma.

## NATURAL HISTORY

Local pain at the site of tumor, worse at night, begins the clinical course of nearly all bone sarcomas. It results from tension placed by the expanding tumor on the periosteum. Mild fever may occur with Ewing's sarcoma and reticulum cell sarcoma. As the tumor enlarges, disability in an extremity, muscle wasting, pathologic fractures leading to a bedridden state, and weight loss may develop. Spread to lungs generally occurs as the first distant metastasis, except in multiple myeloma. Malignant giant cell tumors, however, as a rule, follow a prolonged locally destructive course without metastasizing. Other bones may suffer metastatic involvement. Death stems from pulmonary complications or emaciation from unrelieved pain; in multiple myeloma, hypercalcemia or renal failure may bring on demise.

## DIAGNOSIS

**History and physical examination.** Pain occurs at the site of a bone tumor. It is mild and intermittent at first, persists, and grows steadier and more severe during the succeeding weeks. The patient often associates the onset of pain with a trivial injury. Pain is usually worse at night with subsequent complaints of disability of the limb. Examination may reveal little if the bone lies covered by soft tissue as in the upper femur, pelvis, and spine, but a tender swelling can generally be felt around the knee or in ribs, arms, or skull. The physician can now make an educated guess about the type of tumor by noting the above symptoms and signs in addition to noting the age and sex of the patient.

**X-ray studies.** The next and *essential* step is x-ray films of the affected bone.

Experienced radiologists have achieved a high degree of accuracy in diagnosing bone tumors from careful radiographic studies—70% to 80% accuracy—and practicing physicians rely heavily on their judgment. In these films one can see normal anatomy of the bone and its reaction to the tumor as well as the growth characteristics of the tumor, features that appear only at operation or at autopsy with soft part cancers. Certain x-ray features characterize each bone cancer; however, they are too numerous for listing here, and would mean little without illustrative films. Arteriography has recently helped diagnostic accuracy by showing vascular patterns of the various tumors. Strontium bone scanning is rapidly developing into a useful method of early diagnosis of bone defects not large enough to be seen on conventional x-ray films. However, bone scans only demonstrate lesions that have a reactive normal bone process going on around them.

**Biopsy.** The pathologist remains the final authority. We need a biopsy. Malignant bone tumor diagnosis is difficult and often means the loss of limb by amputation; therefore it demands full cooperation and consultation between clinician, radiologist, and pathologist—a complete pooling of information on each patient. *Bone biopsy* must follow the x-ray films no matter how certain everyone may feel about the diagnosis. Often a special bone-penetrating needle (Turkel or Craig) can secure a small core of tissue and result in adequate material for diagnosis, especially where the histologic features fit the clinical and radiographic picture or in inaccessible sites such as the pelvic bones or vertebra. Where doubt exists about the adequacy of the needle core, in small tumors, or where amputation of an extremity hinges on accurate diagnosis, open biopsy is indicated. One takes a generous wedge of tissue. Because of the danger of seeding cancer cells in the deep soft tissue wound needed to approach many bone tumors, a clean-cut single wedge of tumor and careful hemostasis become doubly important. Only harm results from the rough scooping out of the necrotic, central bulk of a malignant tumor. The pathologist can most easily make an accurate diagnosis from the actively growing edge of the tumor. Frozen section diagnoses are possible in some laboratories with some pathologists.

**Laboratory studies.** Serum calcium, phosphorus, alkaline phosphatase, and protein electrophoresis studies help to confirm opinions as to the true nature of most tumors and yield specific findings in a few. Serum electrophoresis pinpoints the abnormal globulins of multiple myeloma, as does Bence Jones proteinuria. The alkaline phosphatase remains normal in multiple myeloma. An elevated acid phosphatase is pathognomonic of metastatic prostatic cancer. Alkaline phosphatase levels rise in Paget's disease of bone and also with osteoblastic tumors; hypercalcemia and hypercalcuria occur whenever tumors destroy bone rapidly.

### Differential diagnosis

Considering all bone growth, primary and secondary, the most common bone tumor is *metastatic cancer*. Age differences between most primary bone cancers (the young) and most metastatic tumors (the older) give us our first lead. The majority of metastases to bone will be accompanied by an obvious primary cancer in prostate, lung, breast, colon, rectum, and kidney, or a lymphoma; the occasional thyroid cancers spread to bone quite often, and the differentiated ones may take up radioactive iodine. X-ray features of both primary and metastatic bone tumors may be similar, although breast and prostatic cancer favor spine, ribs, and pelvis, not the common sites of primary bone sarcoma. Neuroblastoma with bone metastasis in children will confuse the diagnosing physician if the primary tumor is small. The main differential diagnosis in older patients lies between multiple myeloma, osteosarcoma in Paget's disease of bone, and metastatic cancer. The finding of the primary carcinoma usually resolves the problem.

Several benign self-limiting growth irregularities, without any danger of malignant potential that occur during the growing years, may mimic osteosarcoma and Ewing's sarcoma. Even the radiologic features of the following small lesions can look like bone sarcoma: (1) nonossifying fibroma, (2) metaphyseal fibrous defect, (3) simple bone cyst, (4) eosinophilic granuloma, (5) aneurysmal bone cyst, and (6) fibrous dysplasia. All of these have x-ray characteristics but bone biopsy usually has to be done for complete assurance.

The following benign tumors with clinical beginnings exactly like bone sarcoma demand careful x-ray study and often biopsy to exclude malignant possibility: (1) benign giant cell tumor versus malignant giant cell tumors; (2) osteoid osteoma versus osteosarcoma, Ewing's sarcoma; (3) osteochondroma (exostosis), the most common benign bone neoplasm, can easily be defined by x-ray appearance and location on the outside of the cortical surface of metaphyses of long bones; malignant change is unusual, heralded by symptoms and x-ray changes in the cartilaginous cap; (4) enchondromas are often multiple, frequently in a small bone of hands and feet, in central shaft of bone as opposed to external cortical osteochondromas; they have slight malignant potential; and (5) rarely chondroblastomas and chondromyxoid fibromas of bone may be confused with giant cell tumors.

The following miscellaneous bone lesions may cause diagnostic difficulty: (1) *myositis ossificans*—previous history of trauma and resemblance on x-ray film to parosteal osteosarcoma; (2) *osteomyelitis*—signs of acute inflammation locally, blood picture denoting infection, and, in some patients, a draining sinus; (3) bone *tuberculosis*—usually found with an active or healed tuberculous lung lesion; a positive guinea pig culture solves the uncertainty; and (4) *healing fractures* may cause confusion also.

## PREVENTIVE MEASURES

Obviously we can only prevent bone sarcomas with our present knowledge by protecting people against exposure to radioactive, bone-seeking isotopes. This effort will involve ever more sophisticated studies of the body "burdens" of the various isotopes that populations and special industrial workers can safely carry.

The careful, periodic, follow-up x-ray examination of patients with the various benign bone lesions that occasionally become malignant constitutes an early diagnostic effort rather than true prevention.

## TREATMENT PRINCIPLES

1. The conscientious orthopedist does well to take time to secure a biopsy and have another expert consultant before making a treatment decision. Many combinations of x-ray therapy and surgery are possible; to select the best for

each individual patient demands consideration of as accurate a histologic classification as possible, of the dysfunction or deformity involved (often amputation), of the age of the patient, and the likelihood of complete control. Automatic amputation for all bone sarcomas of extremities constitutes an indefensible oversimplification of a complex problem.

2. *Osteosarcoma* and *chondrosarcoma* usually indicate an amputation of the extremity; the principle in technique is to remove the joint above the lesion so as to have adequate margin around the entire involved bone. Preoperative high dose x-ray therapy has a few advocates. Wide local resection may succeed in small lesions in the ribs and scapula, especially with *chondrosarcomas*. The trend is to treat the majority of *peripheral* (secondary) *chondrosarcomas* by radical local excision. Parosteal osteosarcoma is a much better behaved tumor than the others and this may influence the surgeon toward a wide local resection, depending upon other considerations besides histology.

3. *Giant cell tumors* in general respond to conservative surgery for the definitely benign, accessible lesions where no dysfunction is involved, for children, and for those in whom x-ray treatment has failed. Particularly, x-ray therapy must be avoided in the rare childhood tumors. Radical surgery or a combination of irradiation and surgery may be needed for malignant giant cell tumors. Radiotherapy generally applies when dysfunction would result from surgery, as in the spine or pelvis.

4. The occasional periosteal fibrosarcoma may yield to wide local resection rather than amputation.

5. *Multiple myeloma* responds readily to x-ray therapy in particular loci, but chemotherapy with various drugs must help control the systemic spread of the disease (Chapter 33).

6. *Reticulum cell sarcoma* of bone generally responds well to radiation, similar to the soft tissue lymphomatous varieties, but older reports cite good results from preoperative x-ray and amputation. Certainly nodal and soft tissue metastases are x-ray problems.

7. For *Ewing's sarcoma,* most experts agree that irradiation serves as the best treatment.

## COMMON ERRORS

1. Overreliance on x-ray diagnosis without biopsy.

2. A pathologist's misdiagnosis of biopsy material, a natural failing because most pathologists only see occasional bone tumors.

3. Blind irradiation of skeletal lesions without a sound diagnosis.

4. Amputation without histologic diagnosis. Many benign lesions simulate osteosarcoma.

## PROMISING DEVELOPMENTS FOR THE FUTURE

Preliminary clinical trials with combined x-ray therapy and systemic chemotherapy for Ewing's sarcoma show considerable promise for improved survivals in this disease.

## PROGNOSIS

1. Osteosarcomas have only a fair to poor chance for survival. Parosteal types do well—75% 5-year survival has been reported. However, the second 5-year period often includes many failures because of primary inadequate treatment. The type developing in Paget's disease has a poor prognosis. Chondrosarcomas fare better.

2. Malignant giant cell tumors remain localized for long periods and the outlook is generally good.

3. Fibrosarcomas of bone fare moderately well.

4. The outlook for multiple myeloma is poor—a 10% relative 5-year survival rate.

5. Reticulum cell sarcoma of bone, in contrast to the soft tissue variety, has a fairly good survival rate—almost half are alive at 5 years.

6. Ewing's sarcoma has the poorest survival of all, although one recent report shows 20% of patients alive at 5 years as a crude rate.

### REFERENCES


Ackerman, L. V., and del Regato, J. A.: Cancer, ed. 3, St. Louis, 1963, The C. V. Mosby Co., pp. 1133-1180.

Ackerman, L. V., and Spjut, H. J.: Tumors of bone and cartilage. In Atlas of tumor pathology, Sect. II, Fasc. 4, Washington, D. C., 1962, Armed Forces Institute of Pathology.

Barnes, R., and Catto, M.: Chondrosarcoma of bone, J. Bone Joint Surg. **48B:**729-764, 1966.

Borges, E. J., Paymaster, J. C., and Bhansali, S. K.: Primary malignant tumors of bone, Amer. J. Surg. **113:**225-231, 1967.

Coley, B. L.: Neoplasms of bone, ed. 2, New York, 1960, Paul B. Hoeber, Inc.

Cutler, S. J.: End results in cancer, Report no. 3, Washington, D. C., 1968, U .S. Department of Health, Education and Welfare, p. 191.

Dahlin, D. C., and Coventry, M. B.: Osteogenic sarcoma, J. Bone Joint Surg. **49A:**101-110, 1967.

Enneking, W. E.: Local resection of malignant lesions of the hip and pelvis, J. Bone Joint Surg. **48A:**991-1007, 1966.

Falk, S., and Alpert, M.: Five-year survival of patients with Ewing's sarcoma, Surg. Gynec. Obstet. **124:**319-324, 1967.

Hartman, J. T.: Needle biopsy of bone, J.A.M.A. **200:**201-203, 1967.

Hems, G.: The risk of bone cancer in man from internally deposited radium, Brit. J. Radiol. **40:**506-511, 1967.

Hems, G., and Mole, R. H.: The relative toxicities of radium 226, plutonium 239 and strontium 90 for bone tumor induction, Brit. J. Radiol. **39:**719-726, 1966.

Hutter, R. V. P., Worcester, J. N., Jr., Francis, K. C., Foote, F. W., Jr., and Stewart, F. W.: Benign and malignant giant cell tumors, Cancer **15:**653-690, 1962.

Jaffe, H. L.: Tumors and tumorous conditions of the bones and joints, Philadelphia, 1958, Lea & Febiger.

Johnson, R., and Humphreys, S. R.: Past failures and future possibilities in Ewing's sarcoma, Cancer **23:**161-166, 1969.

Lichtenstein, L.: Bone tumors, ed. 3, St. Louis, 1965, The C. V. Mosby Co.

Marcove, R. C., Miller, T. R., and Cahan, W. C.: The treatment of primary and metastatic bone tumors by repetitive freezing, Bull. N. Y. Acad. Med. **44:**532-544, 1968.

Markowa, J., and Marek, A.: Experimental bone tumors caused by common viruses, Nature **213:**831-833, 1967.

Martland, H. S.: The occurrences of malignancy in radioactive persons, Amer. J. Cancer **15** (Part III):2435-2516, 1931.

McKenna, R. J., Schwinn, C. P., Soong, K. Y., and Higginbotham, N. L.: Sarcomata of the osteogenic series, J. Bone Joint Surg. **48A:**1-26, 1966.

Phillips, R. F., and Higginbotham, N. L.: The curability of Ewing's endothelioma of bone in children, J. Pediat. **70:**391-397, 1967.

Raven, R. W.: Bone. In Raven, R. W., and Roe, F. J. C., editors: Prevention of cancer, New York, 1967, Appleton-Century-Crofts, pp. 333-337.

Schajowiez, F., and Dorqui, J. C.: Puncture biopsy in lesions of the locomotor system, J. Bone Joint Surg. **21:**531-548, 1968.

Stradford, H. T.: Bone Tumors. In Rubin, P., editor: Clinical oncology for medical students, Rochester, N. Y., 1967, University Rochester School of Medicine and Dentistry, pp. 191-199.

Tapp, E.: Beryllium induced sarcomas of the rabbit tibia, Brit. J. Cancer **20:**778-783, 1966.

Van der Heul, R. O., and Von Ronnen, J. R.: Juxta-cortical osteosarcoma, J. Bone Joint Surg. **49A:**415-439, 1967.

Vaughn, J.: The effects of skeletal irradiation, Clin. Orth. **56:**283-303, 1968.

Chapter 29

# Lymphoma

Solid neoplasms of lymphoid tissues may conveniently be grouped under the generic term *lymphoma.* All of the reticuloendothelial neoplastic diseases (mainly lymphomas and leukemias) ultimately originate from the pluripotential primitive reticular cells (stem cells). These cells are thought to give rise to many differentiated forms such as red cells, lymphocytes, platelets, monocytes, granulocytes, histiocytes (phagocytes), fibroblasts, and osteoblasts. Lymphomas comprise about half of such diseases that come from the reticular cells per se, from their *lymphocytic* or *histiocytic* derivatives, or from *combinations* of these cells. Such primitive precursor cells are concentrated in lymphoid organs (nodes, bone marrow, spleen, and thymus), but in the adult some primitive reticular cells probably lie hidden and fixed in all tissues. This arrangement accounts for the multitude of reticuloendothelial neoplasms and particularly for the occasional orgin of lymphoma in nonlymphoid organs and tissues. Many authorities believe that the small lymphocyte acts as the precursor cell for lymphoma, possessing the same pluripotentiality as the reticular cell, but this idea seems less well established than the one we present here (Rappaport).

Because the lymphocytic and histiocytic derivatives of the reticular cells serve mainly to generate immune defenses against foreign antigens, neoplasms of these tissues naturally involve immunologic defects of various sorts. In this chapter we will consider the tumors commonly called Hodgkin's disease, lymphosarcoma, reticulum cell sarcoma, and Burkitt's tumor. More accurate terms for lymphosarcoma, giant follicle lymphoma, and reticulum cell sarcoma will be substituted, as explained later, since they reflect a newer understanding of the close association and common origin of lymphomas.

## INCIDENCE AND DISTRIBUTION

Lymphomas account roughly for 3% of all cancers, with a male-female ratio showing a slight male predominance. The incidence figures have remained steady over the past few decades. Hodgkin's disease, which constitutes nearly half of the lymphoma population, is a tumor of young adults with an age peak between 20 and 30 years; most Hodgkin's patients are under 50. By contrast, the lymphocytic lymphomas (lymphosarcoma)—one third of the lymphomas—and the histiocytic and undifferentiated lymphomas (reticulum cell sarcoma)—one sixth of lymphomas—occur almost entirely at older ages with peaks at 60 to 70 years. Therefore we are speaking of adult disease. By contrast, when the lymphocytic cells of children become neoplastic they tend to take the fluid form of leukemia rather than the solid one of lymphoma.

The incidence appears lower in Negroes. A relatively high incidence of Hodgkin's disease occurs in Holland and in Denmark. One rare lymphoma, the recently discovered Burkitt's tumor (African lymphoma), possesses a marked geographic limitation in distribution. Nearly all cases occur within a sharply defined climatic belt in central equatorial Africa where mosquitoes propagate with ease and carry, among other diseases, the virus of yellow fever. Naturally, much interest has recently centered on attempts to identify an insect-vectored virus as the cause of Burkitt's tumor.

## ETIOLOGY

### External initiating agents

Because of the special susceptibility of lymphoma patients to infections, numerous attempts have been made through the years to incriminate an infectious agent as the primary cause of lymphoma; all attempts have failed. Hodgkin's patients are particularly susceptible to tuberculosis and fungal infections. The histologic picture of this tumor may often resemble that of an infectious granuloma. Still the many studies with various spirochetes, protozoa, cocci, and bacilli, including tubercle bacilli, have not uncovered a causative relation. Today many workers expect a virus to be identified as the initiating factor in lymphoma and work to find the viral cause of Burkitt's tumor proceeds rapidly. One author states that the definite space-time clustering of this tumor makes the odds 1000 to 1 in favor of the disease being due to an infectious agent. A herpes type of virus (EB virus), apparently common but nonpathogenic for most humans, has recently been taken from Burkitt's tumor tissue culture, injected into a human volunteer, and produced infectious mononucleosis; the latter condition resembles lymphoma in many respects.

During the last few years a handful of the several thousand patients receiving kidney transplants and intensive immunosuppressive drugs have developed lymphomas. Observers believe the origin of the tumors postdated the drug treatment. Induction of lymphoma by other chemicals remains possible, since lymphomas frequently appear, along with carcinomas, in laboratory animals treated with well-known carcinogenic hydrocarbons.

### Predisposing factors

A number of investigations point up the coincidence of immunologic defect and reticuloendothelial neoplasia; they suggest an underlying abnormal immune state as the basic stage setting for the neoplastic process. The clinical signs of abnormal immunity and of the neoplastic tendency frequently appear together or in varying sequences. For example, one third of a large group of patients with autoimmune hemolytic anemia also had lymphoma; disturbances of delayed hypersensitivity (tuberculin test) commonly occur in Hodgkin's disease, and these patients often show tolerance to allogenic skin grafts; allogenic disease in mice can progress to malignant lymphoma. These connections become understandable when we remember that one of the principal functions of the lymphocyte is to become sensitized against foreign antigens and proliferate sufficiently to inactivate them. Thus a deficiency of normal lymphocytes produced by overgrowth of the abnormal would account for delayed hypersensitivity and delayed homograft rejections.

Immune disturbances may also be conceived to stem from abnormal antigenic responses of the neoplastic cells themselves. In either event it makes some sense to picture an initial immune deficiency state from whatever cause, permanent or temporary, that somehow provides a stimulus to normal lymphoid tissue to "overperform" its normal function and thus progress toward neoplasia. We have speculated in Chapters 10, 21, and 26 with the same concept about endocrine gland tumors that seem to follow prolonged overstimulation by their corresponding trophic hormones.

## PATHOLOGY

As stated before, varying degrees of lymphocytic or histiocytic (or a combination) differentiation from the primitive reticular cell accounts for the varieties of lymphoma. A classification expressive of the clinical varieties but reflecting the similarities of lymphomas is given below (each type may be *nodular* [more benign] or *diffuse* [less benign]):

I. *Hodgkin's disease**
   A. *Lymphocyte predominance*
   B. *Nodular sclerosis*
   C. *Mixed cellularity*
   D. *Lymphocyte depletion*

II. *Lymphocytic lymphoma*† (lymphosarcoma)
   A. Well-differentiated (nodular form—giant follicle lymphoma)
   B. Poorly differentiated (lymphoblastic)

III. *Mixed, lymphocytic, and histicytic*† (usually nodular)

IV. *Histiocytic lymphoma*† / *Undifferentiated lymphoma* (rarely nodular) } (reticulum cell sarcoma)

V. *Burkitt's tumor*

The familiar subdivisions of Hodgkin's disease, developed by Jackson and Parker in 1944, are as follows: (1) Hodgkin's *paragranuloma* (8%), roughly comparable to lymphocyte predominance; (2) *Hodgkin's granuloma* (90%), roughly including most nodular sclerosis and mixed cellularity types; and (3) Hodgkin's sarcoma (2%), which in general corresponds to lymphocyte depletion. The reason for using the newer Lukes and Butler subdivisions is that they successfully break up the 90% majority in the granuloma group and enable the new class of nodular sclerosis to be identified as a separate subgroup with a much better prognosis than the other Hodgkin's granulomas.

---

*Simplified from Lukes, R. J., and Butler, J. J.: The pathology and nomenclature of Hodgkin's disease, Cancer Res. **26**:1063-1081, 1966.

†Rappaport, H.: Tumors of the hematopoietic system. In Atlas of tumor pathology, Sect. III, Fasc. 8, Washington, D. C., 1966, Armed Forces Institute of Pathology.

Most lymphomas seem to begin in one *lymph node* or node group, usually in the neck. In some cases the rapid spread to distant nodes and organs gives the impression of systemic, multicentric origin for lymphoma, and additional support for this view comes from the fact that many lymphomas have become generalized throughout the body when first diagnosed. But, as Craver maintained, lymphoma probably begins, just as does carcinoma, at a single site, and then its cells invade and metastasize from there. We do not imply origin from one cell necessarily, but from one node or group of nodes.

After the original node group enlarges, its cells spread to adjacent nodes; these involved nodes remain more or less discrete in Hodgkin's disease but merge and are densely adherent in the other lymphomas. Adjacent nodal regions then undergo invasion—the opposite neck, axilla, or mediastinum—and spread below the diaphragm to retroperitoneal and inguinal nodes follows. This orderly pattern of adjacent nodal spread seems more typical of Hodgkin's disease; other lymphomas frequently skip to distant nodes or sites. Accompanying the early stages we often find a selective loss of delayed sensitivity responses on skin testing (Hodgkin's disease).

After varying intervals of time—often only a few weeks in the reticulum cell sarcoma group—nonlymphoid organs become involved, with consequent obstruction or other dysfunction. Mediastinal node masses may invade the trachea, bronchi, pleura, or lung parenchyma; retroperitoneal masses may obstruct ureters or invade vertebral bodies. Almost all organ systems of the body can succumb quickly to this secondary spread—bone marrow from contiguous invasion or metastases, especially the vertebrae, ribs, sternum, and upper femora; the spinal cord from external compression (herpes zoster frequently accompanies cord involvement); the liver and usually the spleen as well, since it is the body's largest lymphoid organ, from nodular or diffuse invasion. The ease with which all lymphoid tissues become involved seems explainable by the behavior of the normal lymphocytes, which circulate freely among lymphocyte depots. Thus the path of metastasis for the abnormal lymphocyte is accessible and ready for rapid transport. Skin dermatoses that probably reflect abnormal immune responses to tumor antigens appear often, and actual skin metastases may occur.

At times lymphocytic lymphoma, but not Hodgkin's disease, will begin in a nonlymphoid organ such as the stomach or intestines, and on rare occasions it seems to start in the breast, thyroid, or lung.

Pathologists agree that the reticular cell exists, although they sometimes disagree on its exact description. Thus there is often disagreement and difficulty in classifying lymphomas. *Hodgkin's disease* requires the detection of the *Reed-Sternberg* cell for diagnosis. This large cell has a characteristic polylobulated nucleus, or multiple nuclei. It may not be the truly malignant cell of the disease, but it serves as the hallmark of diagnosis. The bulk of the Hodgkin's node is composed of an inflammatory reaction, probably due to the malignant cells; varying amounts of eosinophilia, fibrosis, and necrosis appear.

In general the aforementioned histologic classes of Hodgkin's disease can be considered sequential stages in the worsening and progression of the disease, although nodular sclerosis often may not participate in this progression. Lukes and

Butler conceive of the following four subdivisions as representing increasing immunologic defect as the normal host immune responses degenerate: (1) *lymphocyte predominance*—a favorable, "early" stage in which Reed-Sternberg cells are few, lymphocytes are many, and only a highly selective immune defect exists; (2) *nodular sclerosis*—the most frequent picture of the disease, especially when it starts in the mediastinum, with a relatively promising outlook and moderate amounts of both types of cells; (3) *mixed cellularity*—a stage containing a mixture of cells with a poor prognosis, representing disease likely to spread in discontinuous patterns to distant sites; (4) *lymphocyte depletion*—the end stage with few lymphocytes, lymphopenia, and anergy of both cellular and humoral immune responses, which leads quickly to death.

*Lymphocytic lymphoma* (lymphosarcoma) generally exhibits a nodular or diffuse infiltration of lymphocytes throughout a lymph node with destruction of the usual nodal architecture. The nodular pattern generally indicates a more benign type of disease. The well-differentiated nodular lymphocytic lymphoma follows the most benign course of all; this form has generally been called giant follicle lymphoma or Brill-Symmers disease. When the lymphocytic lymphoma cells appear quite undifferentiated and immature, the lymphoma is classified as lymphoblastic in type, and it follows a correspondingly more aggressive course.

As indicated in our classification, malignant histiocytic or undifferentiated lymphoma commonly bares the label reticulum cell sarcoma, rarely assumes the nodular form, and spreads diffusely, rapidly, and in an unpredictable irregular fashion.

Burkitt's tumor may have tumor cells resembling those of poorly differentiated lymphocytic lymphoma, but the other features of the disease, such as origin in nonlymphoid tissue of the face, jaw, neck, or abdominal organs of children, serve to identify it. Cases resembling Burkitt's tumor are now being reported occasionally from other parts of the world.

### Precancerous lesions

No lesions of lymph nodes qualify as precancerous.

## NATURAL HISTORY

Although there are differences in clinical evolution among the lymphomas, in their early stages similarities predominate. As stated before, the majority of lymphomas show a painless, persistently enlarged *neck node* as the first clinical sign. Occasionally an enlarged mediastinal node initiates the clinical course, and sometimes anemia or bone pain may present first. Lymphocytic lymphoma can also start as a lump in the tonsil or elsewhere in Waldeyer's pharyngeal lymphoid ring, but Hodgkin's disease seldom does so. Strangely, the spleen, which is the largest single lymphoid depot, is seldom the site of a primary lymphoma.

In the previous section we described the orderly progression pattern, particularly in *Hodgkin's disease*—node-to-node and nodal region to adjacent nodal region, then spread below the diaphragm to enter clinical Stage III, and finally spread to nonlymphoid organs (Stage IV). At any stage in this theoretical pattern, *systemic symptoms of malaise, fever, itching, night sweats, and weight loss* may begin. The progress of the other lymphomas does not ordinarily follow this se-

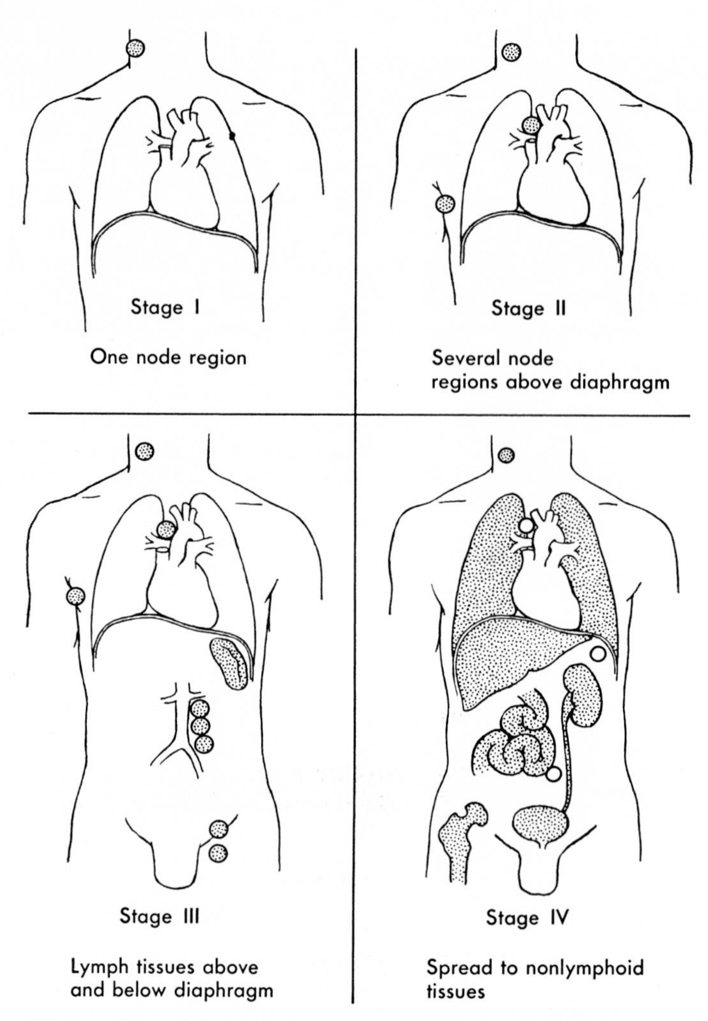


**Fig. 22.** Simplified version of four clinical stages of lymphoma designed especially for Hodgkin's disease. The concept of this type of lymphomatous progression often fits with other lymphomas as well. (Modified from Geller, W.: Hosp. Med. **4**:11, 1966.)

quence as closely; it may proceed irregularly and discontinuously. In all lymphomas, however, progression varies widely from patient to patient, and periods of exacerbation and quiescence may alternate irregularly and spontaneously without treatment. Progression from one stage to another may vary from periods of weeks to years.

The great variety of clinical pictures in Stages III and IV, caused by organ compression, invasion, or obstruction, makes advanced lymphomas hard to characterize. Situations one can find are as follows: spinal cord compression with the full assortment of peripheral nerve dysfunctions, depending on the location of the mass; ureteral obstruction with hydronephrosis and pyelonephritis; superior vena caval obstruction, tracheal compression, and pleural effusion; jaundice from extrahepatic portal area blockage; peripheral edema from major limb vein and lymphatic obstruction; and intestinal disturbances from mesenteric invasion or pathologic fractures from bone metastases. Hepatosplenomegaly usually appears, especially toward the end of the course. Anemia may supervene from bone marrow replacement by tumor or from an autoimmune hemolytic anemia. Brain invasion is rare. Secondary infections frequently develop, particularly fungal infections, intestinal moniliasis, and tuberculosis in patients with Hodgkin's disease; bacterial infections predominate with the other lymphomas.

*Lymphocytic lymphomas* may follow quite a different course from Hodgkin's disease; a minority will finally develop a leukemic blood and bone marrow picture—a type in well-differentiated lymphocytic lymphomas that resembles chronic lymphocytic leukemia—but the condition is not identical with leukemia. Also these patients frequently show agammaglobulinemia, which probably accounts for the susceptibility to pneumococcal and staphylococcal infections. A few cases begin in the stomach or bowel, presumably from patches of lymphoid cells in those organs. Well-differentiated lymphomas with a nodular pattern run a uniquely indolent clinical course at first, with remissions lasting for years. Sooner or later, however, 75% of them change into a diffuse pattern, which worsens the prognosis.

The *reticulum cell sarcoma group* usually progresses rapidly, recurs quickly, and spreads to distant sites without sequential node region involvement as in Hodgkin's disease, although the rare nodular form may behave less malignantly. Older persons particularly succumb more quickly to this most lethal of the major groups of lymphoma. A terminal leukemic phase is rare.

*Burkitt's tumor* shows a peak age between 6 and 7 years: half of the patients first exhibit disease in the face and half first exhibit disease in the abdomen. Without treatment all patients succumb within 1 year. Bone involvement and hemolytic anemia occur frequently.

We have mentioned the common progression pathway of Hodgkin's disease, of giant follicle lymphoma, and of diffuse lymphocytic lymphoma. Occasionally the poorly differentiated and mixed lymphomas, and even Hodgkin's disease, will progress to a terminal histologic picture of reticulum cell sarcoma. However, lymphocytic lymphoma does not evolve into Hodgkin's disease, and the reticulum cell sarcoma group, along with Hodgkin's disease, seldom if ever leads into leukemia.

Death in most lymphomas results from overwhelming infection, often pneumonia, inanition, vital organ invasion, or uncontrollable bleeding associated with thrombocytopenia. When chemotherapeutic drugs are pushed too far in the later stages of lymphoma, they may be responsible for the terminal state.

## DIAGNOSIS

**History.** A careful history can be rewarding if vague complaints arouse a suspicion of lymphoma in the physician's mind. But really early diagnosis of Stage I lymphoma comes from a careful *physical examination*—the detection of an abnormally large, asymptomatic lymph node.

**Biopsy.** Lymph node biopsy constitutes the main definitive method of making a diagnosis in lymphoma. This means the whole node with capsule intact. Misdiagnosis often results from selecting an uninvolved node adjacent to a tumorous one because it comes out easier or from taking one of the seldom involved, accessible inguinal nodes that commonly show chronic inflammation. Any painless node that enlarges and remains so for more than 3 weeks, without an infectious explanation or without response to an appropriate antibiotic, demands removal. Needle biopsy does not usually give adequate material for diagnosis. When node biopsy reveals only nonspecific lymphadenitis but adenopathy persists, the patient needs to be observed closely and have a second or third biopsy later to be sure that an atypical, slow-growing lymphoma is not the ultimate cause. When lymphocytic lymphoma begins in the stomach or intestine, a laparotomy and incisional biopsy become necessary.

**X-ray studies.** X-ray films of lungs, long bones, spine and pelvis will disclose invasion in half of lymphoma patients in the stages at which we presently diagnose them. Osteoblastic lesions suggest Hodgkin's disease whereas purely osteolytic ones favor lymphocytic lymphoma. Intravenous pyelography may be used, but by far the most accurate way to find retroperitoneal nodal spread is by *lymphangiography*. This study has become a necessity in lymphoma, since at least one third of patients have the deep-seated disease revealed only in this manner. Bone scanning with radioisotopes may reveal metastases when conventional bone films are negative.

**Laboratory studies.** Valuable information is added to the patient's work-up by laboratory studies. Blood abnormalities vary widely, but they seldom show changes that distinguish one lymphoma from another. Pancytopenia from bone marrow replacement seldom develops, but granulocytosis and slight normocytic, normochromic anemia occur commonly. Lymphopenia alone may appear; a variable degree of eosinophilia accompanies some cases of Hodgkin's disease. Hemolytic anemia as well as thrombocytopenia may be present. One may differentiate circulating cells of a poorly differentiated lymphocytic lymphoma in the leukemic phase from the blast cells of acute leukemia, but in the case of well-differentiated lymphocytic lymphoma the picture in the peripheral blood remains indistinguishable from chronic lymphocytic leukemia.

The cells of malignant lymphoma can sometimes be identified in bone marrow aspirates, but this is a nearly useless gesture in Hodgkin's disease. In view of the frequency of bone involvement in lymphoma we often find an *elevated alkaline phosphatase,* but this may also result from spread of tumor to the liver. Gammaglobulins are sometimes elevated, but hypogammaglobulinemia develops more often in the later stages of disease.

**Skin tests.** As stated before, *anergic* reactions to skin testing with various antigens (tuberculosis, mumps, streptokinase, monilia, for example) commonly accompany Hodgkin's disease and sometimes other lymphomas as well.

## Differential diagnosis

Any disease presenting as a *lump in the neck* can mimic Stage I lymphoma (Chapter 9). A generalized lymphadenopathy, however, suggests lymphoma rather than Hodgkin's disease. *Metastatic cancer* in the neck from *oral, pha-*

*ryngeal, laryngeal, nasopharyngeal,* or *thyroid cancer* needs a tissue diagnosis, and this comes easier from the *primary tumor.* When such biopsy is positive, then the neck lump is presumed to be metastatic without further diagnostic surgery. However, if no oropharyngeal or other primary cancer turns up, then node removal becomes necessary.

*Anaplastic lung cancer* metastatic to a supraclavicular node may closely resemble lymphoma clinically and histologically. Low lying lymphomatous nodes may simulate a nodular goiter. When the adenopathy of chronic lymphocytic leukemia imitates lymphoma, blood and marrow studies decide the matter.

In instances where no primary cancer exists, nodules from *chronic infectious lymphadenitis, branchial cysts,* or *tuberculous adenitis* may require removal for differentiation. Nodules that show calcification on x-ray film suggest tuberculous adenitis. *Acute lymphadenitis* usually has an accompanying throat infection that should respond to antibiotics.

*Infectious mononucleosis* often simulates lymphoma but the hetrophile antigen reaction will identify mononucleosis. *Cat-scratch fever* with adenopathy, *post-vaccinial lymphadenitis,* toxoplasmic lymphadenitis, and lymphogranuloma venereum demand careful clinical appraisal or tissue study to distinguish them from lymphoma. *Boeck's sarcoid* may give great diagnostic difficulty when it presents as a mediastinal mass, which could as well be Hodgkin's disease or other lymphoma. If skin lesions or peripheral adenopathy are also present, the histology of these tissues may clarify the matter. The various rheumatoid disorders may also resemble lymphoma.

Bone lesions of lymphoma may resemble the bone *metastases* that frequently occur from carcinomas of *prostate, breast, lung, kidney,* or *thyroid.* They also need differentiation from *primary bone lesions* (Chapter 28). Radiologic analysis of good x-ray films usually suffices, although one must perform an open biopsy of bone when the bone defect is the only sign of disease.

Primary lymphoma of the stomach or small bowel looks like a primary carcinoma on x-ray films; only laparatomy and biopsy can detect the difference.

## PREVENTIVE MEASURES

Little positive action appears possible in the area of prevention. We can remember in a tentative way the possibility that immunosuppressive drugs, such as azathioprine, may take part in the induction of lymphoma. The intense lympholytic effect of the chemotherapeutic agents also suggests their review as potential carcinogens now that their use is being extended to diseases less serious than cancer.

## TREATMENT PRINCIPLES

1. *Staging* of the disease constitutes the first step in treatment (Fig. 21). The simplified diagram of the staging system used by most therapists for Hodgkin's disease can help in picturing the stages of the other lymphomas as well.

2. *Radiotherapy* constitutes the treatment of choice. Lymphocytes succumb to x-ray therapy more readily than almost any other cell in the body.

3. Optimal x-ray treatment, particularly in early Hodgkin's disease, means *megavoltage field therapy,* to a dosage considered destructive of the tumor—3500

to 4000 rads in 3 to 4 weeks, applied to the entire involved and adjacent nodal regions. For example, in Stage I Hodgkin's disease in a neck node the mediastinum and axillae also receive prophylactic irradiation. Such a plan now promises hope of permanent cure in Stages I and II of Hodgkin's disease. This thorough, wide x-ray treatment of regions should preclude local recurrence.

4. *Chemotherapy* plays an adjunctive role in the early stages and a major role in the later stages of lymphoma. Four specific indications for its use bear mention: (a) *acute* forms of lymphoma; (b) *systemic* symptoms; (c) *scattered tumor* at multiple sites—Stages III and IV; and (d) in *combination* with radiotherapy in early stages at the discretion of the therapist. Most long-term survivors have received some chemotherapy as an adjunct to x-ray treatment, but chemotherapy alone has not succeeded in permanent arrest.

The alkylating agents prove the most effective drugs, especially nitrogen mustard for its rapid effect. A number of other drugs will also yield good responses; *methotrexate, cyclophosphamide, chlorambucil* (as oral maintenance therapy), and *vinblastine*. Corticosteroids kill tumor cells in lymphomas and they usually help in instances of bone marrow suppression or hemolytic anemia.

5. *General medical management,* if careful and intensive, may prolong useful life. Such measures as adrenal steroids for hemolytic anemia, antibiotics and gamma globulins for infections, combined chemotherapy and irradiation for spinal cord compression or vena caval compression or for skin or bone lesions, and chemotherapy for systemic symptoms may palliate successfully if indications for their use are promptly detected. In addition to treating a disease, however, the physician also has the challenging task of managing the complications of drug therapy.

6. *Surgery* must accomplish the node biopsy for diagnosis. Resectional surgery for the occasional gastrointestinal primary lymphoma may succeed very well indeed; postoperative irradiation usually follows this surgery. Splenectomy for "hypersplenism," for a painful large spleen, or for hemolytic anemia proves worthwhile on rare occasions. Surgical resection has also achieved what amounts to cures in a few small series of Stage I lymphomas confined to the neck.

## COMMON ERRORS

1. Inadequately low x-ray dosage, using small ports, has been a common practice in the past when only palliation was the aim in Stages I and II and when gross disappearance of the lump was the end point. With the possibility of real cure in Hodgkin's disease now gaining acceptance, undertreatment will tend to disappear.

2. Some clinicians push chemotherapy too hard in the late stages of lymphoma, thus substituting a devastating drug toxicity for the complications of the disease.

## PROMISING DEVELOPMENTS FOR THE FUTURE

A chemical measurement of occult tumor activity would give the treating physician a guide to continued therapy in the face of clinical remission. When such chemical indicators have been found in other cancers, survivals improved

**Table 2.** Actuarial 5-year survivals in Hodgkin's disease*

| | Stages I and II | All stages |
|---|---|---|
| All types | 70% | 57% |
| Nodular sclerosis | 76% | 71% |
| Mixed cellularity | 49% | 37% |

*Based on data from Keller, A. R., Kaplan, H. S., Lukes, R. J., and Rappaport, H.: Correlation of histopathology with other prognostic indicators in Hodgkin's disease, Cancer **22:**487-499, 1968.

markedly. One possible clue in lymphomas is the *serum copper level,* recently found to reflect microscopic tumor activity. Another such possibility is the measurement of the *leukocyte alkaline phosphatase* activity in Hodgkin's disease.

## PROGNOSIS

**Hodgkin's disease.** The survival rate in large studies (Cutler) has increased steadily during the past 25 years. The cause may be more aggressive radiotherapy.

A crude figure of *30%* 5-year survivals appears in some reports.

Clinical staging offers the best initial guide to prognosis; histologic classes can also be of great help. We show Keller and associates' latest figures in Table 2 because they seem to represent a carefully studied group of patients treated aggressively for possible cure.

Kaplan (1968) produces evidence to show that if a patient has no recrudescence of Hodgkin's disease for 5 years, the patient has a 95% chance of permanent cure; the chances after 3 disease-free years are almost as good.

**Lymphocytic lymphoma (lymphosarcoma).** Roughly one in four survives 5 years. Giant follicle lymphoma carries an outlook two or three times better than the whole group.

**Reticulum cell sarcoma group.** Twenty percent generally survive 5 years despite the widespread impression that all patients die in 2 years.

### REFERENCES

Ackerman, L. V., and del Regato, J. A.: Cancer, ed. 3, St. Louis, 1962, The C. V. Mosby Co., pp. 1218-1242.

Aisenberg, A. C.: Hodgkin's disease, New Eng. J. Med. **270:**508-513, 565-570, 617-622, 1964.

Bakemeier, R. F.: Malignant lymphomas. In Rubin, P., editor: Clinical oncology for medical students, Rochester, N. Y., 1967, University of Rochester School of Medicine and Dentistry, pp. 200-213.

Bennett, J. M., Nathanson, L., and Ruthenburg, A. M.: Significance of leukocyte alkaline phosphatase in Hodgkin's disease, Arch. Intern. Med. **121:**338-341, 1968.

Burchenal, J. H.: Summary of informal discussion on immunology of Hodgkin's disease, Cancer Res. **26:**1170-1175, 1966.

Craver, L. F.: Malignant lymphomas and leukemias, New York, 1952, American Cancer Society Inc.

Cutler, S. J.: End results in cancer, Report no. 3, U. S. Department of Health, Education and Welfare, Washington, D. C., 1968, pp. 171-187.

Cyr, D. P., Geokas, M. C., and Worsley, G. H.: Mycosis fungoides: hematologic findings and terminal course, Arch. Derm. **94:**558-573, 1966.

Davidson, J. W., Saini, M., and Peters, M. V.: Lymphography in lymphoma. Radiology **88:** 281-286, 1967.

Diamond, H. D.: The medical management of cancer, London, 1958, Grune & Stratton, Inc., pp. 1-50.

Franssila, K. O., Kalima, T. V., Voutilainen, A.: Histologic classification of Hodgkin's disease, Cancer **20:**1594-1601, 1967.

Gall, E. A., and Mallory, T. B.: Malignant lymphoma, Amer. J. Path. **18:**381-429, 1942.

Geller, W.: Diagnosis and treatment of Hodgkin's disease, Hospital Med. **4:**6-20, 1968.

Grace, J. T.: Quoted in Medical Tribune, Oct. 31, 1968, from address given at the Clinical Congress of American College of Surgeons, Atlantic City, Oct., 1968.

Hartsock, R. J.: Postvaccinial lymphadenitis, Cancer **21:**632-649, 1968.

Henle, W.: Evidence for viruses in acute leukemia and Burkitt's tumor, Cancer **21:**580-586, 1968.

Hrgovcic, M., Tessmer, C. F., Minckler, T. M., Mosier, B., and Taylor, G. H.: Serum copper levels in lymphoma and leukemia, Cancer **21:**743-755, 1968.

Jackson, H., Jr., and Parker, F., Jr.: Hodgkin's disease, I. General considerations, New Eng. J. Med. **230:**1-8, 1944.

Kaplan, H. S.: Prognostic significance of the relapse free interval after radiotherapy in Hodgkin's disease, Cancer **22:**1131-1136, 1968.

Kaplan, H. S.: Role of intensive radiotherapy in the management of Hodgkin's disease, Cancer **19:**356-362, 1966.

Karnofsky, D. A.: The staging of Hodgkin's disease, Cancer Res. **26:**1090-1094, 1966.

Keller, A. R., Kaplan, H. S., Lukes, R. J., and Rappaport, H.: Correlation of histopathology with other prognostic indicators in Hodgkin's disease, Cancer **22:**487-499, 1968.

Lee, B. J., and Martin, R. S.: Indications for lymphangiography in lymphomas and carcinomas, Med. Clin. N. Amer. **50:**675-688, 1966.

Lukes, R. J., and Butler, J. J.: The pathology and nomenclature of Hodgkin's disease, Cancer Res. **26:**1063-1081, 1966.

MacMahon, B.: Epidemiology of Hodgkin's disease, Cancer Res. **25:**1189-1200, 1966.

Miller, D. G.: Immunological deficiency and malignant lymphomas, Cancer **20:**579-588, 1967.

Mittleman, A., Stutzman, L., and Grace, J. T., Jr.: Splenectomy in malignant lymphomas and leukemia, Geriatrics **23:**142-149, 1968.

Moquin, R. B., and Dameshek, W.: Leukemia and malignant lymphomas. In Nealon, T. F., Jr., editor: Management of the patient with cancer, Philadelphia, 1966, W. B. Saunders Co., pp. 969-981.

Musshoff, K., and Boutis, L.: Therapy results in Hodgkin's disease, Cancer **21:**1100-1113, 1968.

Peters, M. V.: Radiation therapy in localized Hodgkin's disease, J.A.M.A. **191:**122-123, 1965.

Pirofsky, B.: Autoimmune hemolytic anemia and neoplasia of the reticuloendothelium, Ann. Intern. Med. **68:**109-121, 1968.

Rappaport, H.: Tumors of the hematopoietic system. In Atlas of tumor pathology, Sect. III, Fasc. 8, Washington, D. C., 1966, Armed Forces Institute of Pathology.

Rosenberg, S. A., Diamond, H. D., and Craver, L. F.: Lymphosarcoma, survival and effects of therapy, Amer. J. Roentgen. **85:**521-532, 1961.

Rubin, P., Schwarz, G., Lukes, R. J., and Skimkin, M. B.: Hodgkin's disease, J.A.M.A. **190:** 910-917, 1964.

Schwartz, R. S., and Beldotti, L.: Malignant lymphomas following allergenic disease: transition from an immunological to a neoplastic disorder, Science **149:**1511-1514, 1965.

Scott, R. M., and Brizel, H. E.: Time-dose relationships in Hodgkin's disease, Radiology **82:** 1043-1049, 1964.

Starzl, T. E.: Remarks at Sixth National Cancer Conference, Denver, Colo., Sept., 1968.

Toth, B., and Shubik, P.: Studies with malignant lymphomas: possible interaction problems between chemical and viral inducing agents, Monograph no. 22, Washington, D. C., 1966, National Cancer Institute, pp. 313-328.

White, L. P.: Treatment of tumors of the hematopoietic system, Mod. Treat. **3:**706-761, 1966.

Wright, D. H.: Burkitt's tumor and childhood lymphosarcoma, Clin. Pediat. **6:**116-123, 1967.

Chapter 30

# Leukemia

Just as common but less controllable than the lymphomas are the "fluid" forms of reticuloendothelial neoplasia called leukemia. Since the function of leukocytes is to circulate and react against foreign antigens and bacteria, the character of leukemia naturally evolves as a blood and lymph system disease, associated with abnormal circulating cells, susceptibility to infections, and various other immunologic dysfunctions. Leukemia of myeloid origin starts in the bone marrow where granulocytes are produced; leukemia of lymphoid origin probably can start in any organ with lymphoid depots. Rarely blood cells other than leukocytes escape from normal controls to attain an abnormal degree of proliferation, for example, erythroleukemia, erythremic myelosis, and "megakaryocytic leukemia."

## INCIDENCE AND DISTRIBUTION

Roughly 3% of all cancers are leukemias, and the disease accounts for 5% of cancer deaths. Proportions of the various types and of the acute and chronic forms vary with age and sex. Leukemia constitutes the *most common childhood cancer,* occurring usually in the *acute lymphoblastic* form wherein males predominate slightly over females. Chronic myelocytic and acute myeloblastic leukemia develop in the young and middle-aged adult (male equal to female), whereas the chronic lymphocytic type occurs in older adults. In the latter, males develop it twice as often as females. Lymphoid and myeloid forms occur with equal frequency. Acute types may develop at any age, but the acute lymphoblastic type peaks in early childhood, whereas the acute myeloblastic type does so at an older age. True monocytic (monoblastic) leukemia is a rarity; it concentrates in older people, also without sex predilection.

Epidemiologists in the United States, Europe, and the Far East believe leukemia has increased over the past few decades. However, in 1967 the leukemia mortality rate in the United States white population dropped slightly for the first time. Although some variations in incidence rates occur over the world, only the relatively low incidence in most oriental countries seems significant. Recent reports of clusters of leukemia cases in certain American communities now appear to lack importance. Negroes have been less susceptible than whites in this country.

## ETIOLOGY

### External initiating agents

No etiologic study of cancer excites more current interest than the recent intensive work of the large task force working on the "probable" viral factor in the carcinogenic complex of leukemia. Many animal leukemias now emerge as dependent on a virus, such as those discovered by Gross, Rauscher, Moloney, Friend, and Gaffi. Dmochowski has found a viruslike particle in the node of a human leukemic victim; others have detected *Mycoplasma.* But no causative relation between viruses and human leukemia has been demonstrated to date.

One agent that definitely induces leukemia, when conditions of susceptibility and dosage are right, is *ionizing radiation.* The causative role of excessive x-ray exposure receives support from the older studies on uranium miners and on pioneer radiologists, who had significantly increased risks. More recently the tenfold increase of leukemia among persons exposed to the atom bomb in Hiroshima and Nagasaki adds more conclusive evidence. The bomb exposure produced mainly the myelocytic type and reached a peak about 6 years after the radiation exposure in 1945.

In animals a variety of agents produce leukemia on occasion, such as the polycyclic hydrocarbons. Benzene has been incriminated in human leukemia. Indeed all compounds that produce a toxic effect on the bone marrow and hemopoietic mechanism (chemotherapeutic drugs and immunosuppressive drugs) must be considered suspect.

### Predisposing factors

Some investigators report a high correlation of the occurrence of leukemia in monozygotic twins. The disease develops more commonly in mongolism, Klinefelter's syndrome, and other genetic disorders. One epidemiologist suggests that these hereditary disorders associated with cytogenic defects may predispose to leukemia. Others believe similarly that these inherited chromosomal breaks and other genetic abnormalities have a patterned grouping in one group of chromosomes that sets the stage for the proliferation of clones of fully leukemic cells, arising *because of* the genetic defect. Most likely some combination of the above external and internal factors needs to occur, and in proper sequence, to bring on leukemia.

## PATHOLOGY

A simple classification by cell type serves best. The degree of leukemic cellular differentiation corresponds roughly to the degree of acuteness or chronicity of the disease—the less differentiated the cells, the more acute the course.

I. *Lymphocytic* leukemia (48%)
   A. Acute lymphoblastic, childhood
   B. Chronic lymphocytic, older ages

II. *Myelocytic (granulocytic)* leukemia (43%)
   A. Acute myeloblastic,* adult
   B. Chronic myelocytic, adult

*The term myelomonocytic leukemia fits easiest as a variant of acute myeloblastic leukemia; see Amromin, G. D.: Pathology of leukemia, New York, 1968, Paul B. Hoeber, Inc., p. 10.

III. *Monocytic* leukemia (rare)
  A. Acute monoblastic

IV. Other systemic proliferative diseases of hematopoietic tissues
  A. Erythremic myelosis } Di Guglielmo's syndrome
  B. Erythroleukemia }
  C. Megakaryocytic leukemia
  D. Idiopathic thrombocythemia
  E. Plasma cell "leukemia"

The first and typical alteration in leukemia occurs in the *bone marrow,* the seat of normal hemopoiesis. Marrow changes often take the form of a hyperplastic pattern in the normal elements. Acute leukemic marrow shows immature white cells, so primitive as to resemble "stem" cells. Large numbers of these abnormal "blasts" replace the normal hemopoietic activity, and normal phagocytic and immune defense mechanisms thereby suffer. Involvement of the rest of the reticulo-endothelial system varies with the type of leukemia. Chronic lymphocytic leukemia often produces lymphadenopathy and hepatosplenomegaly, findings that may persist for years. Lymphadenopathy rarely occurs in myelocytic leukemia but splenomegaly does.

The second category of leukemic alteration includes involvement of non-lymphoid tissues, producing various syndromes that simulate many other diseases. Sheets and blocks of leukemic cells infiltrate, replace, or displace normal organs and tissues; they plug capillaries and disrupt lymphatics. This affects normal tissue circulation, metabolism, and oxygenation. It has been estimated that it requires a trillion ($10^{12}$) leukemic cells, weighing roughly 640 grams, to kill a human being.

Microscopically, replacement of normal marrow structure by abnormal lymphocytes or lymphoblasts is typical of acute lymphoblastic leukemia. In the acute myeloblastic type there is a shift in the normal myelocytic series toward blastic and immature forms. Auer bodies (cytoplasmic rods), if present, are pathognomonic of this type. Marked replacement of erythroid activity occurs in the acute leukemias. Megakaryocytes are often increased in chronic myelocytic leukemia. In the latter disease an extra chromosome, the Philadelphia chromosome ($Ph^1$) appears in the marrow (and often in the peripheral blood); this chromosome may show up in megakaryocytes or in erythroid cells as well as in the myelocytic cells.

Peripheral white blood cell counts may be normal or low; acute leukemic patients often show leukopenia. The highest counts develop in the chronic lymphocytic form, running as high as 1 million white blood cells per cubic millimeter. Anemia may be absent in early stages but when it appears, it is usually normocytic and normochromic.

*Leukemic skin* lesions and changes occur frequently in a multitude of appearances—elevated reddish purple papules, furuncles, petechiae, and ecchymoses (from thrombocytopenia or excess of fibrinolysins)—and occasionally herpes zoster results from the disturbance in immune defenses. Immune deficiencies can result from the disease, from the drugs used in treatment, or from both.

The *lungs* may become affected by leukemic infiltrates, and hemorrhages may block off bronchioles to produce distal atelectasis, infection, and pneumonitis. In this respect, patients suffer from secondary infectious processes due to bronchial blockage just as they do with primary lung cancer. The *kidneys* often enlarge from leukemic infiltrates, especially in acute leukemia, as frequently evidenced by hematuria. Hydronephrosis can develop from nodal blockage of a ureter and hyperuricemia may arise in acute leukemia, in chronic myelocytic, and after treatment in chronic lymphatic leukemia; this results from leukemic cell breakdown and leads to renal uric acid stones and renal failure.

In 50% of the cases the *heart* succumbs to leukemic invasion in the terminal stages. Valvular and great vessel obstructions, pericarditis, pericardial effusion, or pericardial hemorrhage with tamponade can be found. The entire gastrointestinal tract is subject to invasion, and depending upon the segment involved, patients may experience nausea, vomiting, pain, diarrhea, hematemesis, or melena. The *mouth* shows signs in acute leukemia in most of the cases; gums become red and hypertrophied, and bleed readily. Tonsillar, nasopharyngeal, and sinus masses may appear; epistaxis is common. *Bone* and joint swelling from hemorrhages develop most often in children, which is accompanied by considerable bone pain from periosteal involvement. Spinal cord compression syndromes and cerebral signs may develop as they do with the lymphomas.

The three main derangements from these tissue and organ infiltrates are (1) *hemorrhages* from thrombocytopenia or thrombocytosis, fibrinolysin excess, or capillary disruptions; (2) *anemia* from lowered red cell production and shorter red cell life-span, sometimes from autoimmune hemolytic anemia in chronic lymphocytic leukemia, or from combinations; (3) *infection* from lack of normal white blood cells caused by the disease, by the toxicity of the treatment drugs, or from the hypogammaglobulinemia found in chronic lymphocytic leukemia. Such infections as boils, mouth and gum ulcerations, streptococcal and staphylococcal pharyngeal tonsillitis, pneumonia, and perianal and perirectal abscesses may be found. *Escherichia coli* and *Pseudomonas aeruginosa* frequently cause these infections; *Candida* and *Aspergillus* are also frequent pulmonary pathogens.

### Precancerous lesions

No definite preleukemic changes exist today, despite frequent retrospective references to "preleukemic phases." This phrase usually refers to patients whose diagnosis remains uncertain in the early stages. Many adults with chronic refractory anemia in time will develop acute leukemia.

## NATURAL HISTORY

As a general rule, untreated acute leukemia comes on rapidly with few prodromal signs or symptoms and follows a quick downhill course in a matter of weeks or months, with bleeding phenomena, fever, and extreme malaise, if untreated. Chronic leukemia, on the other hand, evolves gradually; it may smolder undetected for months or years before a diagnosis is made. Symptoms and signs may be few or absent. *Anemia, hemorrhage,* and the signs of *hypermetabolism* constitute the common features of acute and terminal leukemia.

*Acute leukemia of childhood* is nearly always lymphoblastic in type, with blast forms in the peripheral blood; the peripheral white blood cell count may be low, normal, or high. Anemia and thrombocytopenia commonly accompany each other from the considerable blastic infiltration of the bone marrow. As we would expect, ecchymoses and petechiae show up frequently in the oropharynx and skin; epistaxis, fatigue, fever, and bone and joint pains usually appear. The spleen and the peripheral lymph nodes are enlarged in more than half of the cases. If untreated, the patient deteriorates rapidly and dies of circulatory collapse or infection. "Stem cell," myeloblastic, or monoblastic leukemia in childhood occurs on rare occasions with similar clinical pictures.

*Acute leukemia* in the adult is generally myeloblastic in type. A severe, refractive anemia may be the only initial finding. Symptoms and signs may be milder than those in children, but, in general, these patients show the same bleeding tendency, hypertrophy and bleeding of the gums, gastrointestinal ulcerations, thrombocytopenia, hypofibrinogenemia, and frequent central nervous system involvement from intracranial hemorrhages that result in nerve palsies and signs of meningeal irritation. Various infections, fever, and moderate splenomegaly also characterize acute myeloblastic leukemia. Once the diagnosis is established, these patients respond poorly to treatment and die of bleeding or infection within a matter of weeks or months.

*Chronic lymphocytic leukemia* occurs most frequently after the age of 50. Mature lymphocytes cause a peripheral lymphocytosis, with counts running from slight leukocytosis up into the hundreds of thousands. The clinical picture is frequently characterized by an insidious onset, malaise, a palpable spleen, and varying degrees of anemia. Lymphadenopathy is common. The disease may be static and asymptomatic for many years, even without treatment. This type almost never progresses to an acute terminal blastic phase. Many patients develop agammaglobulinemia, hypogammaglobulinemia, and/or autoimmune hemolytic anemia. (By contrast, no defect in immunoglobulins or immunologic responses appear in acute lymphoblastic leukemia.)

*Chronic myelocytic leukemia* attacks adults between 25 and 50; it is first heralded by an increase in peripheral neutrophils, metamyelocytes, myelocytes, nucleated red cells, and platelets—a general hyperactive response of the marrow. Splenomegaly may be quite marked, and this form of leukemia frequently terminates in an acute blastic, leukemic crisis.

*Monocytic* leukemia usually presents as an acute disease, with swelling, redness, and ulceration of gums, ulceration and bleeding from the throat, sternal tenderness, and scattered ulcerations in other parts of the gastrointestinal tract as well as frequent skin lesions.

Temporary, spontaneous remissions in leukemia are rare and short lived.

## DIAGNOSIS

**History and physical examination.** Leukemia can be suggested, but not diagnosed, by history and physical examination. Bleeding gums, ecchymoses in skin or oropharynx, infiltrations around the eyes, as well as signs and symptoms of anemia and peripheral nerve or central nervous system involvement often obtain in acute leukemia. Usually we find an excessive tenderness of the sternum. In chronic lymphocytic leukemia the only sign may be lymphadenopathy.

**Hematologic and other laboratory studies.** An unexplained leukocytosis in the *peripheral blood* often first alerts the physician to the possibility of leukemia. Acute leukemia, however, frequently presents as leukopenia. Typically, this form also shows peripheral blast cells, anemia, and thrombopenia.

In chronic lymphocytic leukemia one also sees peripheral leukocytosis, anemia, and thrombopenia, but the frequent additional findings of autoimmune hemolytic anemia or hypogammaglobulinemia point more specifically toward this chronic form.

Chronic myelocytic leukemia is suggested by an increase of peripheral nucleated red cells and in platelets and by immature neutrophils. The *Philadelphia chromosome* nearly always appears in typical cases.

All patients with unexplained persistent leukocytosis, leukopenia, abnormal peripheral white blood cells, unexplained anemia, or a low platelet count need marrow studies to help make the diagnosis, be it leukemia or another disease.

*Bone marrow* examination constitutes an essential maneuver unless the diagnosis of leukemia is certain on peripheral blood studies. One can aspirate satisfactory marrow specimens from manubrium, sternum, vertebral process, or iliac crest. The details of cellular structure of the primitive leukemic cells constitute the main diagnostic criteria. Most specific, if present, are the Auer rods in myeloblastic leukemic cells and the Philadelphia chromosome in the myelocytic form.

Elevated *serum* uric acid and reduced globulins on electrophoresis are confirmatory findings for most types of leukemia; low globulins do not obtain in acute lymphoblastic leukemia. A positive-direct Coombs' test denotes autoimmune hemolytic anemia and occurs in 20% of chronic lymphocytic leukemias. Elevated levels of vitamin $B_{12}$ in the serum occur only in myelocytic and monocytic leukemias, not in the lymphocytic forms. A negative leukocyte alkaline phosphatase stain tends to favor a diagnosis of chronic myelocytic leukemia.

**X-ray studies.** Radiographic studies serve mainly to survey the degree of leukemic spread to mediastinal nodes, lungs, or bone. In the acute leukemia of children, bone involvement is the rule; typical radiolucent bands next to epiphyseal lines appear in most such patients.

**Biopsy.** Node biopsy can also help in diagnosing leukemia. But a well-differentiated, diffuse, lymphocytic lymphoma looks identical to chronic lymphocytic leukemia in a node. Biopsies of the gum can give diagnostic aid in acute leukemia, but skin biopsies are not reliable.

## Differential diagnosis

The lymphocytes of *infectious mononucleosis* can be distinguished from leukemia cells by experienced observers on study of the peripheral blood smear. Also, mononucleosis usually shows the typical heterophile agglutination reaction.

*Infectious lymphocytosis in children,* a self-limited disease of unknown etiology, causes much confusion with leukemia; the only reliable difference between the two is the course of the disease.

*Aplastic anemia* may simulate acute leukemia. But the former differs from leukemia by often having a pancytopenia, a dry marrow tap, no splenomegaly or sternal tenderness, and often a low reticulocyte count. If one obtains a dry marrow tap, open marrow biopsy must follow to ascertain the true marrow status.

*Leukemoid reactions* also cause confusion. These reactions arise from a number of processes that stimulate or irritate the marrow, such as tuberculosis, massive hemorrhage, poisons, some drugs, other severe infections, septicemia, or widely spread deposits of metastatic carcinoma in the marrow. Myelofibrosis with extramedullary erythropoiesis is closely related to chronic myelocytic leukemia and may engender a leukemoid peripheral blood picture. *Bone marrow biopsy* becomes the most reliable study in diagnosing leukemoid reactions.

As mentioned before, a diffuse, well-differentiated *lymphocytic lymphoma* closely resembles chronic lymphocytic leukemia in the node biopsy picture. Diagnosis rests on peripheral smear findings.

Several groups of disease cause *purpura* on the basis of thrombocytopenic-dysproteinemic states such as Waldenström's macroglobulinemia, multiple (plasma cell) myeloma, the various primary anemias, and also idiopathic thrombocytopenic purpura and drug-induced purpuras. Combinations of serum electrophoretic, blood, and marrow studies will usually clarify the diagnosis. Hemorrhagic thrombocythemia can pose great difficulties in differentiation from chronic myelocytic leukemia; one gains some help from blood and marrow studies, a negative leukocyte alkaline phosphatase stain, and the Philadelphia chromosome found with this leukemia.

*Polycythemia vera* can produce marked hyperplasia of granulocytic and megakaryocytic cells in the marrow in addition to its high peripheral red blood cell count and hematocrit. The more common secondary polycythemia results from other disease states when relative tissue hypoxia causes erythropoietin overproduction (presumably in the kidney) with excessive stimulation of erythropoiesis in the marrow. Here the differential problem is easier.

Leukemia may produce joint symptoms like those of *acute rheumatic fever*.

*Neuroblastomas* sometimes cause retroocular masses and leukemic-like hemorrhages in childhood, requiring biopsy, coupled with negative blood studies, to identify the true cause.

## PREVENTIVE MEASURES

In our present state of knowledge we can ensure people against unnecessary radiation exposure. We have nearly quit the leukemogenic practice of irradiation for thymic and tonsillar enlargement and for ankylosing spondylitis; radiologists and dentists probably receive adequate protection from excess x-ray exposure. The use of radioactive substances for the treatment of noncancerous diseases also seems on the wane. X-ray exposure of the fetus in utero especially should be kept to an absolute minimum. Avoidance of uncontrolled exposure to benzene and of the optional use of marrow toxic drugs would seem worthwhile.

## TREATMENT PRINCIPLES

1. *Chemotherapy* constitutes the mainstay of treatment in acute leukemia and usually in the chronic forms as well. Combinations of drugs have recently been

proved more effective than single drugs alone. Generally the combinations that induce remissions differ from the combinations or single drugs that maintain remissions. Combinations employ drugs from different groups (alkylating agents, hormones, antimetabolites, and antibiotics), whose toxic effects differ, thereby allowing each one to be employed at nearly top dosage. Theoretically, in this way one achieves an immediate additive, tumor cell–killing effect, compared to the effect of one drug alone. But time-dose relationship in drug therapy seems quite vital to success. Short, intensive, high-dose courses of drugs seem more effective than long-term, low-dose courses.

For the first time in the history of cancer chemotherapy a truly specific chemical difference in a cancer cell has been found and exploited for treatment. The leukemic cell of acute lymphoblastic leukemia in both children and adults lacks the ability to synthesize asparagine, whereas normal cells are able to synthesize this amino acid. Since leukemic cells are therefore dependent upon the extracellular pool of asparagine, the administration of L-asparaginase, which binds asparagine, kills leukemic cells by depriving them of this extracellular pool. Remissions in acute leukemics are reported in about one half of the cases treated with L-asparaginase.

Most of the progress in the treatment of leukemia has occurred in *acute lymphoblastic leukemia of childhood.* Seven drugs have so far proved their effectiveness in inducing remissions or in maintaining them—vincristine, methotrexate, 6-MP, prednisone, Cytoxan, arabinoside cytosine, and daunomycin. Experts employ two or more of these drugs in *combination* at the start, at relatively high doses, in a crash effort to attain remission. Once attained, remission can be maintained by one drug, often a different one from those used to induce remission. When a maintenance drug becomes ineffective, another drug is tried. *Dosage* of each drug becomes of crucial importance to obtain maximal leukemic "cell kill" with tolerable toxicity. The *timing* of drug regimens makes a considerable difference also.

Remissions generally take place in 1 to 3 weeks after the onset of treatment. Maintenance regimens of drugs are administered for 6 to 12 weeks as a rule, with equal resting intervals free of drugs. One gauges drug effectiveness by following the peripheral blood and bone marrow pictures; reversion to normal of each of these constitutes complete remission.

New and better drugs and their combinations are coming to light every year. The alert physician will keep an open mind about any drug regimen; it may be outdated by the time he hears of it.

The brain harbors leukemic cells in 80% of the acute forms in children. This presents a real obstacle to treatment because most drugs will not penetrate the peculiar capillary walls of the brain, the *blood-brain barrier.* One solution to this problem is the intrathecal route of administration of drugs such as methotrexate; a still experimental and highly toxic drug, BCNU, has the ability to cross the barrier. Irradiation can also relieve central nervous system complications.

*Chronic leukemia* is quite a different treatment problem. In the chronic lymphocytic form, one generally withholds all treatment until symptoms appear or laboratory studies indicate a worsening or progression of disease, such as an enlarging tumor mass of any source, thrombocytopenia, or progressive anemia. One often treats chronic myelocytic leukemia according to the peripheral white blood count and usually begins treatment if the count is over 30,000.

*Chronic myelocytic leukemia* almost always responds to *busulfan* (Myleran). Once a blastic crisis occurs, however, the response is minimal.

*Chronic lymphocytic leukemia* may follow the most benign course of all, showing only peripheral leukocytosis or lymphadenopathy and requiring no treatment. When symptomatic, these patients generally gain a remission with *chlorambucil, Cytoxan,* or prednisone, but there is little evidence that survival is significantly prolonged by treatment in this form of the disease.

2. *X-ray therapy* can play a significant role in the management of chronic lymphocytic leukemia. Small doses will usually palliate symptomatic foci of leukemic infiltration, such as spots of bone pain, orbital proptosis, a very large spleen, focal infiltrate in the brain or spinal cord, or areas causing bladder hemorrhage. Fractionated total body irradiation has produced remissions, according to recent reports, that equal or exceed the remission rate of drugs.

3. The autoimmune hemolytic anemia of chronic lymphocytic leukemia often responds to cortisone, hydrocortisone, or azathioprine.

4. Multiple metabolic, anatomic, and functional disturbances affect acute leukemic patients, either as a result of the primary disease or its complications, or as a result of the toxic effects of treatment. Supportive care and specific treatment for the two common secondary complications of leukemia, infection and hemorrhage, loom large in the total management of the patient. Since normal granulocytes comprise the body's main defense against bacterial and fungal infections (mainly moniliasis), the leukemic patient with a low supply of normal cells falls easy prey to these forms of sepsis. A constant search for infectious foci, the use of cultures and sensitivity studies, regularly repeated blood counts, and the prompt use of appropriate bactericidal antibiotics or immune globulins, all must be applied with skill and without delay.

5. *Hemorrhages* generally result from thrombopenia that arises from leukemic destruction of megakaryocytes or similar damage from chemotherapeutic drugs. *Platelet transfusions* are now available to tide patients over acute thrombopenic periods. Anemia may require corticosteroids or transfusions; hyperuricemia with renal calculi and their urinary complications will demand *allopurinol* to interrupt uric acid formation by inhibiting xanthine oxidase.

6. *Objective criteria* of response to a particular type of treatment merits the physician's close attention, since subjective responses or impressions are unreliable. Such criteria include (a) reduction in size of tumorous masses; (b) reduction in abnormal organ size; (c) reversion toward normal of blood and marrow pictures; (d) weight gain; (e) return toward normal of pathologic serum globulins; and (f) disappearance of fever.

7. Removal of a large painful spleen by surgery is occasionally preferred to splenic radiation as a palliative effort.

## COMMON ERRORS

1. Some physicians still believe that leukemia is too fatal to be worth treating at all.

2. Most physicians cannot keep abreast of current advances in the combina-

tion drug treatment of leukemia. For this reason, acute leukemia probably demands specialty attention in or near a center for such diseases.

3. Secondary infections and the complications of treatment may often remain untreated because the conditions are mistakenly attributed to drug-resistant leukemia itself. At death at least one third of patients show fungal gastrointestinal disease that results from the heavy, widespread use of chemotherapy. Monilial gastrointestinal infection, pneumonia, or drug-induced thrombopenia can usually be successfully, if temporarily, managed when anticipated as common complications.

4. Hyperuricemia may easily escape notice until renal failure occurs.

## PROMISING DEVELOPMENTS FOR THE FUTURE

1. The L-*asparaginase* discovery, although somewhat disappointing in initial clinical results, presages an era of increasingly sophisticated chemical anticancer agents. Better drug combinations will no doubt constantly emerge.

2. The widespread effort to demonstrate a virus as an essential link in the causation of leukemia gives encouragement that antisera can some day be prepared against leukemic cells, if not vaccines for the prevention of leukemia.

3. *Germ-free rooms* for the care of acute leukemic patients may become more widely available in the future.

4. Much hope was held recently for bone marrow transplants in leukemia, often coupled with total body irradiation after marrow removal. So far these trials have not given much patient improvement, probably because of the antihost, antibody producing capacity of the homotransplanted marrow. Further refinements may yet demonstrate a place for this procedure.

## PROGNOSIS

1. In *acute leukemia* roughly 40% of children are living at the end of 1 year, but only 10% at 3 years. Marked increase in longevity has been achieved in the last few years in childhood leukemia with each new type of effective drug. Burchenal now has documented over 150 long-term survivors (5 to 17 years), with one third of the children no longer under treatment. Adults fare poorly with the acute form; only 10% are alive at 1 year, and 1% to 3% at 3 years.

2. *Chronic leukemic* patients live an average of 2½ to 3 years. The lymphocytic form carries the best outlook; Cutler reports a 40% *relative* 5-year survival in chronic lymphocytic leukemia, but only 13% for the chronic myelocytic form.

### REFERENCES


Ackerman, L. V., and del Regato, J. A.: Cancer, ed. 3, St. Louis, 1962, The C. V. Mosby Co., pp. 1243-1267.

Amromin, G. D.: Pathology of leukemia, New York, 1968, Paul B. Hoeber, Inc.

Bakemeier, R. F., and Miller, D. R.: In Clinical oncology for medical students, ed. 1, Rochester, N. Y., 1967, University of Rochester School of Medicine and Dentistry, pp. 220-231.

Beard, M. F.: The liver, radiation and leukemia, Amer. J. Roentgen. **81**:504-508, 1959.

Blair, T. R., Bayrd, E. D., and Pease, G. L.: Atypical leukemia, J.A.M.A. **198**:21-24, 1966.

Bodey, G. P.: Fungal infections complicating acute leukemia, J. Chronic Dis. **19**:667-687, 1966.

Boggs, D. R., Sofferman, S. A., Wintrobe, M. D., and Cartwright, G. E.: Factors influencing the duration of survival of patients with chronic lymphocytic leukemia, Amer. J. Med. **40:**243-254, 1966.

Brady, J. I., and Beizer, L. H.: Immunologic incompetence of neoplastic lymphocyte in chronic lymphocytic leukemia, Ann. Intern. Med. **64:**1237-1245, 1966.

Burchenal, J. H.: Long-term survivors in acute leukemia and Burkitt's tumor, Cancer **21:**595-599, 1968.

Comen, P. E.: Chromosome studies in leukemia, J. Canad. Med. Ass. **96:**1599-1605, 1967.

Cutler, S. J.: End results in cancer, Report no. 3, U. S. Department of Health Education and Welfare, Pub. Health Ser., NIH, Washington, D. C., 1968, pp. 193-214.

Damashek, W., and Unz, F.: Leukemia, ed. 2, New York, 1964, Grune & Stratton, Inc.

Diamond, H. D.: The medical management of cancer, New York, 1958, Grune & Stratton, Inc., pp. 51-83.

Farber, S.: Concluding remarks, Cancer Res. **27**(part I):2657-2660, 1967.

Fraumeni, J. F., Jr., and Miller, R. V.: Epidemiology of human leukemia: recent observations, J. Nat. Cancer Inst. **38:**593-605, 1967.

Galton, D. A. G.: Pathogenesis of chronic lymphatic leukemia, Canad. Med. J. **94:**1005-1010, 1966.

Holland, P., and Holland, N. H.: Prevention and management of acute hyperuricemia in childhood leukemia, J. Pediat. **72:**358-366, 1968.

Horsfall, F. L., Jr.: Leukemia in man and mouse, Acta Med. Scand. **445**(supp.):304-311, 1966.

Kaplan, H. S.: On the natural history of the murine leukemias, Cancer Res. **27:**1325-1340, 1967.

Krauss, S.: Chronic myelocytic leukemia with features simulating myelofibrosis with myeloid metaplasia, Cancer **19:**1321-1332, 1966.

Moquin, R. B., and Damashek, W.: Leukemia and malignant lymphomas. In Nealon, T. F., Jr., editor: Management of the patient with cancer, Philadelphia, 1965, W. B. Saunders Co., pp. 969-1011.

Rall, D. P.: Pharmacologic aspects of selective chemotherapy of leukemia and Burkitt's tumor, Cancer Res. **27:**2650-2655, 1967.

Rappaport, H.: Tumors of the hematopoietic system. In Atlas of tumor pathology, Sect. III, Fasc. 8, Washington, D. C., 1966, Armed Forces Institute of Pathology.

Research Report, Progress against leukemia, rev., Public Health Service Pub. no. 960, National Cancer Institute, Bethesda, Md., 1968, U. S. Department of Health, Education and Welfare.

Sandberg, A. A.: The chromosomes and causation of human cancer and leukemia, Cancer Res. **26**(part I):2064-2081, 1966.

Viner, E. D., and Richardson, F. M.: The etiology of leukemia, Med. Sci., pp. 55-63, March, 1966.

Zarafonetis, C. J. D., editor: Proceedings of the International Conference on Leukemia-Lymphoma, Philadelphia, 1968, Lea & Febiger.

Zubrod, C. G.: Acute leukemias and Burkitt's lymphoma, Cancer **21:**553-557, 1968.

Chapter 31

# Tumors of the adrenal

The adrenal gland contains numerous sets of endocrine-producing cells. When retaining the hormone-making function of the normal cells of origin, tumors from these various cells exhibit a wide variety of clinical syndromes correlated with the physicochemical action of their secretory products. One embarks on a fascinating study of adrenal physiology in trying to understand and to diagnose these tumors. Diagnosis is seldom so simple as the palpation of a tumor mass; it requires careful analysis of the multiple clinical and laboratory abnormalities presented by these adrenal endocrinopathies.

Each individual tumor of the adrenal gland occurs rarely; as a group they are uncommon, far less than 1% of all cancers. Most cortical tumors develop in females, but they often develop in children and adolescents. Of the medullary tumors, neuroblastomas usually occur in early childhood, whereas pheochromocytomas are found at all ages.

Five major types of neoplasms or hyperplasias of the adrenal gland occur—primary aldosteronism, Cushing's syndrome, the virilizing (adrenogenital) syndrome, pheochromocytoma, and neuroblastoma (Table 3). We may clarify the subject by deviating somewhat from the format of previous chapters to discuss each tumor syndrome separately.

## PRIMARY ALDOSTERONISM

This endocrinopathy develops, as described by Conn, from adrenal cortical adenomas that appear round, well-demarcated, bright yellow, and very vascular; it is composed of cells from the outer layer of the cortex, the zona glomerulosa. Conn has contended that the small cortical adenomas often found incidentally at postmortem are in fact "aldosteronomas" that, if looked for, could have been found by appropriate antemortem studies of the metabolic imbalances they produce. Other authorities have not accepted this viewpoint, regarding the adenomas as a cause of hypertension without hypokalemic alkalosis.

These adenomas secrete varying amounts of excess aldosterone, a mineralocorticoid regulating body water and electrolyte balance. One finds hypertension (probably from salt and water retention) and usually a persistently low serum potassium with an elevated bicarbonate and high pH *(hypokalemic alkalosis),* plus concomitant high urinary potassium and a fixed urine specific gravity (isos-

**Table 3.** Adrenal tumors

| | Possible types of tumor | | Normal cells and their hormones | Clinical tumor syndromes | Associated tumor types | A few suggested abnormal tests |
|---|---|---|---|---|---|---|
| Cortex | Hyperplasia<br>Adenoma<br>Carcinoma | STEROIDS | 1. *Zona glomerulosa*<br>Aldosterone (C-21, mineralocorticoid) | 1. Primary aldosteronism (Conn's syndrome) | 95% adenoma | Serum K↓, Na normal or↑, $NaHCO_3$↑ urine K↑, sp. gr. fixed |
| | | | 2. *Zona fasciculata*<br>Cortisol (C-21, 17-OHCS* glucocorticoids) | 2. Cushing's syndrome | 70% hyperplasia<br>30% adenoma, or carcinoma | Urine 17-OHCS↑, often 17-KS↑; ACTH and dexamethasone responses often + |
| | | | 3. *Zona reticularis*<br>Androgens and estrogens (C19, 17-KS†) | 3. Virilizing (adrenogenital syndrome) | 65% hyperplasia<br>35% carcinoma (?) | Urine 17-KS↑, pregnanetriol↑ |
| | | | | 4. Mixed Cushing's and virilizing | Variable | Variable |
| | | | | 5. Feminizing (rare) | 75% carcinoma<br>25% adenoma | Urine 17-KS↑; ACTH and dexamethasone responses usually negative |
| Medulla | Benign<br>Malignant | CATECHOLAMINES | Chromaffin and ganglion cells<br>Epinephrine and norepinephrine | 1. Pheochromocytoma (hypertension, etc.) | 90% benign | Urinary free catecholamines or vanillylmandelic acid (VMA)↑ |
| | | | | 2. Ganglioneuroma (no endocrine effects) | 100% benign | Serum and urine metabolites of tyrosine and catecholamines↑ |
| | | | | 3. Neuroblastoma (no endocrine effects) | 100% malignant | |
| | | | | 4. Mixed | Variable | Variable |

*OHCS = Hydroxycorticosteroids.
†KS = Ketosteroids.

thenuria) from impaired renal tubular function. On finding such changes one tries first to establish that this imbalance does not represent secondary aldosteronism, which occurs in advanced cirrhosis, nephrosis, and congestive heart failure. Other causes of increased aldosterone secretion are sodium depletion, dehydration, and hemorrhage and the use of thiazide diuretics.

In the total clinical picture of primary aldosteronism, where the secretory activity of the tumor is high, one finds *hypertension* in every instance, and usually *muscle weakness, polyuria, headache,* and *polydipsia. Paresthesias, visual disturbances,* transient paralyses, fatigue, and occasionally tetany can also be found. In the smaller tumors with a lower excess of aldosterone secretion only an elevated blood pressure may be present, thus simulating a mild to moderate case of essential hypertension.

Physical findings include, of course, hypertension, mild retinopathy, and cardiomegaly; the patient is usually between the ages of 30 and 50. The diagnosis rests upon a combination of clinical and laboratory findings.

Proteinuria is usually present, as well as an abnormal glucose tolerance test. Since the principal effect of aldosterone is on the kidney, where it acts on the distal convoluted tubule, causing reabsorption of sodium and excretion of potassium, hydrogen, ammonia, and magnesium, most diagnostic laboratory studies consist of measurements of abnormalities related to these electrolytes. Excess urinary potassium and abnormal responses to the dietary administration of excess potassium and to sodium restriction suggest aldosteronism. Extracellular fluid volume and plasma volume are generally elevated with primary aldosteronism and an exaggerated response to sodium infusion appears, as it does with Cushing's syndrome and in excessively hydrated normal persons. Measurements of aldosterone excretion and renin-angiotensin levels in the blood are difficult and not always available.

Hypertensive patients who show hypokalemia after the administration of the thiazide diuretics carry a high suspicion of having "aldosteronomas." Renal angiography does not usually show the vascular pattern of the small aldosterone producing tumor itself, but it will give information about the kidney vasculature; occasionally vascular obstruction of the kidney will produce secondary aldosteronism. Renal biopsy showing hypertrophy and hypergranularity of the juxtaglomerular cells may also help with diagnosis; the patient with primary aldosteronism should show a marked decrease in the number of such cells and no granularity.

Several of the conditions producing secondary aldosteronism have been mentioned above. In addition, there may exist an essential hypertension treated with thiazide diuretics that exactly simulates primary aldosteronism, since some of these patients develop hypokalemia. Such patients, however, usually have normal extracellular fluid and plasma volumes. Other differential diagnoses include severe essential hypertension, renal vascular disease, overdosage with exogenous steroids, renal disease, and occasionally congenital aldosteronism in children.

Since nearly all of these are autonomously secreting adenomas, surgical removal becomes the treatment of choice. One explores both adrenals carefully, searching for multiple tumors. Occasionally one must segmentally resect one gland, and then the other, to find tiny adenomas.

Surgery abolishes the syndrome successfully in most patients, obtaining relief of hypertension and of metabolic abnormalities. Occasionally a mineralocorticoid insufficiency will require some time to return to normal.

## CUSHING'S SYNDROME (HYPERCORTICISM)

Cushing's syndrome occurs more often than the other syndromes; it stems from a hyperplasia, an adenoma or a carcinoma, of the middle zone of cortical cells, the zona fasciculata. When extra-adrenal in origin, this syndrome can arise from exogenously administered cortisol, excess adrenocorticotropic hormone (ACTH) stimulation of the adrenal from pituitary tumor or hyperfunction, or from the occasional ACTH-like secretions of other cancers (lung, pancreas, and carcinoids). Hyperplasias are often tiny, usually bilateral, and sometimes multiple; adenomas are generally unilateral and cause atrophy of the opposite adrenal cortex. These middle zone cortical cells secrete cortisol (hydrocortisone) and other glucocorticoids in response to ACTH. The excess circulating cortisol produces Cushing's syndrome. Hyperplasias remain responsive to ACTH, whereas neoplasms of these cells respond to ACTH less often and to varying degrees. The rare carcinomas, which are usually the cause of Cushing's syndrome in children, posses ssuch autonomy as seldom to be stimulated by trophic substances; they do produce excess corticoids, however, and hence also cause the clinical syndrome.

The classic Cushing's syndrome from excess circulating cortisol develops typically in young adult females. It consists of a unique *central adiposity, hypertension, osteoporosis, weakness, kyphosis, ecchymoses, amenorrhea,* impotence in the male, polycythemia, and abdominal pain. These symptoms may be present for many months or years, sometimes stationary but eventually progressive. If unchecked, they result in death in an average period of 9 years.

Often associated with the excess cortisol production of Cushing's syndrome is an oversecretion of androgens; these accumulate, especially in carcinoma, and result in virilizing signs and symptoms that cause a mixed syndrome. When Cushing's syndrome arises from adenoma or carcinoma rather than from hyperplasia, the clinical picture may be the same but the underlying hormonal imbalance differs. There is no ACTH excess, rather there is a deficit; the drive comes autonomously from the cortical tumor cells free of feedback controls, and the excess cortisol produced inhibits ACTH production, which results in atrophy of the opposite adrenal gland.

Only about one third of patients with Cushing's syndrome harbor adrenal neoplasms; two thirds have cortical hyperplasias or pituitary tumors or show no morphologic pathology. The determination of urinary metabolites of adrenal hormones has generally been the mainstay of laboratory diagnosis. Excess circulating cortisol results in elevated urinary 17-hydroxycorticosteroids (17-OHCS); excess androgen-like compounds yield increased urinary 17-ketosteroids (17-KS). To distinguish cortical hyperplasia (from excess ACTH stimulation) from true neoplasm can be difficult and may depend upon numerous laboratory studies. A marked increase in urinary 17-OHCS after the administration of *ACTH* or *Metopirone,* plus a decrease in 17-OHCS after large doses of *dexamethasone,* all point toward hyperplasia of the adrenal from a primary pituitary disturbance.

The opposite reactions with these three tests suggest adrenal neoplasm. Very high urinary 17-KS suggests carcinoma rather than adenoma, since malignant cortical tumors often produce a diversity of steroids. Carcinoma is more likely when (1) patients are very young children or infants, (2) the symptoms are of short duration, (3) both urinary 17-OHCS and 17-KS are very high, and (4) tumors are large.

Skull x-ray films help often in establishing pituitary adenomas as a cause of hypercorticism by showing widening of the sella turcica. Visual field abnormalities may help likewise.

Cortical hyperplasia from pituitary excess ACTH generally responds best to adrenalectomy, even though treatment of the pituitary disorder or tumor may be required months or years later. Pituitary treatment can be delivered either by surgery, by the implantation of radioactive substances, or by x-ray therapy. Long-term results in these cases cannot yet be assessed. Adrenal tumors need surgical removal after a thorough, bilateral, adrenal exploration, generally through the transabdominal route. The resection should be done in tissue planes widely outside the gland because doubt as to the malignant character of the neoplasm always exists until after removal and histologic study. Results in adenomas are uniformly good; carcinomas improve but usually recur. At this stage a relatively specific drug, dichlorodiphenyldichloroethane (*o,p′*-DDD), may offer some palliation.

## VIRILIZING (ADRENOGENITAL) SYNDROME

A virilizing syndrome can arise from congenital adrenal hyperplasia or from a virilizing adrenocortical tumor of the middle and inner zones of the cortex. A feminizing cortical tumor is rare.

*Congenital adrenal hyperplasia,* the most common cause, arises from an inborn error of metabolism due to a recessive mutant gene; the central defect consists of an enzymatic deficiency occurring at one of four levels in steroid synthesis. One end product, cortisol, is thereby reduced in the circulation and ACTH becomes excessively produced, resulting in adrenocortical hyperplasia. The enzymatic defect results in a shunting off and accumulation of intermediate and alternative products that have androgenic clinical effects causing the clinical syndrome, and these products then cause a high excretion of urinary 17-KS. The virilizing signs begin in fetal life and show at birth as anomalies of the genital tract.

Two forms of congenital adrenal hyperplasia predominate: (1) the *simple virilizing type* called "female pseudohermaphroditism," characterized by clitoral enlargement and a persistent urogenital sinus (the defect is less frequent and hard to recognize in male infants); and (2) the *salt-losing form,* which presents as an acute adrenal insufficiency—apathy, diarrhea, vomiting, hyperkalemic acidosis. In the laboratory the use of the ACTH stimulation test on urinary pregnanetriol, 17-KS, and 17-OHCS can usually differentiate hyperplasia from tumors. Treatment of hyperplasias in these infants and young children consists of cortisone; later, at the age of 2 or 3 years, surgical correction of the pseudohermaphroditism may be necessary.

A second cause of the virilizing syndrome is an *adrenocortical tumor.* These are less common than tumors producing Cushing's syndrome. They occur most often in adolescent and young adult females and cause an obvious clinical picture, including *clitoral hypertrophy, hirsutism, precocious pubic* and *axillary hair, rapid growth, premature closure of epiphyses,* and premature bone maturation. In these young women there is no family history of adrenal tumor and the youngsters have undergone normal development prior to the onset of virilization. Anomalies of the genitalia are not seen at birth with these tumors. In adult females, hirsutism, deepening of the voice, clitoral hypertrophy, atrophy of the breast, and amenorrhea are quite obvious. Virilization of the adult male can seldom be recognized quickly, but in the preadolescent male, premature pubertal changes and enlargement of the penis and prostate may be noted.

At any age, clitoral hypertrophy reliably indicates androgenic overproduction and many observers find that in the adult, hypertrophy of the clitoris often indicates cortical carcinoma. Other virilizing and mixed syndromes without clitoromegaly generally come from a benign tumor.

Higher urinary 17-KS levels are usually present, the greater the virilization, the higher the level. As a rule ACTH administration does not raise, nor does dexamethasone suppress, the urinary 17-KS in patients with these autonomously secreting tumors. Excretion of 17-OHCS may be elevated in patients with carcinoma or in mixed Cushing's–virilizing syndromes.

Most virilizing adrenocortical tumors are benign by clinical criteria but malignant histologically. They must be differentiated from congenital adrenal hyperplasia, as outlined above, from "acquired" hirsutism in young women, and from the Stein-Leventhal syndrome, wherein patients have normal 17-KS levels and normal responses to ACTH stimulation and dexamethasone suppression tests; they also may resemble arrhenoblastoma of the ovary. In the latter tumor the clinical and laboratory pictures may simulate a virilizing adrenal tumor closely, and diagnosis may depend upon pelvic palpation of an ovarian mass.

Treatment consists of surgical excision of the affected gland; results are good. One performs a wide resection if one suspects cancer in large tumors. Recurrences may respond to *o,p′*-DDD.

*Feminizing adrenal tumors* occur rarely, attract notice most easily in males (gynecomastia and testicular atrophy), and are usually malignant. They need differentiation from other excess estrogen-producing conditions; "idiopathic" gynecomastia in males, patients undergoing estrogen treatment for prostatic cancer, cirrhosis of the liver, estrogen-producing testicular tumors (interstitial cell tumors of the testis), and other estrogen-secreting tumors (granulosa cell and theca cell tumors).

## PHEOCHROMOCYTOMA

Composed of chromaffin tissue, this generally benign adenoma secretes excess amounts of epinephrine and/or norepinephrine in a somewhat intermittent fashion. A pheochromocytoma generally starts in the adrenal medulla, but in 10% of cases occurs in extra-adrenal locations—periaortic, periadrenal areas or along the sympathetic chain. Ten percent of these tumors are multiple, either bilateral in the adrenal or in extra-adrenal sites. The excess catecholamines produced by a pheochromocytoma yields a clinical picture characterized mainly by hypertension, which over the years leads to severe cardiovascular and cerebrovascular damage. However, if these tumors are diagnosed, treatment regularly succeeds in arresting the process. It is estimated that roughly one half of 1% of all hypertensive persons harbor pheochromocytomas.

The *symptomatology* of pheochromocytoma can be summarized as follows: (1) persons under 50; (2) paroxysmal hypertension in one half of the cases; (3) constant hypertension in the other one half; (4) very high blood pressure with wide fluctuations; (5) recent origin of hypertension or hypertension that begins in pregnancy; (6) hypertension in young persons; (7) hypertension associated with diabetes or an increased metabolism; (8) some kind of intermittent attack occurring almost daily that begins suddenly and is of short duration; (9) sudden, severe headaches; (10) excess sweating, either in paroxysmals or steadily; (11) palpitations; (12) pallor; (13) nausea; (14) tremors; and (15) weakness. Children have peculiar tendencies in regard to this symptomatology when they harbor pheochromocytomas. More children have persistent hypertension, visual complaints, high blood sugar, elevated metabolism, and multiple tumors than do adults.

Pharmacologic and biochemical tests usually make the diagnosis of these tumors once it has been thought of and the proper studies have been ordered. These studies are numerous and require exacting detail in preparation and performance. The easiest lead to diagnosis is to find elevated free catecholamines and vanillylmandelic acid (VMA) in the patient's urine. If these tests are within normal range (as they are in one fifth of all cases) and suspicion is high, then other tests need to be done. Plasma catecholamine levels may be elevated; cold pressure–histamine provocative tests generally raise the blood pressure in pheochromocytoma. The tyramine test to release *l*-norepinephrine from body stores, where it lies in excess amounts in pheochromocytoma, may be helpful. The Regitine test to depress blood pressure may also aid in diagnosis. Combinations of these laboratory studies are necessary in some cases. Extra-adrenal tumors secrete norepinephrine exclusively, rather than epinephrine, whereas medullary pheochromocytomas secrete both.

Intravenous pyelography and chest, bone, and skull films need to be done to complete the diagnostic survey. Aortography, gas insufflation in the retroperitoneal area, and venography have special hazards that prevent their routine use.

Pheochromocytomas vary greatly in size from a few centimeters to 15 or 20 cm. in diameter. In children, one in five occur bilaterally. They appear brownish and may show cystic areas, hemorrhage, necrosis, and capsular invasion; the latter characteristic imitates but does not prove that the tumor is malignant. Only 3% of these tumors will metastasize. Histologically, the Henle stain identifies the catecholamine content of these tumor cells and so confirms the diagnosis.

A hypertensive patient under the age of 50 with any kind of episodic symptoms needs study for a pheochromocytoma. Essential hypertension or coronary artery disease with episodic hypertension plus chest pain can simulate the pheochromocytoma syndrome. Regitine should only reduce blood pressure with pheochromocytoma. If an elevated metabolism suggests hyperthyroidism, normal radioiodine uptake and normal protein-bound iodine in the serum plus elevated serum pressor levels should indicate pheochromocytoma.

These tumors need surgical excision by the abdominal route because only one half can be lateralized before operation by x-ray studies. Long incisions and wide exposure help the surgeon carry out a thorough retroperitoneal exploration for extra-adrenal, multiple, or bilateral tumors. The surgeon resects widely through the periadrenal fat rather than enucleating the gland closely. As stated before, results of this adrenalectomy are uniformly good if all tumor tissue has been detected and removed.

## NEUROBLASTOMA

This tumor constitutes the most frequent, solid, metastasizing neoplasm of childhood, along with its less common variant, ganglioneuroblastoma. It is also the most frequent malignant abdominal tumor in children as well as the most common cancer of the adrenal gland at all ages. Presumably it begins in the fetus from embryonic neural crest cells, which normally differentiate into sympathetic ganglion cells or chromaffin cells. Although these are the cells that constitute the adrenal medulla, unaccountably only one half of these tumors begin in the adrenal. The other half start in other sympathetic nerve locations along the spinal column. The benign tumor of sympathetic tissue, ganglioneuroma, occurs rarely in the adrenal gland and seldom in the very young child.

Neuroblastoma may be present at birth, but usually comes to diagnosis under the age of 4; the average age of patients is 3 years.

All sympathetic tissue has the capacity to synthesize catecholamines from tyrosine. The most common catecholamines are homovanillic acid (HVA) and vanillylmandelic acid (VMA). Although a few patients show hypertension, diarrhea, and excessive perspiration, usually no symptoms from increased circulating catecholamines ensue from adrenal neuroblastoma, in contrast to the other tumor syndromes described above. Clinical findings arise either from a huge primary tumor mass that may interfere with bowel function or from the very frequent metastases to bone (especially femur and skull). Occasionally spinal cord invasion and cord compression occur. Patients experience bone pain and very frequently a unilateral exophthalmos from skull metastases. Generally one finds a palpable mass in the abdomen or flank.

Many neuroblastoma patients show an anemia. Despite extensive bone marrow replacement by tumor the true cause of the anemia is not known. Bone marrow aspirations frequently aid in the diagnosis by revealing malignant cells. A majority of children with neuroblastoma have an elevation of one or more catecholamines or their metabolites, usually VMA or HVA, in the urine. Measurements of 24-hour urine catecholamines not only help in diagnosis but also help measure response to treatment; reappearance of such substances in the urine may be the first indication of relapse. One needs to remember, however, that elevated urinary VMA may also occur in retinoblastoma, pheochromocytoma, leukemia, the carcinoid syndrome, chemodectoma, cystic fibrosis, pulmonary insufficiency, paroxysmal tachycardia and burns.

X-ray films often help diagnosis; there is a characteristic calcification in most neuroblastomas. On intravenous pyelography the kidney will be dislocated downward and a few patients actually show renal parenchymal invasion by the tumor simulating the picture of Wilms' tumor. Chest films may show involvement of mediastinal or hilar nodes and occasional lung metastases appear. Bone metastases occur in lytic, blastic, or mixed varieties.

The primary tumor has usually attained a large size by the time of diagnosis; it grows quickly, breaks through its pseudocapsule with ease, and soon invades the surrounding structures. Generally a soft, friable, dark tumor, it commonly shows areas of hemorrhage or necrosis within it. Microscopically "rosettes" of malignant cells typify neuroblastoma, since apparently the first sign of differentiation of primitive sympathetic cells is the formation of these "rosettes."

One must distinguish neuroblastoma from Wilms' tumor. Generally no intrinsic deformity presents on intravenous pyelography with neuroblastoma; calcifications are present and metastases usually become evident on x-ray films of bones and on bone marrow aspiration. If one is not certain on clinical and laboratory evidence, open biopsy of the primary tumor constitutes a last resort. Ewing's bone sarcoma and occasionally lymphoma may suggest neuroblastoma and require biopsy for differentiation.

Several reports indicate that neuroblastoma may on rare occasion "mature" into a ganglioneuroma, both spontaneously and after treatment, thereafter behaving like a benign tumor composed of mature ganglion cells. This has been reported only in extra-adrenal neuroblastomas.

Treatment needs to be individualized. Occasionally a clean surgical resection of a purely localized tumor may prove to be enough for permanent control. In most instances palliative subtotal resection with postoperative x-ray therapy constitutes the treatment plan. X-ray treatment usually produces good regression in the primary tumor as well as in metastatic disease, and it can take much credit for the successes reported in neuroblastoma. Chemotherapy also adds to the percentage of survivors when combined with surgery and irradiation. Cyclophosphamide, vincristine, and daunomycin are the preferred drugs being used at the present time. Distant metastases frequently regress under such chemotherapy. Many experts give courses of chemotherapy for 6 months to 2 years in curable patients, even those with initially localized disease. For far advanced disease with bone metastases (positive marrow smears), subtotal surgical removal may be omitted and equal palliation achieved with only x-ray therapy and chemotherapy.

Prognosis in neuroblastoma is better if the child comes to diagnosis under the age of 2 with a localized tumor. The few neuroblastomas occurring in the thorax have the best prognosis. Conversely, children coming to diagnosis over the age of 2 years with tumors in the adrenal medullary location, or with tumors that have spread to bone, carry the worst prognosis. One encouraging report in patients with liver metastases states that two thirds of a small group have been controlled with radiation to the liver, plus appropriate treatment for the local tumor. Roughly 40% of children survive free of disease over the long term.

## COMMON ERRORS

The failure to think of adrenal tumors as a possible cause of these many symptom complexes has denied patients the benefits of control. Also many surgeons in the past have failed to appreciate the need for complete exploration of both retroperitoneal areas in most cases of suspected adrenal tumors.

**REFERENCES**

Ackerman, L. V., and del Regato, J. A.: Cancer, St. Louis, 1963, The C. V. Mosby Co., pp. 900-921.

Conn, J. W.: Primary aldosteronism, a new clinical syndrome, J. Lab. Clin. Med. **45:**3-17, 1955.

El-Bolkainy, M. H., Pierce, G. B., Jr., and French, A. J.: Regression of an adrenal cortical carcinoma by estradiol treatment, Cancer Res. **27:**1846-1852, 1967.

Goldfine, A.: Treatment of pheochromocytoma, Mod. Treatm. **3:**1360-1376, 1966.

Hotckkis, R. C., Davidson, A. C., Messina, E. J., and Redisch, W.: Pheochromocytoma, Ann. Surg. **166:**1021-1028, 1967.

Hutter, A. M., and Kayhoe, D. E.: Adrenal cortical carcinoma, Amer. J. Med. **41:**572-592, 1966.

Karsner, H. T.: Tumors of the adrenal. In Atlas of tumor pathology, Sect. VIII, Fasc. 29, Washington, D. C., 1950, Armed Forces Institute of Pathology.

Lipsett, M. B.: Treatment of adrenal carcinoma, Mod. Treatm. **3:**1377-1388, 1966.

Mahesh, V. B., Greenblatt, R. B., and Coniff, R. F.: Urinary steroid excretion before and after dexamethasone administration and steroid content of adrenal tissues and venous blood in virilizing adrenal tumors, Amer. J. Obstet. Gynec. **100:**1043-1054, 1968.

Marchant, J.: Development of adrenal cortical carcinoma in $C_{3H}$ mice following castration and the administration of 7,12-dimethyl benz(a)anthracene, Brit. J. Cancer **21:**750-754, 1967.

Migeon, C. J.: Treatment of congenital adrenal hyperplasia, Mod. Treatm. **3:**1348-1359, 1966.

O'Neal, L. W.: Surgery of the adrenal glands, St. Louis, 1968, The C. V. Mosby Co.

Rhamy, R. K., McCoy, P. M., Scott, H. W., Jr., Fishman, L. M., Michelakis, A. M., and Liddle, G.: Primary aldosteronism, Ann. Surg. **167:**718-727, 1968.

Schimke, R. N., Hartmann, W. H., Prout, T. E., and Rimoin, D. L.: Syndrome of bilateral pheochromocytoma, medullary thyroid carcinoma and multiple neuromas, New Eng. J. Med. **279:**1-7, 1968.

Scott, H. W., Jr., Foster, J. H., Liddle, G., and Davidson, E. T.: Cushing's syndrome due to adrenocortical tumor, Ann. Surg. **162:**505-516, 1965.

Sjoerdsma, A., Engelman, K., Waldmann, T. A., Cooperman, L. H., and Hammond, W. G.: Pheochromocytoma: current concepts of diagnosis and treatment, Ann. Intern. Med. **65:** 1302-1326, 1966.

Smithwick, R. H., Sherwin, R. P., Carr, H. E., Jr., Curtis, G. W., Thorn, G. W., Robertson, C. W., and Harrison, J. H.: The adrenal glands. In Nealon, T. F., Jr., editor: Management of the patient with cancer, Philadelphia, 1967, W. B. Saunders Co., pp. 828-864.

Zintel, H. A., and Schuh, F. D.: Surgical disease of the adrenal glands, Amer. J. Gastroent. **44:**515-535, 1965.

# Chapter 32

# Cancer in children

Separate consideration of childhood cancers seems appropriate because the predominant types of cancer in children differ so markedly from the predominant types in adults. A study of this difference should help us to understand cancer as a whole. A few instances of each of the adult types of carcinomas have been reported in children, but they are so rare as to be medical curiosities. Childhood cancer gains additional importance, also, because its control results in many more years of normal life salvaged than does control of an adult cancer.

Some of the more frequent malignant neoplasms of youngsters have already been described—leukemia, Wilms' tumors, and neuroblastomas. Central nervous system tumors will not be described in this synopsis. We will try to avoid unnecessary repetition, but describe important additional tumors and at the same time emphasize the progress in salvage of children with cancer by recent, improved methods of treatment.

## INCIDENCE AND DISTRIBUTION

Despite being a leading cause of death in children, second only to accidental death, childhood cancer seldom comes to the attention of most physicians. Altogether these cancers account for 1% to 2% of all cancer deaths. Most reports come from concentration of childhood tumors in children's hospitals. The peak age incidence of these neoplasms lies between birth and 5 years of age; it then falls to half this level by the age of 15. During the late teens there is a slow but steady rise again, continuing on throughout adulthood. Leukemias compose the largest single group of these early childhood cancers; others, such as neuroblastomas, Wilms' tumors, teratomas, and retinoblastomas might be termed "embryomas," since they are found in infancy and early childhood and probably have initiation in embryonic tissue before birth. Brain tumors come to diagnosis at all ages during childhood. Bone sarcomas, Hodgkin's disease, and miscellaneous adult types predominate between the ages of 5 and 15. When adult types of carcinoma occur, they tend to be found late in childhood. Brain tumors show little or no age concentration in children.

Outside the characteristic location of Burkitt's tumor (African lymphoma) in central equatorial Africa (Chapter 29), no significant geographic variations in distribution have been noted.

## ETIOLOGY

### External initiating agents

No doubt exists today in the minds of experts that childhood cancers often undergo their initiation process before birth, during embryogenesis. X-rays constitute the one fairly certain agent in causation; MacMahon documented that fetuses exposed in utero to diagnostic x-rays of the mother's pelvis suffered a significantly higher death rate from cancer before the age of 10. But obviously this factor can only account for a small percentage of childhood cancers. Other external prenatal factors no doubt await identification. Stewart suggests that the rapid formation of newly differentiating cells during the process of embryogenesis, with numerous cells in mitosis at any given time, constitute a special cancer hazard. Cells of laboratory animal embryos are more susceptible to carcinogenic agents than adult cells in vivo and in vitro. Weller proposed some years ago that external carcinogenic agents ingested by the mother passed the placental barrier to initiate the fetal cancerous process, but little work has been done to enlighten us on this point.

Postnatal x-ray therapy has already been mentioned (Chapter 10) as a causative agent in papillary carcinoma of the thyroid, which often becomes evident before the age of 15.

### Predisposing factors

Hereditary and genetic factors influence many childhood cancers. Familial multiple polyposis of the colon, retinoblastoma, and xeroderma pigmentosum are outstanding examples. Two types of retinoblastoma have been described—the familial one controlled by a single dominant, abnormal gene in the germ cell and the sporadic one occurring at a slightly older age, perhaps caused by a somatic mutation of the same gene. Linkage of cancer susceptibility to other congenital defects occurs—mongoloid children carry 30 times the normal risk of developing leukemia.

Siblings of children with cancer show an increased risk of having cancer themselves; the concordance of childhood leukemia in monozygotic twins runs as high as 25%. Also first born children and children of older mothers (35 and over) run a significantly higher risk of leukemia.

## PATHOLOGY

The types of childhood cancers and rough estimations of their percentage contribution to the whole group (a composite of several large studies) are given below.

| | |
|---|---|
| Leukemia | 35% |
| Central nervous system (brain) | 20% |
| Lymphoma | 10% |
| Sarcoma (soft part and bone) | 10% |
| Neuroblastoma | 10% |
| Wilms' tumor | 5% |
| Retinoblastoma | 3% |
| Teratomas | 3% |
| Miscellaneous | 4% |

Leukemia has been described in Chapter 30, lymphoma in Chapter 29, soft part sarcoma in Chapter 27, bone sarcoma in Chapter 28, neuroblastoma in Chapter 31, and Wilms' tumor in Chapter 24. Brain tumors fall outside the scope of this synopsis. We will attempt to deal here with two unusual cancers of childhood not yet covered, retinoblastoma and the teratomas, and add some information on neuroblastoma. Common benign tumors and tumorous conditions will be mentioned only where appropriate to differential diagnosis.

*Retinoblastoma* arises from the retina as a flat or as a projecting, pink-white mass (exophytic and endophytic varieties) that may frequently be noted at birth. With enlargement it invades the choroid, then the other soft tissues of the orbit and then the bony orbit; it spreads frequently along the optic nerve to the meninges, subarachnoid space and brain. The exophytic kind may present as a necrotic, infected mass replacing the eye. Metastases occur late to lungs, liver, bones, or nodes. Fine calcifications may be present in the tumor. Immature cells called retinoblasts, which often form "rosettes," compose this highly malignant tumor.

*Teratomas* are relatively common in the newborn. They frequently occur in the sacrococcygeal region, but may also present in the ovary and occasionally in the testicle, retroperitoneum, or neck. Composed of tissue from all three of the embryologic cell layers, teratomas differ from the more common "dermoid" tumor that contains only two embryologic cell types. They occur in cystic or solid forms; the solid teratomas are more likely to harbor malignant elements. The malignant portion usually comes from only one tissue. Epidermis, brain tissues, intestinal and respiratory mucosa, cartilage and bone, and striated and smooth muscle can frequently be identified in them. All of these tissues should be examined carefully and suspected of being malignant. When cancerous, the malignant component spreads in all ways—by local invasion and via lymphatics and the bloodstream to distant sites. In the sacrococcygeal site they usually present as an obvious bulge at one side or the other of the intergluteal fold; a few may grow inside the sacrum in a retrorectal position.

Ovarian teratomas may be present at birth but seldom become diagnosed until later in childhood or in adult life, since most are benign (Chapter 31). When found early they are discovered accidentally at laparotomy done for more commonly suspected illness such as appendicitis. *Dermoid* tumors of childhood occur in subcutaneous, superficial locations over the body, especially in the head lateral to the orbit; they are invariably benign.

*Hemangiomas* of infants, seldom malignant, probably represent a developmental anomaly more than a true neoplasm, and nine out of ten regress spontaneously as growth slows and tissues mature during the first year or two of life. Melanomas seldom exhibit metastasizing ability before puberty (Chapter 5).

The soft part sarcoma most common in childhood is the *embryonal rhabdomyosarcoma,* often occurring in the head and neck and genitourinary system; it is somewhat akin to the sarcoma botryoides of the uterovaginal tract in the infants. The most common location for embryonal rhabdomyosarcoma is in the orbit. Abdominal desmoids (fibromatosis) also occur.

### Precancerous lesions

All fetal and neonatal tissues should be regarded as cancer prone when subjected to any known carcinogenic stimulus. Intestinal polyposis in children is potentially cancerous but the isolated, juvenile, colorectal retention type of polyp (a distinct pathologic variant) is not. Skin keratoses in xeroderma pigmentosum carry a high cancerous risk, and, of course, so does the entire skin of these children when exposed to ultraviolet light.

## DIAGNOSIS

**History and physical examination.** *Retinoblastoma* may first cause a squint of the affected eye in the infant or child; an opaque light reflex can soon be noted in the normally dark pupil, along with inequality of the pupils and, later, with loss of vision. Study of the eyegrounds will help reveal a tumor. The tumor mass may produce a painful secondary glaucoma. About one fourth of these children harbor bilateral tumors. Fine calcifications on an x-ray film will point strongly toward a diagnosis of retinoblastoma, as will enlargement of the bony optic nerve canal. Biopsy and frozen section may be indicated, since this neoplasm can be confused with pseudotumors of unknown, possibly infectious origin, retrolental fibroplasia, retinal fibrosis, lymphoma, hemangioma, or neurofibroma. Parasitic infections can also produce an opaque, light pupil.

*Sacrococcygeal teratomas* should be suggested externally if any asymmetry or bulge of the gluteal area is evident. A digital rectal examination becomes especially important to detect retrorectal masses or extensions. Most of these tumors do not destroy the bony sarcum, but if bone erosion appears on an x-ray film, the lesion must be considered malignant. Teratomas may, but generally do not, disturb bladder or bowel function or impair lower limb motion. This clinical feature helps distinguish them from *sacral meningomyelocele;* the latter usually does cause motor disturbances, is more commonly cystic without calcification, expands when the baby cries, and causes widening of the neural arch on x-ray films. One usually can make this diagnosis on clinical grounds without biopsy.

**Biopsy.** A wedge biopsy of the growing edge of any nonabdominal mass in children, however, is a good general rule of diagnosis.

**X-ray studies.** Diagnostic x-ray films must be used with caution in children because of the danger of injuring these highly susceptible growing tissues.

**Laboratory studies.** Bone marrow aspirations may yield malignant cells in an appreciable number of *neuroblastomas,* but negative studies, of course, mean little.

## DIFFERENTIAL DIAGNOSIS

The most frequent diagnostic problem in the young child concerns the abdominal mass, which, of course, lies deep and is not easily accessible for biopsy. Decisions regarding procedure must be based on clinical and laboratory findings. The differential usually lies between Wilms' tumor and neuroblastoma. Table 4 listing common differences may help.

Often differential diagnostic problems involve the common hemangioma as a possibly malignant tumor of undetermined nature. The hemangioma is superficial, soft, bluish or reddish, compressible, and often on the trunk as well as in many

**Table 4.** Common differences between Wilms' tumor and neuroblastoma

| Findings | Wilms' tumor | Neuroblastoma |
|---|---|---|
| Calcification | No | Yes |
| Catecholamines in urine | No | Yes |
| Bone metastases (films and marrow smears) | Seldom | Often |
| Intrinsic calyceal distortion (intravenous pyelogram) | Yes | Seldom |

other locations, and may increase in size during the first 6 months or year of life. The commonest type of bright red capillary-cavernous hemangioma regresses spontaneously during the first few years of life. One should diagnose this lesion by the clinical signs to avoid the profuse hemorrhage that ensues with open biopsy.

Unusual, accessible solid masses require open wedge biopsy.

Cystic masses in childhood are relatively frequent and may suggest malignant tumors. Congenital cysts are very common such as those in the neck (cystic hygromas), branchial cleft cysts, thyroglossal duct cysts, mediastinal cysts, and lung, pancreatic, mesenteric, and umbilical cysts: such cystic masses generally represent developmental anomalies.

## PREVENTIVE MEASURES

Recent improvements in radiologic techniques have reduced the total number of rads of exposure delivered to the fetus by x-rays of pregnant mothers. Still an x-ray film must be ordered with highly adequate reasons in view of the possible risk to the fetus.

Healthy parents who have one child affected with cancer may safely have another child; but if two children are so affected, the risk of additional cancerous children is too great to take knowingly. It also seems wise for any person cured of an embryonal cancer to avoid having children; this statement applies mainly to retinoblastoma.

Mothers would have fewer cancerous children if they are under the age of 35, but the risk is not great enough to advise women against childbearing because of age alone.

## TREATMENT PRINCIPLES

1. As a rule, one chooses *surgery* as the first step in treating most solid childhood cancers, either for diagnosis only or for both diagnosis and treatment together at one operation. Surgery secures a firm diagnosis and, if carefully planned, avoids permanent structural damage; it may result in control of many localized cancers. But the surgeon needs a constant awareness of the adult growth end result from each tiny bit of tissue or structure removed in a small child to avoid unnecessary mutilation. Neuroblastoma patients appear to profit from the removal of 95% of the tumor when it is nonresectable (Koop).

2. Preoperative *radiation* may help with some large, highly malignant tumors—sarcomas, lymphomas, Wilms' tumors, or neuroblastomas. Surgery has been traditionally the treatment for retinoblastoma, but preoperative radiation becomes

more frequently used each year in this tumor also. *Postoperative radiation* should yield good control in Wilms' tumors, retinoblastoma, and neuroblastoma if bits of tumor remain after resection and in metastatic lesions of all sorts; if the patient survives x-ray therapy, he carries a high risk of permanent bone and soft part "hypodevelopment."

3. *Chemotherapy* in conjunction with the above two modalities seems to increase survivals in Wilms' tumors and in neuroblastomas and is generally employed after operation. In initially widespread cancers, chemotherapy can achieve worthwhile regressions. Actinomycin D proves the most effective of the various agents, followed by cyclophosphamide and vincristine. Newer agents (daunomycin and BCNU) often secure regressions in most of the highly undifferentiated primitive cell types of cancer, such as the sarcomas.

4. Vitamin $B_{12}$ still has some advocates for inhibiting neuroblastoma.

## COMMON ERRORS

Misdiagnosis is easy in these pleomorphic, anaplastic cancers because their spectrum is so wide, their occurrence is so infrequent, and they develop in unfamiliar sites of the body as compared to our more or less standardized concepts of cancers in adults.

## PROMISING DEVELOPMENTS FOR THE FUTURE

1. We need more children's hospitals for these specialized problems.
2. Education of parents will help in earlier diagnosis and more cooperative accomplishment of treatment plans.
3. Genetic counseling no doubt will become more and more useful and widely available.
4. Careful monitoring of, and refinements in, x-ray machines will continue to reduce x-ray exposure of the fetus in utero when films are needed.
5. Studies of maternal, prenatal carcinogenic factors that may initiate or promote cancer should bear fruit in the future.
6. Newer laboratory diagnostic aids are emerging; one study suggests that the variations in serum nerve growth factor are related to the activity of neuroblastoma.

## PROGNOSIS

**Neuroblastoma.** With the more recently employed combinations of treatment (surgery, x-ray therapy, and chemotherapy), a crude 2-year survival rate of 50% in these infants has been demonstrated. The location of the primary tumor seems most important prognostically, those in the thorax surviving best whereas tumors above the clavicle do worst. The younger the child, the better the prognosis. Also, the more differentiated the tumor, the better the prognosis. Spontaneous remission has been reported in 28 cases of neuroblastoma. Today about one third of all patients treated by all methods survive. Koop has found that in neuroblastoma there is no relation between the adequacy of excisional surgery and survival.

**Wilms' tumor.** Here also the younger patients (under 1 year) have a much better prognosis. Ninety percent of these patients survive, whereas only 60% of all patients at all ages are salvaged. One report on survivals in a group of patients treated with aggressive surgical, radiotherapeutic, and chemotherapeutic modalities shows three fourths of the patients alive and well at 2 years.

Collins' constant growth rate concept, based on "doubling time," seems to apply to Wilms' tumors and to neuroblastomas as well as to the leukemias. Thus if a child survives a length of time equal to its age at original diagnosis plus 9 months, it can be presumed cured. With the increasingly intensive use of chemotherapy in these tumors, however, we are now seeing late recurrences, which limit the usefulness of the concept.

**Retinoblastoma.** Since recent knowledge and ophthalmologic technical skill diagnose most of these when still localized, at least 80% of the patients now obtain control of the disease in the large centers. As an overall figure, about half are salvaged.

**Teratomas.** Prognosis worsens with age here also, either because the malignant components of these teratomas develop quickly after birth and become invasive and metastasize within the first 6 months, or because one can solve the technical problem of clean removal easier in the newborn than in the older infant or child.

## REFERENCES

Bill, A. H., Jr.: A study of the nerve growth factor in the serum of neuroblastoma patients, J. Pediat. Surg. **3**:171-172, 1968.

Bolande, R. P., Brough, A. J., and Izant, R. J., Jr.: Congenital mesoblastic nephroma of infancy, Pediatrics **40**:272-278, 1967.

Collins, V. P.: The treatment of Wilms' tumor, Cancer **11**:89-94, 1958.

Collins, V. P., Loeffler, R. U., and Tevey, H.: Observations on growth rates of human tumors, Amer. J. Roentgen. **76**:988-1000, 1956.

Cutler, S. J.: End results in cancer, Report no. 3, Bethesda, Md., 1968, U. S. Department of Health, Education and Welfare.

Dargeon, H. W.: Tumors of childhood, New York, 1960, Paul B. Hoeber, Inc.

Grant, R. N.: The challenge of childhood cancer, C.A. **18**:35-39, 1968.

Gross, R. E.: The surgery of infancy and childhood, Philadelphia, 1953, W. B. Saunders Co.

Holder, T. M.: Tumors peculiar to infants and children. In Nealon, T. F., Jr., editor: Management of the patient with cancer, Philadelphia, 1966, W. B. Saunders Co., pp. 1012-1039.

Iriarte, P. V., Hananian, J., and Cortner, J. A.: Central nervous system leukemia and solid tumors of childhood, Cancer **19**:1187-1194, 1966.

Kissane, J. M., and Smith, M. G.: Pathology of infancy and childhood, St. Louis, 1967, The C. V. Mosby Co.

Koop, C. E.: Factors affecting survival in neuroblastoma, J. Pediat. Surg. **3**:113-115, 1968.

Koop, C. E., and Hernandez, J. R.: Neuroblastoma: experience with 100 cases in children, Surgery **56**:726-733, 1964.

Mahorner, H.: Two rare malignancies, Amer. Surg. **34**:53-56, 1968.

Michael, P.: Tumors of infancy and childhood, Philadelphia, 1964, J. B. Lippincott Co.

Stanley-Brown, E. G., and Dargeon, H. W.: Presenting symptoms of neuroblastomas and Wilms' tumors, Clin. Pediat. **5**:681-682, 1966.

Stewart, A.: Epidemiology of childhood cancers. In Raven, R. W., and Roe, F. J. C., editors: The prevention of cancer, New York, 1967, Appleton-Century-Crofts, pp. 352-358.

Tan, C., Tasaka, H., Yu, K. P., Murphy, L. M., and Karnofsky, D. A.: Daunomycin, an antitumor antibiotic in the treatment of neoplastic disease, Cancer **20**:333-353, 1967.

Tefft, M., and Wittenborg, M. H.: Radiotherapeutic management of neuroblastoma in childhood, J.A.M.A. **205**:159-166, 1968.

Chapter 33

# Chemotherapy

In view of the fact that approximately two thirds of all cancers are incurable and eventually kill the patient, chemotherapy that seeks to control systemically spread cancer naturally assumes a growing importance as the total volume of cancer in our population increases. Today chemotherapy permits all physicians, not just surgeons and radiotherapists, to participate actively in managing the cancer patient. Therefore a basic outline of available data in this field must be part of each physician's background of knowledge. Whereas most doctors have little need for acquaintance with the technique of a neck dissection, nor for the details of dosimetry in planning to irradiate a cervical cancer, they have an absolute obligation to know that choriocarcinoma of the uterus (trophoblastic disease) can now be cured in most instances by intensive administration of methotrexate or actinomycin D.

Compared to the naïve hopes aroused in all minds when drug therapy of cancer first became available, the day-to-day use of drugs for the common solid human cancers has proved disappointing. Drugs have been overused and deaths have resulted; they have been misused in patients when no benefit could be expected. The fact that a drug is of benefit in an occasional case of a certain cancer has been falsely used as a sufficient reason to try it in all such cancers. Anticancer drugs still benefit only the minority of patients. Nevertheless advances are being made every year in this field.

Physicians who jump to the conclusion, after a few trials, that chemotherapy offers nothing forget the rapidity of anticancer drug development. The increasing number of useful drugs, the growing knowledge of when in the course of the disease to use them and of how to arrange dosage schedules and courses of treatment, newer understanding of what to expect (for example, knowing the population percentage of tumor cells killed per dose), widening of technical skill in routes of administration so as to increase tumor dose but decrease toxicity, advancing knowledge of the various combinations of drugs and of combining drugs with x-ray therapy and surgery, and better knowledge of the occasional selective toxicity of drugs for special cancer cells—all of these contribute small improvements that together add up to significant progress in chemotherapy. There are so many types of cancer, discovered in different stages, treated by so many drugs and dosage schedules, and treated with so many different possible combinations that the whole field becomes complex. With this complexity in mind, we will try to outline in this chapter only a convenient current classification of chemotherapeutic drugs with some basic facts about each, plus mention of the common cancers for which various drugs have proved useful. The reader needs to remember that much in this field is still experimental.

We will not discuss hormones; they have been dealt with in appropriate chapters on certain cancers. Corticosteroids will be mentioned. We do not present a guide to the details of therapy, but merely a statement of fundamentals that each doctor must have in mind when considering the total treatment plan for each cancer patient. Dosages will only occasionally be given. Objective response rates will be stated when available; such a response usually means a decrease in measurable tumor size by 50% that lasts for at least 2 months.

At the present time roughly thirteen commonly used drugs exist that can be divided into four categories according to mechanism of action. These drugs have a demonstrable effect on about twenty types of human cancer. But the list of drugs and neoplasms affected grows each year; the reader must consult the references and new papers each year to cover the field.

## PRINCIPLES OF DRUG ACTION AND THERAPY

1. Since anticancer drugs mainly affect cells that are actively multiplying, all tissues that multiply at a fast rate succumb to the drugs to some extent; those with the highest rate are the most sensitive. Thus toxicity seldom occurs in tissues with a low cell turnover—brain, muscle, kidney, and liver. However, toxicity is frequent in tissues with high cell turnovers—the bone marrow, oral and intestinal mucosa, hair follicles, ovarian cortex, and testicular tubules. Similarly, fast-growing neoplasms are susceptible, whereas slow-growing neoplasms are not. Drugs attack most actively the fast-growing leukemias and lymphomas in healthy hosts, and they attack least the slow-growing solid cancers in debilitated hosts.

2. One should rely on drugs only after the usefulness of surgery, x-ray therapy, and, in a few cases, the hormones has been exhausted. One exception to this rule of thumb is in planned combination therapy with drugs and x-ray therapy or drugs and surgery.

3. In general, one must administer chemotherapeutic agents until mild or moderate toxicity occurs to obtain maximum benefit for the patient. There are exceptions to this in a few cancers where maintenance drug regimens are of proved value or in some breast cancers where adjuvant chemotherapy after surgery provides benefit.

4. One should try hard to find a measurable parameter to gauge the effect of the drug on the patient—a peripheral mass, masses demonstrated by x-ray in the lungs, or abnormal blood or urinary chemistry studies. Subjective improvement is not a reliable guide to therapy.

5. Close monitoring, with complete blood counts, selected blood chemistry studies, platelet counts, and occasional bone marrow and reticulocyte determinations, becomes a necessity with all anticancer drug administration. With a number of the more toxic drugs one soon learns to stop the drug quickly if an abnormal trend appears in any of these determinations.

6. Very close surveillance of the patient becomes necessary for maximum benefit. The physician needs to detect drug resistance of malignant cells at an early stage and be prepared to change drugs promptly should resistance occur.

7. In general, once the physician begins drug administration it is wise to continue if there is any suspicion that viable cells persist, as long as toxicity does not contraindicate this course.

8. Deaths from chemotherapy usually occur from uncontrolled, unopposed infection in the patient who is made severely leukopenic by the drugs.

9. The potential chemotherapy patient must have as complete a hospital study as one would have prior to a major surgical operation because these patients are going to be severely stressed. As Brennan emphasizes, the agents are not pharmacologically selective like hormones and antibiotics, but are overall cell poisons much like chemosurgery.

10. In addition to selecting those patients in whom the much more effective and controllable means of surgery and irradiation (and hormones) have been fully used, one also selects patients with definitely progressing disease. "Prophylactic" use of drugs over a long period to prevent recurrence or destroy microscopic metastases has not been of proved value and at present does not constitute a legitimate expectation or objective. One must not turn to drugs in desperation after months of medical neglect on the premise that the patient will die soon anyway. Here drugs do more harm than good.

11. Do not expect to prolong life. Drugs may reduce tumor size to ease pain, relieve mechanical obstruction of a hollow viscus, or reduce vascular and lymphatic compression; they may allow areas of ulceration to heal and permit lytic bone lesions to reossify. But added longevity is usually slight, as a general rule.

## ALKYLATING AGENTS

These cytotoxic, mutagenic, radiomimetic drugs destroy cells by distorting and breaking deoxyribonucleic acid (DNA) molecules (and to a lesser extent, disrupting other cell constituents); they do this by joining active alkyl groups to active sites in purines and pyrimidines of the DNA chain. They also interfere with a number of enzymatic reactions. Any suggestion of selective tumor toxicity is due to the vulnerability of the more readily dividing groups of tumor cells as compared to division rates of normal cells. Alkylating drugs are the oldest of modern chemotherapeutic agents.

**Mechlorethamine (nitrogen mustard, Mustargen, $HN_2$).** Hodgkin's disease constitutes the tumor for which mechlorethamine is most commonly employed, although x-ray therapy will generally be used first and achieve the greatest total benefit for the patient. This drug plays a role when the disease spreads systemically or when the spinal cord compression or superior vena caval compression occurs. It also helps in the patient who has had x-ray therapy to tolerance. Mechlorethamine works more quickly than x-ray therapy. Dameshek and associates claim 80% of patients respond, about half with complete remissions, half with partial remissions. Another use for the drug lies in patients with anaplastic, small cell (oat cell) *carcinoma of the lung;* half of the patients show objective regressions of tumor size, but this lasts only 2 to 6 weeks and life is not prolonged. However, the drug finds frequent use in *malignant effusions*—especially in the *pleural* cavity. The drug is diluted somewhat and injected directly into the space where its mild vesicant action produces an adhesive pleuritis and obliterates the space, preventing future effusions. Fairly prompt nausea and vomiting develop with the use of mechlorethamine, but these symptoms pass quickly. Bone marrow depression develops later, particularly leukopenia. Deaths related to the drug now run less than 1% and occur from infection.

**Cyclophosphamide (Cytoxan).** Several tumors respond to this agent—*acute leukemia, "reticulum cell sarcoma," multiple myeloma,* and *malignant tumors* of early *childhood.* It is the only alkylating drug that will produce remissions in childhood leukemia, although it is actually less effective than 6-MP, methotrexate, steroids, or vincristine. It may be as effective as mechlorethamine in Hodgkin's disease. Impressive prolongation of life occurs in multiple myeloma—a median survival of 32 months. One can give Cytoxan orally or by injection.

Toxicity to bone marrow from Cytoxan equals that from other alkylating agents; in addition, temporary alopecia occurs in most cases. Bladder toxicity in children constitutes a unique problem with this drug alone. Nausea and vomiting are milder than with mechlorethamine.

**Chlorambucil (Leukeran).** Primarily useful in *chronic lymphocytic leukemia* and in *ovarian cancer,* chlorambucil comprises one of the least toxic and most widely used of the alkylating agents, perhaps because it is administered orally and is reliably absorbed. It acts *slowly* and rarely produces lethal toxicity. Objective remissions in chronic lymphocytic leukemia occur in over half of patients; its use is indicated when the patient feels weak and fatigued and when lymphadenopathy or splenomegaly causes symptoms. Thrombocytopenia does not respond to this drug. Remissions from 4 to 6 months are common in "lymphosarcoma" patients who exhibit systemic symptoms, anemia, etc. Short-lived responses also occur in "reticulum cell sarcoma."

So many patients with *ovarian cancer* have incurable spread of tumor that palliation only can be sought for them. Most of these cancers respond to x-ray therapy and to drugs. Long-term chlorambucil therapy produces worthwhile remissions in many cases; we are just learning how to use the drug in relation to surgery and x-ray therapy. Perhaps an initial course of drug before the fibrosis from the other therapies can occur and then maintenance use after surgery and x-ray therapy will prove most effective. Dosage must be somewhat lowered for patients undergoing x-ray therapy and for those in the immediate postoperative period. Marrow depression may develop after a few weeks, usually a pancytopenia, with neutropenia occurring first. Biweekly blood counts and occasional marrow aspiration will suitably monitor a particular dosage schedule.

**Thio-TEPA (triethylenethiophosphoramide).** Another relatively safe, widely used drug, thio-TEPA has had its greatest usefulness in *ovarian cancer* (in which chlorambucil now supersedes it). A 60% remission rate has been reported. It has proved of value also as an *adjuvant measure to surgery in breast cancer*—premenopausal women undergoing radical mastectomy who show several positive axillary nodes are the only patients benefited. Noer speculates that the lowering of the local recurrence rate after radical mastectomy in this group results from reduction of ovarian estrogen by a direct effect of the drug on the ovary. This agent was favored also for advanced breast cancer until 5-fluorouracil replaced it. Experimentally, some centers employ thio-TEPA instilled into the *bladder* to eradicate small superficial tumors, mostly papillomas. Administered intravenously in a loading dose of 10 to 15 mg. in 5 days, the drug should then be withheld for 2 weeks to determine the effect on the marrow. After this, repeated courses or weekly maintenance dosages may be given to keep the white blood count between 5000 and 2500 and the platelets between 200,000 and 100,000. Toxicity develops in the form of bone marrow depression—neutropenia, thrombocytopenia, and, after prolonged dosage, red cell depression.

**Busalfan (Myleran).** This anticancer agent plays a major therapeutic role in only one disease—*chronic myelocytic leukemia.* Radiotherapy is equally effective, but inconvenient and more expensive. Four to 6 mg. or more per day given orally will usually begin dropping the white blood cell count within 2 weeks, and within 3 months the count will reach a normal range with few immature forms, at which point the drug may be stopped. Decision on maintenance therapy or resumption of the drug results from following the white blood cell counts. Toxicity is usually mild but varied—amenorrhea, skin pigmentation, gastrointestinal reactions, hyperuricemia from excessive white cell destruction, or testicular atrophy. Agranulocytosis and thrombocytopenia occur commonly and must always be watched for.

**Melphalan (Alkeran, L-phenylalanine mustard, L-sarcolysin).** This mustard-group compound achieves its greatest utility in treating *multiple myeloma* and in *perfusing* extremities harboring *recurrent malignant melanoma.* Acting by lowering the abnormal serum globulins in multiple myeloma, melphalan causes objective improvement slowly, after 2 months on the average, so that prolonged therapy and maintenance therapy are necessary. Dosage has not yet been standardized. Remissions last 3 to 36 months. Toxicity follows the same pattern as with the other alkylating agents and is mainly one of bone marrow depression. Nearly half of extremity melanomas that recur after initial surgery benefit for a period of 4 or more years by melphalan isolation-perfusion (Creech and Krementz).

## ANTIMETABOLITES

This group of compounds interferes with cell reproduction by preventing the synthesis of DNA. As nucleic acid production proceeds at the cellular level, the drug moieties are taken up by the process as though they were the normal metabolites they resemble. But once incorporated into the forming molecule, they stop and distort the process because they are bogus metabolites. Methotrexate inhibits the enzyme dihydrofolic acid reductase and therefore often bears the label of a folic acid antagonist. 5-Fluorouracil binds the enzyme thymidylate synthetase and so inhibits methylation of uridine desoxyribose phosphate; 6-mercaptopurine acts to block DNA synthesis in ways still poorly defined.

**Methotrexate (amethopterin).** Two diseases respond remarkably well to this drug, which accounts for much of the enthusiasm for chemotherapy in recent years. The diseases are *acute leukemia of childhood* and *choriocarcinoma* in women (trophoblastic disease). Farber reports 40% and 70% remissions, half of them complete, in childhood leukemia with a median survival of 14 months. Remissions may require 6 to 8 weeks of therapy. Currently, drug regimens using alternating courses of methotrexate, 6-mercaptopurine, and corticosteroids seem even more effective, based on the concept that drugs are changed before leukemic cells can become resistant. Methotrexate must be used intrathecally for central nervous system damage in acute leukemia because this drug does not pass the blood-brain barrier; otherwise it can be given orally or parenterally. The simultaneous administration of a metabolite, citrovorum factor, when the drug can be regionally concentrated by arterial perfusions or infusions, will protect the bone marrow from systemic, toxic leakage and permit larger local dosage. Most serious toxicity occurs in the bone marrow, but oral and intestinal mucosa, the gonads, skin, and hair follicles show disturbances as well. A sudden drop in the white blood cell count or evidence of impaired renal function can constitute danger signals in giving methotrexate. We must always be on the lookout for kidney damage from high uric acid excretion in acute leukemia, a uricemia aggravated by the rapid cell destruction from drug therapy.

Hertz and associates have produced prolonged remissions that now amount to *cures in half of women* with *choriocarcinoma* (Chapter 20). Surgery plays only an adjunctive role in managing *trophoblastic disease*. Response to drug therapy and recurrences can be easily followed in this disease by urinary chorionic gonadotrophin titers, a fact which may help to explain the success of the drugs; drugs are given intensively until titers remain normal for long periods, which means continuing full doses at a time when only microscopic numbers of cancer cells persist. Drug therapy is titrated in the leukemias according to the bone marrow picture and the blood counts, a more sensitive indicator of active microscopic disease than any test available in common solid tumors. Hence, an ideal combination of circumstances exists in these two conditions—full drug dosages to mild or moderate toxicity when only relatively few viable cancer cells exist as a target. A 5-day course of methotrexate for choriocarcinoma usually causes some toxicity; courses may be given every 1 or 2 weeks, the new course beginning when toxic signs of the previous course disappear. Remissions may require as many as twelve courses, with a median of five.

Methotrexate may achieve short-lived regressions in *squamous cancer of the mouth and throat* in nearly half of patients; it also has value in treating *mycosis fungoides and psoriasis.*

**6-Mercaptopurine (Purinethol, 6-MP).** 6-Mercaptopurine finds a therapeutic place in treating *leukemia*—the *acute leukemias* and *chronic myelocytic leukemia.* The drug accomplishes remissions in childhood acute leukemia more effectively than any other single agent; as mentioned before, most recent leukemic regimens use drug combinations, alternating 6-mercaptopurine with methotrexate and corticosteroids. Adult leukemia does not respond as well, and busulfan actually has proved most effective for chronic myelocytic leukemia. Toxicity of this drug resides almost entirely in bone marrow depression, where it hits particularly the granulocytes. The toxic effects reverse rapidly in 1 week with cessation of the drug. Hepatic necrosis and consequent jaundice may also occur as well as uric acid nephropathy.

**5-Fluorouracil (5-FU, fluorouracil).** The only drug that achieves regressions in gastrointestinal adenocarcinomas (stomach, pancreas, small bowel, and colorectum), is 5-fluorouracil, although only about one patient in five obtains an objective remission. Zubrod believes that despite tumor mass shrinkage, the total patient benefit is small, but Heidelberger and Ansfield report 25% objective remissions for an average duration of 6 months. *Disseminated breast cancer* sometimes responds to 5-fluorouracil, although not as often or for as long a period as it does to hormone therapy; the latter takes precedence in the treatment sequence. Ansfield lists the following conditions as characterizing *poor-responders* among breast cancer patients: liver metastases, pelvic bone metastases that have been irradiated, a previous adrenalectomy or hypophysectomy, advanced age (over 70), resistance from repeated courses of alkylating drugs, and infection. Best results come from treating to slight toxicity with courses 30 days apart until relapse occurs. A course consists of 12 mg. per kilogram of body weight intravenously for 5 days, followed by half of this dose every other day until mild toxicity occurs. Lemon and associates infuse the drug in a glucose and water solution over an 8-hour period with negligible toxicity and almost comparable responses.

A somewhat different toxicity pattern accompanies 5-fluorouracil in that gastrointestinal injury occurs first; this we might expect since the drug has an affinity for intestinal mucosa. Symptoms of stomatitis, a thin watery diarrhea, nausea and vomiting with electrolyte imbalances, or esophagopharyngitis may develop. Marrow toxicity will also occur, and occasionally alopecia, dermatitis, or neurotoxicity. As a guide to management of dosage, mild toxicity consists of visible stomatitis, more than three liquid stools per day, a white blood cell count below 3000, or platelets below 100,000.

A nucleoside derivative of fluorouracil, *floxuridine* (FUDR), which is still unavailable on the open market, promises to yield better responses than 5-fluorouracil based on early testing with a small number of patients.

## ANTIBIOTICS

Two drugs in this group merit study, but only with actinomycin D do we know the mechanism of action. This drug inhibits the manufacture of messenger RNA by DNA.

**Actinomycin D (Dactinomycin, Cosmogen).** Actinomycin D has accomplished an impressive rise in survivals for patients with *Wilms' tumor,* neuroblastoma, and in women with *trophoblastic disease.* In Wilms' tumor the drug is combined with surgery and radiotherapy in a triple, concentrated attack that can cure half of the children with this condition. Complete cures result from actinomycin D alone in choriocarcinoma of the uterus, but best results accrue by using this drug for those women resistant to methotrexate—a 75% survival rate. Combined with local radiotherapy, actinomycin D has produced good effects on the embryonal rhabdomyosarcomas of children as well.

A highly toxic drug, actinomycin D primarily destroys the bone marrow and begins to show toxicity a few days after a course of drug is completed. This rises to maximal toxicity 1 to 2 weeks later. Thrombocytopenia is common and may be

**Table 5.** Summary chart*

| Disease | Marked benefit | Moderate benefit | Slight benefit |
|---|---|---|---|
| Childhood acute leukemia | 6-Mercaptopurine<br>Methotrexate | Corticosteroids<br>Vincristine | Cyclophosphamide |
| Burkitt's lymphoma | Cyclophosphamide (occasional case) | Cyclophosphamide<br>Methotrexate | |
| Adult acute leukemia | | | 6-Mercaptopurine<br>Methotrexate<br>Vincristine<br>Corticosteroids |
| Chronic myelocytic leukemia | Busulfan | 6-Mercaptopurine | |
| Chronic lymphocytic leukemia | | Chlorambucil<br>Cyclophosphamide | Corticosteroids<br>Thio-TEPA |
| "Lymphosarcoma" | | Chlorambucil<br>Cyclophosphamide | Corticosteroids<br>Mechlorethamine |
| "Reticulum cell sarcoma" | | Cyclophosphamide | Mechlorethamine<br>Chlorambucil |
| Hodgkin's disease | | Mechlorethamine<br>Cyclophosphamide<br>Chlorambucil<br>Vinblastine | Vincristine<br>Methylhydrazine |
| Wilms' tumor | | Actinomycin D | |
| Neuroblastoma | | Actinomycin D<br>Vincristine<br>Cyclophosphamide | 5-Fluorouracil<br>FUDR<br>Chlorambucil |
| Multiple myeloma | | Melphalan<br>Cyclophosphamide | Corticosteroids |
| Breast cancer | | | Corticosteroids<br>Thio-TEPA<br>5-Fluorouracil |
| Gastrointestinal cancer | | | 5-Fluorouracil<br>FUDR |
| Choriocarcinoma (trophoblastic disease) | Methotrexate<br>Actinomycin D | | |
| Ovarian cancer | | Chlorambucil | Cyclophosphamide |
| Seminoma of testis | | | Mechlorethamine<br>Thio-TEPA<br>Cyclophosphamide |
| Other testicular cancers | | Mithramycin | Triple combination of actinomycin D, methotrexate and chlorambucil |
| Anaplastic (oat cell) cancer of the lung | | | Mechlorethamine |
| Melanoma | | | Methylhydrazine |

*Modified from Greenwald, E. S.: Cancer chemotherapy, Parts I and II, New York J. Med. **66:**2532-2540, 2670-2681, 1966.

severe; one stops drug therapy if the platelets fall below 150,000. Alopecia, nausea, vomiting, diarrhea, and stomatitis also often develop.

**Mithramycin.** This antibiotic anticancer agent deserves mention as an example of a new drug, not yet on the open market, but one showing great promise for treatment of *embryonal carcinoma of the testis*. Like actinomycin D it exhibits marked toxic effects and demands cautious use.

## MISCELLANEOUS GROUP

Several useful chemotherapeutic agents work in different ways. Among these are the vinca rosea alkaloids that inhibit cell mitosis in metaphase and methylhydrazine that causes chromosomal breaks, resembling the effect of radiotherapy on cells.

*Vinblastine* (Velban) has the capacity to produce remissions averaging 4 to 7 months in most patients with *Hodgkin's disease,* although it is reserved, like alkylating agents, for patients with systemic symptoms or those unable to receive further irradiation. Giving the drug in repeated courses every 1 to 4 weeks as maintenance therapy has proved necessary to sustain remissions. Although it possesses relative safety compared to most drugs, *leukopenia* generally develops and limits therapy.

*Vincristine* (Oncovin, leurocristine) differs from vinblastine in causing only peripheral neuropathy, which is seldom lethal; the drug has no other toxic effects. Since children resist these neurotoxic manifestations, vincristine finds a role as the *safest drug* for the treatment of *acute leukemia in childhood.* Combined with prednisone it has produced an 85% remission rate in these children. Marrow toxicity seldom occurs and it therefore can be used in *leukopenic patients* with other diseases—the only drug that so qualifies. This agent irritates tissue so that one must avoid extravasation; alopecia will occasionally develop.

Several new or experimental drugs excite current interest: (1) *Methylhydrazine* (Natulan, procarbazine) shows promise, even though still experimental, in treating melanoma, since no other drug has an effect on the systemic spread of this disease. It is nearly as beneficial as the alkylating agents or vinblastine in Hodgkin's disease and can also be used in this tumor when marrow depression exists from other therapies. (2) *Arabinosyl cytosine* (Ara-C, cytarabine), reportedly effective against acute childhood leukemia, is an antimetabolite that blocks the formation of deoxycytidylic acid necessary to DNA. (3) *L-asparaginase,* an enzyme that hydrolyzes L-asparagine and thus deprives leukemic cells of this substance that they are uniquely unable to synthesize, is active against acute lymphoblastic leukemia (Chapter 30). (4) *BCNU* (1,3-bis[B-chloroethyl]-1-nitrosourea) helps some Hodgkin's patients who are resistant to other drugs; it acts partly as an alkylating agent.

### REFERENCES

Brennan, M. J.: Chemotherapy of solid tumors, Mod. Treatm. **3:**791-809, 1966.

Burgert, E. O., Jr., and Mills, S. D.: Chemotherapy of malignant lesions unique in children, C.A. **16:**15-20, 1967.

Burkitt, D.: Chemotherapy of African (Burkitt) lymphoma—clinical evidence suggesting an immunological response, Brit. J. Surg. **54:**817-819, 1967.

Creech, O., and Krementz, E. T.: Regional perfusion in melanoma of limbs, J.A.M.A. **188:** 855-858, 1964.

Dameshek, W., Weisfuse, L., and Stein, T.: Nitrogen mustard therapy in Hodgkin's disease, Blood **4:**328-379, 1949.

Farber, S.: Chemotherapy of cancer, antimetabolites and antibiotics, Acta Un. Int. Cancr. **15:**35, 1959.

Frei, E., Ill, Bentzel, C. J., Rieselbach, R., and Block, J. B.: Renal complications of neoplastic disease, J. Chronic Dis. **16:**757-776, 1963.

Funnelly, J. J.: Chemotherapy of inoperable malignancy, Brit. J. Surg. **54:**819-824, 1967.

Greenwald, E. S.: Cancer chemotherapy, Parts I and II, New York J. Med. **66:**2532-2540, 2670-2681, 1966.

Heidelberger, C., and Ansfield, F. J.: Experimental and clinical use of fluorinated phrimidines in cancer chemotherapy, Cancer Res. **23:**1226-1243, 1963.

Hertz, R., Ross, G. T., and Lipsett, M. G.: Chemotherapy in women with trophoblastic disease, Ann. N. Y. Acad. Sci. **114:**881-885, 1964.

Karnofsky, D. A.: Cancer chemotherapeutic agents, C.A. **18:**72-79, 232-234, 1968.

Kennedy, B. J.: Principles of cancer chemotherapy, Mod. Treatm. **3:**685-705, 1966.

Koop, C. E., Hope, J. W., and Abir, E.: Management of nephroblastoma (Wilms' tumor) and abdominal neuroblastoma, C.A. **14:**178-186, 1964.

Lawrence, W., Jr.: Current status of regional chemotherapy. I. Technics, II. Results, New York J. Med. **63:**2359-2382, 2518-2534, 1963.

Lemon, H. M., Modzen, P. J., Mirchandani, R., Farmer, D. A., and Athans, J.: Decreased intoxication by fluorouracil when slowly administered in glucose, J.A.M.A. **185:**1012-1016, 1963.

Luce, J. K., Bradey, G. P., Sr., and Frei, E., III: The systemic approach to cancer therapy, Hosp. Practice, pp. 42-55, Oct., 1967.

Noer, R. J.: Personal communication, 1967.

Papac, R. J., and Calabrisi, P.: Infusion of floxuridine in the treatment of solid tumors, J.A.M.A. **197:**237-241, 1966.

Sullivan, R. D., Miller, E., and Sikes, M.: Antimetabolite-metabolite combination cancer chemotherapy, Cancer **12:**1248-1262, 1959.

Tan, C. T. C., Dargeon, H. W., and Burchenal, J. H.: The effect of actinomycin-D on cancer in childhood, Pediatrics **24:**544-561, 1959.

Veenema, R. J., Dean, A. L., Roberts, M., Fingerhut, B., Chowbury, B. K., and Tarassoly, H.: Bladder carcinoma treated by direct instillation of thio-TEPA, J. Urol. **88:**60-63, 1962.

Vermund, H., and Gollin, F. F.: Mechanisms of action of radiotherapy and chemotherapeutic adjuvants, Cancer **21:**58-76, 1968.

Zubrod, C. G.: In Nealon, T. F., Jr., editor: Management of the patient with cancer, Philadelphia, 1965, W. B. Saunders Co., Chap. 10.

Chapter 34

# End result reporting in cancer

End results help us to give a reliable prognosis in cases of cancer and sometimes aid in deciding between two treatment methods. Several simple, logical requirements exist for tabulating survivals in any series of cancer patients:

1. *All patients seen,* whether treated or not, must be mentioned and classified so the reader will not have to wonder if some unknown or unstated selection process plays a part in the results. This implies a description of the population from which the patients were taken. Such a classification is generally made by sex, age, and clinical stage of disease.
2. The *statistical handling* of the data and a description of method employed in calculating survival rates need to be stated clearly. Patients lost to follow-up and those dying of diseases other than cancer (free of cancer, with cancer present, and unknown if cancer present) must be stated.
3. We must make a clear definition of the *starting time* for the measurement of survival of all patients.
4. One also needs a reasonably accurate, reproducible, and somewhat commonly accepted *system of staging* for each cancer at the time of the patient's admission. Only in this manner can rough comparisons with similarly constructed reports from other centers acquire meaning. Theoretically, staging a cancer in a given patient can involve analysis of many details: clinical evolution, patient delay, pathologic type and grade of tumor, clinical estimate of tumor extent, and type of treatment. For the sake of simplicity and utility, however, clinical estimate of tumor extent, *clinical staging,* alone is used.

Most clinical staging systems are based on the clinical impression of the first qualified examiner or diagnostician. He gives an opinion before any treatment disturbs the natural findings. The importance of staging lies not in accuracy, which is only fair in any clinical assessment, but in *uniformity of method,* which enables rough comparisons between different reports. The oversimplified staging of I (local), II (regional), and III (distant), measuring the extent of the cancer, ignores many important details that help in prognosis. A clinical staging system can be devised for all cancers; pathologic staging methods differ by depending on surgically excised specimen studies, and thus can be applied only to certain tumors that undergo operation.

## TNM SYSTEM OF STAGING CANCER

The TNM system was carefully worked out by a large committee of experts appointed by and representing six national and international medical organizations working primarily in the cancer field. The *T* refers to tumor size, the *N* represents regional lymph nodes, and the *M* stands for distant metastases. Thus, TNM represents each of the factors most influential in prognosis of most types of cancer—initial tumor size, presence or absence of regional node metastasis, and presence or absence of distant metastasis. But it goes farther; usually it also takes into account the varying primary tumor sizes and different degrees of nodal involvement. For example, a woman with a small breast cancer who has nonpalpable axillary nodes might be classified as $T_1N_0M_0$ or a woman with an ulcerating cancer and fixed nodes as $T_3N_2M_0$.

## END RESULT STATISTICAL METHOD

A number of systems exist to calculate survival figures. The most accurate and reliable, as well as the one with a promise of increasing popularity, is called the *life-table,* or actuarial method. The most favored of these methods is the Berkson-Gage type of actuarial end result reporting. The actuarial method used in this system best reflects true survival chances and benefit from treatment. It also has the advantages of using all the information available from well-documented case records and of incorporating results under 5 years, not just 5 years and over, to aid in a comprehensive picture of results of treatment.

Table 6 is a typical Berkson-Gage table giving the end results in a series of patients with glottic or cord cancer of the larynx.

The casual reader cannot gain full understanding of how all figures in each column of Table 6 are reached and treated. Study of the original references only will reveal the details of practical application. But in the last column one can see

**Table 6.** Glottic cancer end results (Berkson-Gage)*

| Interval—years after admission | Alive at beginning of interval | Died cancer during interval | Died other causes during interval | Lost to follow-up during interval | Withdrawn alive during interval | Effective number exposed to risk | Percent dying of cordal cancer | Percent surviving interval | Accumulative percent survival |
|---|---|---|---|---|---|---|---|---|---|
| 1 | 340 | 29 | 21 | 1 | 13 | 322.5 | 9.0 | 91.0 | 91.0 |
| 2 | 276 | 9 | 13 | 1 | 29 | 254.5 | 3.5 | 96.5 | 87.8 |
| 3 | 224 | 10 | 7 | 0 | 37 | 202.0 | 5.0 | 95.0 | 83.4 |
| 4 | 170 | 1 | 9 | 0 | 25 | 153.0 | .7 | 99.3 | 82.8 |
| 5 | 135 | 1 | 8 | 0 | 24 | 119.0 | .8 | 99.2 | 82.1 |
| 6 | 102 | 1 | 5 | 0 | 21 | 89.0 | 1.1 | 98.9 | 81.2 |
| 7 | 75 | 0 | 5 | 1 | 12 | 66.0 | 0.0 | 100.0 | 81.2 |
| 8 | 57 | 0 | 2 | 1 | 18 | 46.5 | 0.0 | 100.0 | 81.2 |
| 9 | 36 | 0 | 2 | 0 | 7 | 31.5 | 0.0 | 100.0 | 81.2 |
| 10 | 27 | 0 | 1 | 1 | 8 | 22.0 | 0.0 | 100.0 | 81.2 |

*From MacComb, W. S.: End result reporting, Amer. J. Surg. **114**:486-488, 1967.

at a glance the rate of dying, and conversely the rate of survival, from glottic cancer over a 10 year period. Deaths from other causes, patients lost to follow-up, and patients entered but not followed long enough in the given interval are all accounted for in computing the cumulative survival percentage; an accurate survival curve can thus be charted by showing a patient's chance of living through this particular disease during each year after treatment.

The *direct method* of calculating survivals is in common use but needs no special mention here since it explains itself. (See James' *Cancer Prognosis Manual.*)

In summary, if one accounts for all patients seen, stages all patients by a common system so the stage composition of each group is clear, and tabulates the end results in a statistically valid, analyzable form, the report of end results will have some significance. Few reports do.

## REFERENCES

Berkson, J., and Gage, R. P.: Specific methods of calculating survival rates of patients with cancer. In Pack, G. T., and Ariel, I. M., editors: Treatment of cancer and allied diseases, vol. I, ed. 2, New York, 1958, Paul B. Hoeber, Inc, pp. 578-589.

James, A. G.: Cancer prognosis manual, New York, 1961, American Cancer Society, Inc.

MacComb, W. S.: Reporting end results, Amer. J. Surg. **114:**486-488, 1967.

MacDonald, E. J.: Criteria for reporting end results, Amer. J. Roentgen. **60:**832, 1948.

Reporting of cancer survival and end results: Booklet no. 3, Chicago, 1963, American Joint Committee for Cancer Staging and End Results Reporting.

# Index

**D**

## M



## N

**Q**



**R**

**T**

**U**



**V**